REVERSE
DIABETES
FOREVER

REVERSE
DIABETES
FOREVER

How to Shop, Cook, Eat, and
Live Well with Diabetes

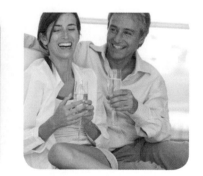
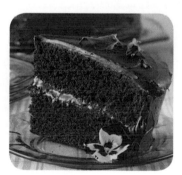
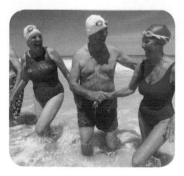
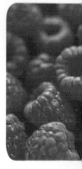

Reader's
digest

New York, NY | Montreal

A READER'S DIGEST BOOK

Copyright © 2016 Trusted Media Brands, Inc.

All rights reserved. Unauthorized reproduction, in any manner, is prohibited.

Reader's Digest is a registered trademark of Trusted Media Brands, Inc.

ISBN 978-1-62145-327-7

Original edition published in 2012; ISBN 978-1-60652-425-1

Names: Reader's Digest, an imprint of Trusted Media Brands, Inc., issuing body.

Title: Reverse diabetes forever newly updated : how to shop, cook, eat and

live well with diabetes / editors at Reader's Digest.

Description: 2nd [edition]. | New York, NY : Reader's Digest [2016] |

Includes index. | Includes indexes. |

Identifiers: LCCN 2016025576 | ISBN 9781621453277 (paperback)

Subjects: LCSH: Diabetes. | Diabetes--Diet therapy--Recipes. |

Low-carbohydrate diet. | Weight loss. | Exercise--Health aspects. | BISAC:

HEALTH & FITNESS / Diseases / Diabetes. | COOKING / Health & Healing /

Diabetic & Sugar-Free.

Classification: LCC RC660.4 .R48 2016 | DDC 616.4/620654--dc23

LC record available at https://lccn.loc.gov/2016025576

We are committed to both the quality of our products and the service we provide to our customers.

We value your comments, so please feel free to contact us.

Reader's Digest Trade Publishing

44 South Broadway

White Plains, NY 10601

For more Reader's Digest products and information, visit our website:

www.rd.com (in the United States)

www.readersdigest.ca (in Canada)

Note to Readers

We pledge that the information and advice inside *Reverse Diabetes Forever* has been checked carefully for accuracy and is supported by leading health experts and up-to-date research. However, each person's health and healing regimens are unique. Even the best information should not be substituted for, or used to alter, medical therapy without your doctor's advice. For a specific health problem, consult your physician for guidance. The mention of any products, retail businesses, or websites does not imply or constitute an endorsement by Trusted Media Brands, Inc.

Printed in China

7 9 10 8

Step forward to put your
diabetes in reverse!

How do you reduce the impact of type 2 diabetes on your life? Some of the answers will surprise you. Inside this newly updated edition of *Reverse Diabetes Forever* you'll discover the many lifestyle tweaks you can make to help stabilize blood sugar and improve your health.

Eat *More* Food

Fill your plate with these fresh, healthy choices, and you can actually eat more food and still reduce weight and stabilize blood sugar!

Sleep Longer

Retrain yourself to sleep a full seven to eight hours per night, and your body chemistry will respond in all the right ways!

Focus on Fun

The exercise prescription for diabetes is mostly about enjoyment: being outdoors, taking long walks, stretching, biking, dancing, and being active. No gyms required!

Enjoy Dessert

Cap off a day of healthy eating with a naturally sweet, nutritionally balanced treat, and your health will only benefit. We provide the recipes!

Sound good? Then turn the page and discover proven ways based on the latest research to stabilize blood sugar and keep your diabetes under control.

Contents

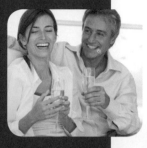

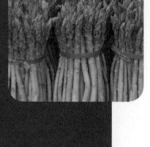

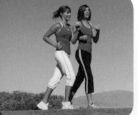

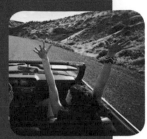

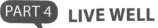

Diabetes: You *Can* Take Control

You can't hop into a car and head out on the highway without first learning how to drive, right? Well, the same is true for managing diabetes. Until you learn how to take proper care of yourself and your condition, controlling diabetes will be as challenging as negotiating a rush-hour freeway without knowing where the brake is.

But here's the good news: Unlike practically any other medical condition on the planet, type 2 diabetes—the type that develops over time, and makes up roughly 95 percent of all cases—puts you in the driver's seat. That's because the best way to manage type 2 diabetes is by making small changes to your everyday lifestyle. No surgery, no hospitals, no tough, mentally exhausting medical regimens are necessary, if you steer your lifestyle properly. Every moment, every day, and every week you have the opportunity to make changes that will help diminish diabetes!

If you have diabetes and aren't taking measures to stop it in its tracks, there's no time to waste. Diabetes is a serious disease, but it's well within your power to control both high blood sugar and the complications it can cause. If you're at risk for diabetes or uncertain whether you have it, get the tests you need. Then get your game on! Steps like eating right, losing some weight, sleeping well, managing stress, and taking medication or insulin to reach your treatment goals will make you feel better physically and mentally—now and over the long haul.

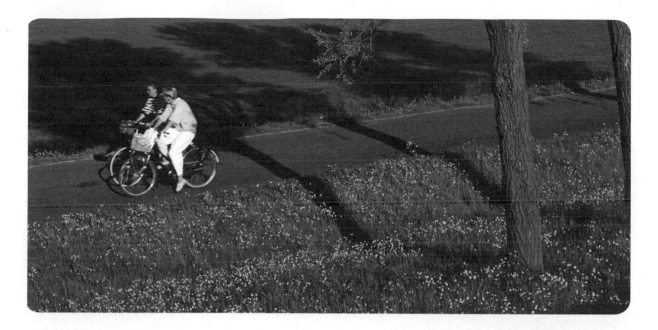

Two Pictures of Diabetes

You can look at diabetes in two ways. One is the big picture, which, frankly, is not very pretty: Across the country (and throughout the world), rates of diabetes have grown to epidemic proportions. Between 1980 and 2014, the number of Americans newly diagnosed with diabetes has tripled; today, roughly 20 million Americans have the disease, or roughly one in every 10 people. Just as alarming, rates among children are climbing as well. Even scarier is that an estimated 86 million Americans aged 20 years or older have prediabetes.

The second way you can look at diabetes is the small-scale picture: the scale of one—you. Here, the news is much brighter: More than ever before, diabetes is a disease you can control and even conquer. And the tools available to help you are getting better all the time.

It's the silver lining in this cloud of gloom and doom—the fact that few serious diseases allow you to fight back as much as diabetes does. If you take the right steps to keep the condition under your control, you can live a full and active life. In fact, some people who successfully turn their diabetes around say that they now feel healthier overall than they have in years.

There is also an upside to the diabetes epidemic: Chronic diseases that threaten huge numbers of people also capture the interest of researchers (not to mention the companies and federal health agencies that fund them). As a result, we've seen significant advances in the way doctors understand, prevent, and treat diabetes. If you need evidence of that, just look at how new findings have improved three key components of diabetes treatment:

Here's where your journey to turn back diabetes begins. You'll learn what you can do

▶ RIGHT NOW

▶ TODAY

▶ THIS WEEK

▶ THIS MONTH

▶ THIS YEAR

▶ AND FOREVER+

to reverse diabetes.

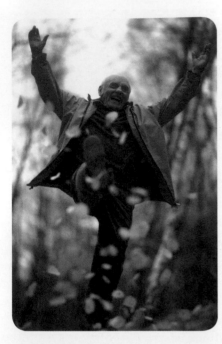

You *can* keep the condition under your control and live a full and active life.

BLOOD-SUGAR CONTROL

Complications of diabetes, such as cardiovascular problems, poor vision, kidney disease, and nerve damage were once thought to be inevitable no matter how hard you tried to manage erratic swings in blood sugar—the core problem of diabetes. But that thinking has changed dramatically. Several major studies from around the world have shown that if you bring blood sugar into a normal range with drugs, insulin, diet, exercise, or a combination of these, you can cut your risk of complications by anywhere from one-third to three-quarters. And if you're diagnosed before you develop complications, it's possible to reverse diabetes-related health problems completely, sometimes with lifestyle changes alone.

LIFESTYLE

Diet and exercise are powerful tools for lowering blood sugar—so powerful, in fact, that they free many people with diabetes from medication and insulin. And using these "power" tools is easier than ever before. Recent research into how foods affect blood sugar has shown that your diet need not be as restrictive as experts once believed. It can include virtually any food you like, as long as you watch your calorie intake. On the exercise side, it turns out that your workouts don't have to be as vigorous as once thought. Even short bouts of activity throughout the day add up to significant benefits to your health. Finally, it takes only a small amount of weight loss (just 7 percent of your body weight) to significantly improve blood sugar.

DRUGS

Earlier generations of diabetes medications have been bolstered by a growing roster of newer drugs that tackle the disease in a variety of ways. In many cases, you can combine these drugs to take advantage of their different modes of operation. The fact that there are also several varieties of insulin (which regulates the body's use of blood sugar) gives you more flexibility in finding a regimen that works for you.

The Reverse Diabetes Forever Formula

The book you're holding in your hands is a tool that will empower you to take control. You'll learn everything from immediate, small changes to help manage blood sugar to plans you can use over weeks, months, and beyond to reverse diabetes forever. We've divided it into key sections of helpful, easy-to-use information:

BE SMARTER

The basics—and more. Discover what causes diabetes, how to reverse its course and the collateral damage, how to marshal an effective healthcare team, and how to harness the latest technology to help you stay on top of your condition.

EAT RIGHT

Though you might have to retool your diet, you'll be delighted to discover that eating for diabetes doesn't mean purging your pantry of delectable food. In fact, you'll learn how to embrace a diet plan that includes plenty of lean proteins, a rainbow of scrumptious fruits and veggies, hearty whole grains, and yes, even tempting desserts.

EXERCISE MORE

Learning how to be physically active is arguably the most important step you can take toward reversing the course of diabetes. But for many people, it's one of the most challenging. In this section, you'll find several different approaches for working activity into your life—and even learning to enjoy it!

LIVE WELL

Beyond eating and exercise are a myriad of choices you can make to ensure that you're doing everything you can to combat diabetes. Take sleep, for example. Your doctor may not even know it, but it turns out that people who sleep well have a much better chance of maintaining blood-sugar control than those who sleep poorly. You'll also discover which supplements can help you—or not—and how to tackle blood sugar–raising stress.

COOK BETTER

Take delight in knowing that cooking for diabetes doesn't mean turning into a kitchen Spartan. From breakfast, lunch, and dinner to holiday favorites, snacks, and party fare, the recipes in this book will satisfy you and delight your family so much that no one will suspect they're diabetes-friendly!

HEALTHY TOOLS

Here you'll find useful food diaries, carb and calorie counters, exercise and blood-sugar logs, and test guides—all designed to chart your progress and make taking control of your diabetes easier than you ever imagined.

Your Forever Plan

We at *Reverse Diabetes* are committed to the notion that making better choices every day will help you be fully healthy. And we're also committed to making it easy to make the choices that will benefit you the most. By incorporating some of the tips this book offers, trying the recipes, and using the food diary, you'll be setting yourself on a path that will take you far away from diabetes and its complications—and toward a lifetime of healthy living.

> You *can* set yourself on a path that will take you far away from diabetes and its complications—and toward a lifetime of healthy living.

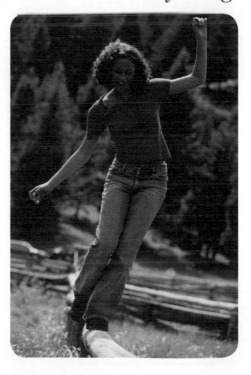

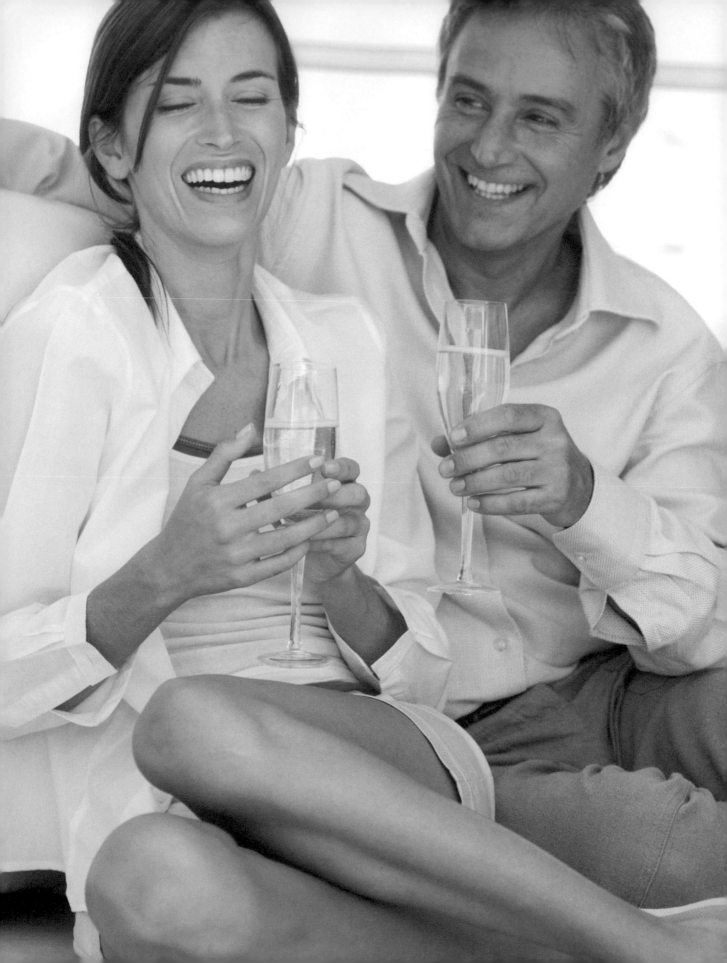

Be Smarter

Breakthroughs. Myths. Insights. What we know about diabetes is constantly evolving. In the pages ahead, you'll discover that a little knowledge can go a long way toward reversing diabetes. There are plenty of good reasons to be smarter about managing the disease. But here are two really great reasons: Controlling diabetes-related high blood pressure cuts your risk for heart disease in half and lowers your odds for kidney disease by 70 percent. Good blood-sugar control can reduce your risk for eye, kidney, and nerve damage by 40 percent or more. Read on to learn more about how to control and even reverse diabetes.

▼▼▼▼▼▼▼▼▼▼▼▼▼

Reverse Diabetes Forever with **a Little Know-How**

Smart lifestyle choices can go a very long way to preventing diabetes or minimizing its effects.

Diabetes is a pandemic, the eighth-most-deadly disease worldwide and the seventh leading cause of death in the U.S. Though genetics plays a role, for the most part you "catch" diabetes from an environment laden with overly processed fatty and sugary foods, too much sitting, 24/7 tension, not enough sleep, and too little fruit, vegetables, and whole grains. All these elements combine to sabotage your body's ability to process blood sugar—and what happens next isn't sweet. Left uncontrolled, diabetes can lead to heart attacks, blindness, kidney failure, amputations, cancer, reproductive problems, and an untimely death.

At the heart of type 2 diabetes is obesity. In fact, almost 90 percent of all people with type 2 diabetes are overweight or obese. If you're a man, your risk of developing the disease jumps 40 times as your BMI, or body mass index, climbs toward the obese end of the BMI scale. The news is even worse for women: Their diabetes risk jumps a whopping 93 times as their weight edges over the obese line on the scale. The good news: Dropping 7 percent of your body weight (15 pounds for a 200-pound person) slashes your diabetes risk by 58 percent. Dropping 10 percent of your weight (20 pounds for a 200-pound person) slashes risks even more, by 8 percent, finds a 2013 study out of John Hopkins.

Diabetes isn't just "a touch of sugar," as our grandmothers once described it. It wreaks life-threatening, body-wide havoc. Diabetes can increase your risk for heart attacks and strokes by as much as four times over that of a person without the disease. Two out of three people with diabetes have high blood pressure; one in three has severe gum disease.

Body-wide inflammation, a hallmark of type 2 diabetes, may help explain why one in four people with high blood-sugar problems is also dogged by depression. Of course, simply staying on top of this health concern is a daily, even hourly, weekly, monthly, and all-year job—one that takes a mental and emotional toll that can lead to burnout and low moods. It's a double whammy. Now there's new evidence that diabetes plus depression further magnifies risk for heart disease.

What's more, the health costs are steep. Diabetes is the leading cause of blindness and kidney failure in the United States. It leads to 73,000 amputations a year. Having diabetes puts you at added risk for 24 types of cancer (including those of the pancreas, liver, kidneys, and thyroid) and a 70 percent higher risk for bone fractures.

Sounds horrid, right? But if there's one lesson in the pages ahead, it's that smart lifestyle choices can go a long way to preventing diabetes or minimizing its effects.

Be Smarter >
Right Now

It's time to commit. Pick one activity to do this moment that will at least symbolically show you're taking a step in the right direction. Fill out a food journal, purge your kitchen of diabetes-unfriendly foods, or simply write yourself a note that you're committed to giving yourself a better life.

Be Smarter >
Today

Taking charge of diabetes doesn't have to be a full-time job, but you have to be mindful of it throughout your entire day, whether you're eating, doing yard work, or getting ready for bed. You'll have a team to help you, but the doctors, nurses, and specialists aren't your primary caregivers—you are. And your success ultimately depends on managing a treatment plan that puts you squarely in charge.

Be Smarter >
This Week

As you begin to manage your condition, you'll find yourself developing a sort of personal expertise in things such as diet, exercise, and blood-sugar monitoring. That kind of mindset will provide you lifelong benefits. So each week pick a different aspect of the disease to study up on. Just a few minutes' reading here and there is all you need. Perhaps you'll dive into the functions of the pancreas, or maybe you can examine how exercise affects blood sugar. The more you know, the better you can control your condition.

Be Smarter >
This Month

Create a game plan for any doctors' visits this month. Make a schedule of the appointments and, with each one, create a goal about what you wish to take from the appointment. Even if it's a routine checkup, you can have a simple goal of getting to know a nurse or practitioner a little better as a way to bolster your healthcare team.

Be Smarter >
This Year

Longer-term goals don't have to be seemingly unscalable mountains. Over the course of a year, if you lose just 7 percent of your body weight, you'll most likely be able to lower your doses of medication and lower your blood sugar. Dealing with ups and downs can be frustrating, but if you have that attainable goal in mind over the course of the year, you'll flip the calendar to a new, better you.

Be Smarter >
Forever+

There's no getting around it: Once you have diabetes, you've got it for life, and no operation, therapy, or drug can cure it—although gastric bypass surgery does put some people into remission. The good news is that controlling it can almost be like a cure in that lowering high blood sugar can stop diabetes in its tracks and reduce your risk of developing the health problems that go along with it. Bringing diabetes under control is an important task—and there's no one better qualified to do it than you.

What Is Diabetes?

You can't see it, you usually can't feel it—so what exactly is diabetes? It's a complex disease that affects your entire body, and it takes healthcare professionals years to learn about its ins and outs. Once you've been diagnosed, though, you won't want to take that long to learn how to take care of yourself. And luckily, you don't have to—you can easily bone up on the basics and prepare yourself for battling your condition right here and now. In fact, education is a cornerstone of care. The more you know about diabetes, the better you'll be able to use all the tools at your disposal to keep blood sugar in check and avoid complications that can compromise your enjoyment of life.

Start Damage Control Immediately

Think about what happens when you spill honey: It gets on your fingers, sticks to everything you touch, and generally gums up your entire kitchen counter. Now imagine a honey spill taking place inside your bloodstream—which is essentially what high blood sugar is. What happens? Cells, proteins, and fats get stickier, slowing circulation, holding back tissue repair, and encouraging material to adhere to your artery walls, where it causes clots and weak spots. In short, excess blood sugar gums up your entire body and sets the stage for all kinds of damage.

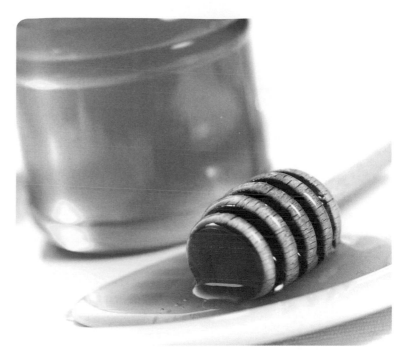

You'd never leave spilled honey on your countertop. Likewise, you should clean up blood sugar as quickly and thoroughly as possible because the "stickiness" only gets worse. Doing so can make you feel better right off the bat. And even if you have no symptoms of diabetes, taking this action will start to reduce your risk of problems, including damage to artery walls, which makes them more likely to snag blood clots and plaque that can cause heart attack, stroke, and high blood pressure.

These complications wreak all kinds of havoc, including impaired healing, infections, lack of sensation that can lead to injury (especially in the feet), loss of vision, swollen ankles, fatigue, sexual dysfunction—the list is long. Fortunately, learning about your condition can help you clean up the excess blood sugar and halt this parade of problems.

Why Glucose Matters

Glucose, also known as blood sugar, is the major source of energy powering your brain, muscles, and tissues—all your body's functions. In fact, glucose is one of nature's great dynamos, providing an almost universal energy source for living things. Scientists know down to the molecule how it's made and what it does, but, interestingly, they've never been able to create it in a lab. Only plants can make glucose through the magic mix of sunlight, water, and other elements and pass this energy along to other creatures through the food chain.

When you eat, your body breaks down the food into smaller, simpler components that move through the small intestine and into the bloodstream. Once in the blood, these nutrients are carried to cells throughout the body.

Different foods break down into different types of nutrients. Protein breaks down into amino acids, which are often used to build or repair tissue. Fat breaks down into fatty acids, which are mostly stored as energy reserves. Carbohydrates (including everything from bread and pasta to fruits and vegetables) mainly break down into glucose, which is used almost immediately for energy. In order to feel your best, you need enough glucose powering your cells at all times.

With diabetes, however, the glucose in your blood doesn't make it into your cells. The cells are deprived of energy, which explains why fatigue is one of the hallmarks of

Imagine a honey spill taking place inside your bloodstream. Essentially, that's what high blood sugar is.

diabetes. And since the glucose can't enter cells, it builds up in the blood. In the short term, excess glucose essentially soaks up water from the bloodstream, creating a paradoxical condition in which you need to urinate more often, while feeling parched with thirst. Too much glucose can also hinder the immune system's infection-fighting white blood cells, making you more vulnerable to illness. Over the long haul, persistently high blood sugar can lead to serious complications, such as damaged nerves, kidneys, eyes, blood vessels, liver, and heart.

A Wild Blood-Sugar Ride

Blood sugar fluctuates normally throughout the day, rising after you eat a meal. In people who don't have diabetes, these fluctuations stay within a span (measured in units of milligrams of glucose per deciliter of blood) that ranges from about 70 to 140 mg/dL. When you have diabetes, though, the patterns become more erratic:

▸ Blood-sugar levels spike to mountainous heights (rather than gentle hills) after meals.
▸ Levels drop more slowly as the body metabolizes the food you've eaten.
▸ Blood-sugar levels are, on average, higher than what is considered to be normal and healthy.
▸ The less you control your diabetes, the more likely your blood sugar is to swing wildly between highs and lows or simply stay high all the time.

Insulin's Inside Job

Glucose may inflict the damage done by diabetes, but it isn't really to blame. Instead, the real troublemaker is the hormone insulin, manufactured by the pancreas. Insulin's job is to "unlock" cells so that glucose can enter. As glucose leaves the bloodstream and enters cells, blood-sugar levels fall. When that happens, insulin levels also plummet so that blood sugar doesn't get too low—a condition called hypoglycemia.

When you have diabetes, the delicate dance of glucose and insulin is thrown out of step, either because the pancreas has trouble manufacturing insulin in the first place or because the body's cells have difficulty letting insulin do its job. The term

What's In a Name?

The term diabetes comes from the Greek word for "siphon"—based on the observation that people with the condition seemed to lose fluids in urine as quickly as they could slake their thirst. The second term in the disease's full name, diabetes mellitus, also comes from Greek and means "sweet," a reference to the sugar in urine that's typical with diabetes. It's said that in ancient times, the sweetness of urine was judged by tasting it—reason to be thankful that blood tests can detect diabetes mellitus today.

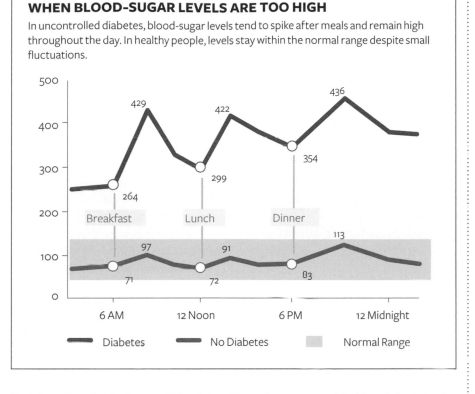

WHEN BLOOD-SUGAR LEVELS ARE TOO HIGH

In uncontrolled diabetes, blood-sugar levels tend to spike after meals and remain high throughout the day. In healthy people, levels stay within the normal range despite small fluctuations.

Diabetes values: 264, 429, 299, 422, 354, 436

No Diabetes values: 71, 97, 72, 91, 83, 113

Times: 6 AM, 12 Noon, 6 PM, 12 Midnight

Meals: Breakfast, Lunch, Dinner

Legend: Diabetes — No Diabetes — Normal Range

that describes this latter condition is insulin resistance—a critical breakdown in the body's ability to utilize insulin properly. Insulin resistance is the underlying cause of the vast majority of diabetes cases.

Scientists are still struggling to understand exactly what goes wrong to cause insulin resistance. It's possible, they suggest, that insulin resistance occurs when problems develop in the normal chain of chemical reactions that must occur to permit glucose to be transported through cell membranes. Or maybe, they speculate, an intricate system of proteins in cells, sometimes called the metabolic switch, loses its ability to sense the presence of insulin and react accordingly.

Even if the biology is still a bit mysterious, however, it's important to remember that the factors known to raise the risk of diabetes are fairly well understood.

Insulin-Blocking Hormones

Insulin isn't the only hormone that can affect blood-sugar levels. A number of others, sometimes called insulin antagonists, have the opposite effect of insulin. These include:

Glucagon. Produced in the pancreas along with insulin, it blocks insulin's ability to lower blood sugar by causing the liver to release stored glucose when the body requires it.

be smarter
this week!

Connect with someone who has diabetes.

Someone you know may benefit from your experiences. Nearly 50 percent of Americans today have diabetes or prediabetes, according to an analysis published in *JAMA* in 2015. Other research finds that peer support (that's you!) can help people better manage their diabetes.

Epinephrine. Also called adrenaline, this so-called stress hormone is released when the body perceives danger. Epinephrine raises blood sugar in order to make more energy available to muscles.

Cortisol. Another stress hormone, it can also raise blood-sugar levels.

Growth hormone. Produced by the pituitary gland in the brain, it makes cells less sensitive to insulin.

Your Pancreas: Small but Mighty

The pancreas is a fist-size organ that resembles an overgrown tadpole. It lies just behind and below the stomach. In its "tail," cells known as beta cells (which are clustered in clumps called the islets of Langerhans) produce insulin and release it when needed. Other cells, called acinar cells, secrete enzymes that help break down proteins, carbohydrates, and fats. Normally, the pancreas acts as a kind of glucose meter, closely monitoring levels in the blood and releasing insulin in spurts to mirror glucose levels. It also helps regulate a process in which the liver stores glucose as glycogen and then releases it back into the bloodstream to raise glucose levels when they fall too low. Certain diabetes drugs work to improve the function of the pancreas.

Symptoms: Silent—or Not So Silent

You may be among the countless people who suspect they have diabetes but have avoided making an appointment to be checked. You're certainly not alone: Denial is an all-too-common response to the subtle symptoms that characterize diabetes—type 1 or 2.

Symptoms or not, the American Diabetes Association recommends that everyone be tested for diabetes every three years after age 45—or more often if they face such risk factors as a family history of the disease. Whatever you do, don't ignore these symptoms; they're a signal that you should make a doctor's appointment ASAP.

Feeling tuckered. When cells can't get glucose and are deprived of energy, you can suffer from both physical and mental fatigue. The brain, in fact, is a glutton for glucose, using far more glucose for its weight than do other types of tissue. Mental fatigue can make you fuzzy-headed and emotionally brittle, while physical fatigue can make your muscles feel weak.

Frequent bathroom breaks. When the body is awash in blood sugar, the kidneys, which recirculate nutrients and filter out waste products, are among the first to know. When overwhelmed by glucose, they try to flush the excess out of your system by boosting urine production, especially after blood-sugar levels reach or exceed about 180 mg/dL.

Unquenchable thirst. As urine is excreted, you lose fluid. To urge you to replace it, the body triggers a persistent thirst.

Snack attacks. The irony of diabetes is that although your body is overflowing with nutritional energy, your cells are starving. Deprived of sustenance, they tell the body's appetite system to send a call for more food, which only creates more glucose that can't be properly used.

Blurry vision. Diabetes can degrade your eyesight in two seemingly contradictory ways. In one, lack of body fluid due to loss of urine can dry out the eyes, constricting the lens and distorting vision. In the other, excess blood sugar can cause the lens to swell, also creating distortion. Both of these effects are temporary, although diabetes can cause other complications that may eventually result in serious visual impairment and even blindness.

More infections. Having too much glucose in your blood makes immune-system cells less effective at attacking viruses and bacteria that cause infection. To make matters worse, some of these invaders actually feed on glucose, making it easier for them to multiply and become an even bigger threat. This can result in frequent upper respiratory illnesses like colds and flu, as well as urinary tract infections, gum disease, and, in women, vaginal yeast infections.

Tingling hands and feet. High blood sugar can damage nerves, a condition that may first become noticeable in the touch-sensitive extremities as a tingling or burning sensation. Damage caused by excess blood sugar can also affect nerves in the digestive tract, provoking nausea, diarrhea, or constipation.

The American Diabetes Association recommends that everyone be tested for diabetes every three years after age 45.

Testing One, Two, Three

Fortunately, a simple blood test can diagnose diabetes. The ADA suggests three tests that measure blood glucose in slightly different ways. Any one of them can give you the information you need.

1. FASTING PLASMA GLUCOSE TEST

If you make an appointment to see your doctor today, this is the test she'll probably schedule for you. And scheduling is definitely necessary, because accurate results depend on your preparing for the test in advance.

▶ How it works:
First, you'll fast for at least eight hours before the test, consuming nothing but water. That way, when blood is

drawn, your gastrointestinal system has long since digested all food. As a result, your blood-sugar levels will be at their lowest ebb, providing the bottom measure of what's typical for you. If you're healthy, your reading will be 100 mg/dL or lower. If the reading is 126 mg/dL or higher, you have diabetes. If it's between 100 and 125, you have prediabetes. If your reading crosses the line into a bad-news diagnosis, your doctor may want to repeat the test on a different day, just to be sure—though if your numbers are through the roof, this may not be necessary.

▶ Why it's used:
The fasting plasma glucose (or FPG) test is the preferred diagnostic tool because it's easy for both patients and doctors, it's relatively cheap, and it generally delivers consistent results—a nearly perfect balance of what you want in a test.

▶ For best results:
Take the test in the morning, not the afternoon. When researchers at the National Institute of Diabetes and Digestive and Kidney Diseases (NIDDK) compared more than 6,000 morning test results with a similar number of afternoon results, the average readings differed by as much as 5 mg/dL. The researchers concluded that up to half the cases of diabetes that would be caught in the morning were being missed in the afternoon. One reason for the discrepancy: People tested in the morning typically go more than 13 hours on average without food, while those tested in the afternoon go only about 7 hours. The NIDDK is now suggesting that different diagnosis standards be developed based on when the test is taken.

2. RANDOM PLASMA GLUCOSE TEST

This test is also referred to as a casual plasma glucose test. Both "casual" and "random" refer to the fact that you can take the test at any time. No fasting is necessary. Because it requires no preparation, the random plasma glucose test is often done as part of routine blood draws. Your first hint at a diabetes diagnosis may emerge as the result of an annual physical and not from any special effort on your part.

▶ How it works:
The procedure is not very different from the fasting glucose test. Blood is drawn and sent to a lab. But when the results come back, the bar for diagnosis is higher because it's assumed you may have had glucose from food in your blood. In healthy people, normal insulin response usually keeps blood sugar under 140 mg/dL even after eating. If a random plasma glucose test shows a blood-sugar level of 200 mg/dL or higher and you have such symptoms as fatigue, excessive thirst, or frequent urination, it's quite likely that you have diabetes.

▶ Why it's used:
Your doctor may use this when you've recently eaten and therefore can't take a fasting glucose test. Don't take a single positive result from a random plasma glucose test as

the final word. Doctors will almost always insist on confirming such results using a more exact test designed specifically to detect diabetes.

3. ORAL GLUCOSE TOLERANCE TEST

This test is regarded as the gold standard for making a clear-cut diagnosis of diabetes, because it assesses blood-sugar levels under highly controlled circumstances and provides extremely reliable results. But because it's so exacting (not to mention expensive and relatively time-consuming), patients and doctors alike sometimes find the oral glucose tolerance test, or OGTT, to be a less desirable one.

▶ How it works:

Like the random plasma glucose test, you first fast for at least eight hours. But this time, that's only the start. When you get to your doctor's office, blood is drawn to provide a point of comparison for additional blood samples that will be drawn again two hours later. After the first blood draw, you drink a super-sweet solution containing about 75 grams of sugar (about three times sweeter than an average soft drink). The subsequent blood draw helps plot out a picture of how your body handles glucose over time. Results are compared with a normal range at each measure, but the two-hour mark is especially critical: If your blood-glucose levels at that point are 200 mg/dL or higher, you have diabetes—final answer. If it's between 140 and 199, you have prediabetes.

▶ Why it's used:

A more exact test is sometimes needed when results from other tests are less conclusive than your doctor would like. Let's say you have a strong family history of diabetes and are experiencing obvious symptoms but neither form of plasma glucose test has confirmed a diagnosis. Or a random plasma glucose test comes back over 200 mg/dL but you have no symptoms. In cases like these, your doctor will fall back on the gold standard for an unequivocal result. A version of the oral glucose tolerance test is also the preferred tool for detecting gestational diabetes, although the diagnostic criteria are slightly different for pregnant women.

▶ What you should know:

Watch what you ingest before the test. Because of the test's sensitivity, OGTT results can easily be skewed by foreign substances in the blood. In particular, let your doctor know if you're taking any kind of medication—including birth-control pills—or herbal or nutritional supplements, since they may boost blood-sugar levels. For ideal results, some doctors recommend that you consume a lot of high-carbohydrate foods for three days before the test in order to mimic a standard diet.

OTHER TESTS YOU MAY NEED

Creatinine. If there are concerns about kidney damage, your doctor may suggest this blood test. Creatinine is a waste product that is normally removed from the body by the kidneys, but as kidney disease progresses, the level of creatinine in the blood increases.

Cholesterol and triglycerides. This blood test, usually done annually, checks your levels of three kinds of fats. LDL, or "bad" cholesterol, is a waxy fat that can build up and harden on the walls of your arteries. Levels of LDL should be 100 mg/dL or less. HDL, or "good" cholesterol, is a healthy fat that actually removes the LDL from your veins and arteries. You want your HDLs to total 45 mg/dL or more. Triglycerides are the circulating storage form of fat, which your body produces from excess glucose or fat. Too much can cause hardening of the arteries. Your levels should be less than 150 mg/dL.

Glycated hemoglobin. Also called the hemoglobin A1C test, this is sometimes used after a diagnosis to get a better idea of your blood-sugar patterns, but it's most commonly used to monitor your condition as you continue living with your disease. Its main benefit: Rather than assess your blood sugar at a specific moment in time, it surveys what's happened with your blood-sugar patterns over two or three months by looking at glucose deposits on a specific type of cell.

Urine. Your urine may also be tested by measuring albumin, a protein whose presence indicates early stage kidney damage. Usually performed annually, this test shows how well your kidneys are functioning.

Finger prick. Tests in which a small drop of blood is squeezed from a fingertip onto a special test strip that's read by a glucose meter are key to daily home monitoring that your doctor will likely recommend once you've been diagnosed. Glucose meter tests are fine for daily tracking but don't offer the kind of precision needed to make a diagnosis that will affect the rest of your life. The American Diabetes Association has stated that do-it-yourself monitoring devices are 10 to 15 percent less accurate than professional laboratory tests. If a healthcare professional gives you a finger-prick diagnosis at a local health fair, take it as a warning, then get to your doctor for follow-up tests to be sure.

The Fattening of America

America's (and the world's) weight gain and diabetes epidemics are so tightly intertwined that they're known collectively as the "diabesity" epidemic. Put simply, nothing influences whether you get type 2 diabetes as much as your weight. Ninety percent of all people with type 2 diabetes are overweight or obese, according to a 2011 study published in the journal *Diabetes Care*. And nothing influences your ability to reverse the condition as much as losing even a few extra pounds.

But the pounds revealed on your bathroom scale aren't the whole story. Federal health surveys show that the average person's waist has enlarged to 38.8 inches from 37.2 inches in 2000. A large waistline boosts diabetes risk regardless of your body weight. That's important information for the 50 percent of normal-weight Americans who are "skinny fat," meaning they're at a "healthy" weight but sporting a tummy pooch.

The most vicious fat in your body lies deep within your abdomen—it wraps around your internal organs and pumps fatty acids and blood sugar–raising hormones into your bloodstream. The take-home message is this: Pay attention to your waist size, not only your weight or body mass index. The best test for visceral fat isn't at your doctor's office. Just wrap a tape measure around your middle. Your odds for diabetes rise if the results are over 35 inches for women, 40 for men. To whittle it, drop pounds via a healthy diet plus regular exercise.

Lack of movement contributes to weight gain. It also shuts down a key enzyme in

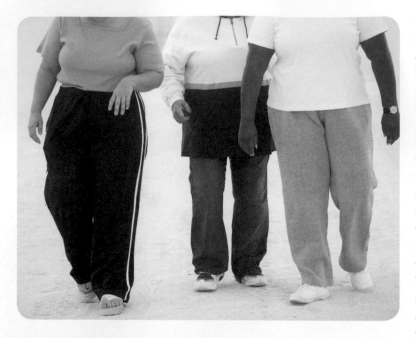

muscle called lipoprotein lipase, which plays a role in blood-sugar regulation. And how does all that fat accumulate? Try these numbers on for size: Five hours of daily TV watching. Two hours of computer scanning. Your job, plus your commute. One 2015 study found that every increase in TV time that offset exercise time resulted in a 0.8 inch increase in waist circumference. And even if you exercise, downtime can still fill you out. Researchers at the Pennington Biomedical Research Center in Baton Rouge, Louisiana, have found that sitting for more than four hours a day nearly doubles the risk for metabolic syndrome, a prediabetic condition. The scariest part? Risk rose even for people with formal exercise routines.

The most vicious fat in your body lies deep within your abdomen—it wraps around your internal organs and pumps fatty acids and blood sugar–raising hormones into your bloodstream.

The Bugs That Fatten Your Gut

In addition to lack of exercise, the types of bacteria that line your intestines may also contribute to weight gain and diabetes. Our digestive tracks are home to tens of trillions of bacteria. There are so many of these microscopic bugs that the bacteria outnumber our cells 10 to 1. Indeed, every single one of us is more microbial than human. More species of gut bacteria exist than do brands of breakfast cereal, with some of these bugs contributing to good health and others to poor health.

The guts of healthy people differ from the guts of obese people as well as from those of people with diabetes. In particular, healthy people have more bacteria that produce a by-product called butyrate as they ferment the food you eat. This fatty acid is thought to boost immunity and drive down health-harming inflammation. People with diabetes, on the other hand, have more of a specific type of bacteria called staph (short for *Staphylococcus aureus*). Staph bacteria produce toxins called "superantigens" that disrupt immunity and lead to chronic inflammation and insulin resistance. Methane—produced by other types of bad bugs—slow the movement of partially digested food through the intestines, giving the body more time to absorb calories and nutrients. If you have a lot of methane-producing bacteria, you'll gain weight more easily and have a much harder time losing weight—no matter how much you exercise or how little you eat.

Scientists are still unraveling the recipe for turning gut health around, but fiber-rich fruits and vegetables (blueberries, Jerusalem artichokes, onions, leeks, dandelion greens, avocado) and bacteria-containing fermented foods (kimchi, sauerkraut, yogurt, kefir, and fermented soy products like miso) seem to be key. Try to consume 1 to 2 servings of each a day.

A low-sugar diet and stress relief may also normalize gut function, so check out Parts 2 and 4 of this book for ways to do both.

Diabetes by the Numbers

About 1.2 million people in the United States have type 1 or "juvenile" diabetes, in which the immune system destroys insulin-producing cells of the pancreas, leading to a lifelong need for insulin injections. But type 1 diabetes isn't the big issue facing the American health system—that would be type 2, or "adult onset" diabetes. This form is caused primarily by lifestyle choices that over time destroy your body's ability to process blood sugar.

How bad is the epidemic? Call it skyrocketing, and you're edging close to the truth. The number of people with type 2 diabetes in the United States has more than tripled in the past 20 years, and the pace is accelerating. As of 2010, more than 10 million Americans had the disease, and that's fast approaching one in ten. Type 2 diabetes used to be a medical problem that arrived with gray hair, retirement dinners, and Social Security checks. No longer. From 1990 to 1998 the incidence of diabetes in people ages 30 to 39 increased by 70 percent.

Most people at risk for high blood sugar don't even know it. According to the American Diabetes Association, of the estimated 86 million Americans with prediabetes, less than 10 percent have been diagnosed. And included among the ranks of the unaware are nearly 7 million Americans who already have full-blown type 2 diabetes.

Then there are millions more who have metabolic syndrome, a cluster of symptoms that raises diabetes risk fivefold. These facts are even more shocking because there's an easy (no overnight fasting required) and accurate blood-sugar test called an A1C that can quickly diagnose the disease.

But the biggest—and scariest—news concerns our kids. Thanks to soaring rates of childhood obesity due to plummeting hours of active play and a penchant for sugary soft drinks, nearly half of children celebrating their eleventh birthday this year will ultimately develop diabetes or prediabetes. In 2015, 208,000 Americans under the age of 20 were estimated to have diabetes.

What causes diabetes? As noted, your refrigerator and your couch. And other things increase your odds. Among them: being over age 45, a history of high blood pressure, a family history of diabetes, low HDLs, high triglycerides, diabetes during pregnancy, polycystic ovary syndrome, and being of African-American, Asian-American, Hispanic, American Indian, or Pacific Islander ancestry. If you have any of these, ask your doctor about a blood-sugar check at your very next visit. And do it today if you've got any warning signs of diabetes, such as unexplained weight loss, excessive urination and thirst, or blurred vision.

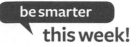

be smarter this week!

Stand every 90 minutes

According to a 2015 study out of the *Annals of Internal Medicine,* a sedentary lifestyle ups your risk of developing type 2 diabetes by a whopping 91 percent. The amount of time most Americans spend sitting: 13 hours a day! So set a timer to remind you to get up and move at least once every 90 minutes.

On the Warning Track:

Prediabetes and Metabolic Syndrome

Wouldn't it be great if your body had an early warning system that signaled you—loud and clear—at the approach of something potentially harmful? Turns out, when it comes to type 2 diabetes, it does. Years before the advent of type 2 diabetes, your body begins quietly alerting you to the fact that you're heading toward an official diagnosis. Trouble is, not everyone listens. Here's what you need to know.

In prediabetes your blood-sugar level is higher than normal, but not within the range of type 2. Even this small rise in blood sugar begins to damage your heart and circulatory system. If you don't take steps to bring your blood sugar down, chances are excellent that you'll develop full-fledged type 2 within the next 10 years or so.

You should see your doctor and ask to be tested if you have any of these prediabetes warning signs:

▸ You're overweight, with a body mass index above 25
▸ You get little or no physical activity
▸ You're over 45
▸ Someone in your family has type 2 diabetes
▸ You're African-American, Hispanic, American Indian, Asian-American, or a Pacific Islander

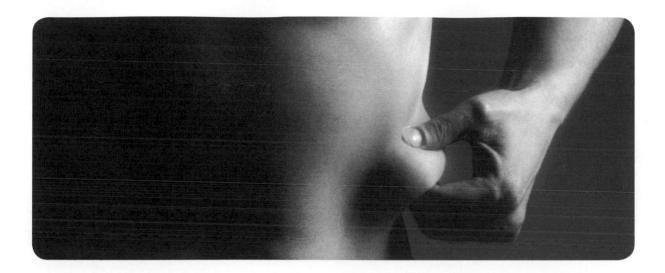

- You developed gestational diabetes when you were pregnant or gave birth to a baby who weighed more than 9 pounds
- You have polycystic ovary syndrome
- You have high blood pressure
- Your high-density lipoprotein (HDL) cholesterol is below 35 mg/dL (0.9 mmol/L) or your triglyceride level is above 250 mg/dL (2.83 mmol/L)
- You regularly sleep fewer than 5.5 hours a night

Though prediabetes can be symptom-free, two minor skin conditions may tip you off that you're a candidate:

Darkened skin patches. You might spot this condition, called *acanthosis nigricans*, as dark-colored skin blotches that show up on the neck, armpits, elbows, knees, or knuckles. It's considered one of the few outward signs of prediabetes.

Skin tags. These small, fleshy colored growths usually hang off the skin. They're harmless, although they might cause irritation depending on their location (often,

It's Costing Us a Bundle

More than $1 out of every $10 spent on healthcare in America covers diabetes, from blood-sugar test strips and drug copays to the price of doctor visits, hospital stays, and surgeries (such as clearing diabetes-related clogged arteries in the heart). The national burden tops $245 billion annually, and the personal burden can be overwhelming: People with diabetes shell out five times more for healthcare than those without it, or about $13,700 per year in healthcare costs.

As a result, just one in four people with diabetes get all of the care they need, a list that includes regular doctor visits, eye exams, medications, and blood-sugar test strips. The disease also results in reduced work productivity and increased absenteeism, costing more than $25 billion a year.

be smarter
today!

Enjoy an extra cup of coffee.

Perhaps you've heard that caffeine raises blood-sugar levels, and that's true. But coffee also contains plant chemical called polyphenols that calms inflammation and oxidation in the body. It's also rich in the minerals magnesium and chromium, both of which may counteract the effects of the caffeine.

That explains why a 2014 study revealed that people who drank an extra cup of coffee a day dropped their risk of developing type 2 diabetes by 11 percent over a four-year period, compared to people who did not increase their coffee consumption. People who drank less coffee—cutting a cup or more out of their daily routine—boosted their risk by 17 percent, found the landmark Nurse's Health Study of more than 100,000 women.

armpits, groin, or skin folds). They are associated with insulin resistance and prediabetes.

TYPE 2 DIABETES SYMPTOMS

If you experience any of these symptoms, it's likely that prediabetes has escalated into type 2 diabetes. Alert your doctor and get a blood test if you notice:

▸ Increased thirst
▸ Frequent urination
▸ Fatigue
▸ Blurred vision

METABOLIC SYNDROME

Even if your blood sugar hasn't edged into type 2 territory, many people have a constellation of conditions, called metabolic syndrome, that left untreated puts them in the huge pool of people who may eventually develop type 2 diabetes. These are classic symptoms:

▸ Obesity (particularly around your waist)
▸ Blood pressure over 120/80
▸ High triglycerides and low high-density lipoprotein (HDL)
▸ Resistance to insulin

You Have Diabetes. Now What?

Hearing that you have a chronic disease is never easy. One day it seems you have a clean bill of health (though you may suspect that something is wrong), and the next you have a problem for the rest of your life. But don't despair. You've probably had diabetes for some time, and now that you know it, you've taken a major step toward being healthier, not sicker.

Still, it can be tough to be optimistic initially. You might feel as if your body has betrayed you or that it's out of control. Some people assume that the worst they've heard about diabetes (accurate or not) lies just around the corner, and they jump to panicky conclusions like "I'll go blind!" or "I can never eat dessert again!" Others are nonchalant, figuring that they've managed to get by up to now with diabetes, so "worrying about it won't get me anywhere." They may also assume that they can treat all aspects of diabetes simply by taking a pill.

You're probably somewhere in the middle of the spectrum between panic and denial. You may even be relieved to finally know why you've been feeling so lousy. All of these emotions are normal. Typically, an I-can't-believe-it phase gives way to feelings of anger and the realization that there's a long road ahead, which can sometimes lead to depression. Here are some ways to deal with the dismay a diagnosis can produce:

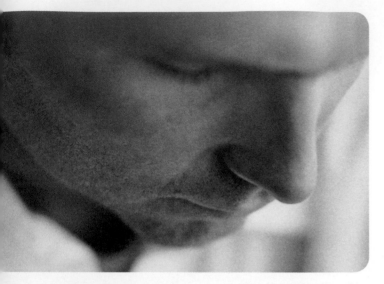

You can anticipate moving through several emotional stages after being diagnosed.

View your emotions as progress. When you accept your feelings as a natural, important part of an ongoing process, it's an indication you're actually working through them and going ahead with the rest of your life.

Think short term. You may feel overwhelmed by all the changes you have to make in your life, the new self-care skills you have to learn, and the sheer volume of medical information you need to absorb. Rest assured that eventually it will all seem second nature. For now, focus on immediate goals ("Today I'll meet my dietitian") that will move you further down the road.

Forge ahead. The key is not to let your diabetes diagnosis paralyze you. The sooner you take action, the sooner you'll feel you've gotten your life back under control—and the sooner you'll start to feel better.

What You Can Expect

When you're diagnosed with diabetes, your doctor will need to cover a lot of ground in a short time. In fact, she'll want to know virtually everything about you: eating patterns, weight history, blood pressure, medications you're taking, whether you smoke or drink, how satisfying you find sex, how many kids you've had, any family history of heart disease, and any treatment you've received for other problems, including endocrine and eating disorders. If you're a woman, you'll even be asked about your children's development. Your doctor isn't prying; all of this information has a bearing on your condition and the management program you'll eventually follow.

Your doctor will also do a thorough physical exam, including a cardiac workup that may involve an electrocardiogram (which records the heart's electrical activity) and a close look at your mouth, feet, eyes, abdomen, skin, and thyroid gland. You'll have a battery of tests, including a blood-lipid test for cholesterol (among other things) and at least two different blood-sugar tests—one that shows what your blood sugar is right now and the other, the A1C, which will show your doctor what your blood sugar has averaged for the past two to three months.

It may seem like a lot to begin with, but this initial assessment is arguably the most important phase of your overall care. Other parts of this phase may include questions that determine how much you know about your disease and how motivated you are to do something about it. Eventually, you'll move on to the next phases, in which you're in charge from one day to the next and your doctor is a resource for follow-up assessments and treatment of any complications.

Will You Need Insulin?

Ask someone who doesn't know much about diabetes how to treat the disease, and chances are they'll say with insulin injections. Insulin generally means needles, and dealing with this one element of care is the single biggest fear for many people with diabetes. Whether you'll actually have to confront the business end of a syringe depends first on which type of diabetes you have. All people with type 1 diabetes need insulin, but the majority of people with type 2 treat their condition without the use of insulin shots.

The good news is that even if you do need insulin, or one of the newer injectable medications developed for type 2 treatment, today's technology means that needles are tinier and hurt less than ever before. Some are just ³⁄₁₆ of an inch long and coated so that they slip painlessly into your skin.

What's more, many oral medications are proven effective at helping to stabilize type 2 blood-sugar swings. And as we just noted, losing weight, eating smarter carbs, and exercising more will have a significant impact on the disease. The type 2 diabetes prescription for the future will focus on smart lifestyle choices, supplemented with a careful mix of oral and possibly injectable medicines. Follow this regimen carefully and the chance that you'll need insulin shots will drop significantly.

If you have type 2 diabetes, your requirement for insulin will depend on a number of factors, including:

How much insulin your body makes on its own. If you have type 1 diabetes, your body doesn't make any insulin; if you have type 2, your body's insulin-making ability is only partially impaired, and the extent of the impairment differs from one person to the next.

How well your body uses the insulin it has. If your cells have trouble using the insulin that's naturally available, you may need supplemental doses.

Your blood-sugar levels. How high above normal your blood-sugar levels tend to be will help guide your doctor in deciding whether insulin is necessary.

How effective other forms of treatment have been. As a rule with type 2 diabetes, insulin is not the first treatment used to bring your blood sugar under control.

Where Do You Stand?

Your doctor looks at a lot of variables when deciding how to treat your diabetes, but she'll pay special attention to two in particular: your blood-sugar readings and your A1C readings. If your blood sugar is sky-high in your initial assessment, you may go straight to drug and insulin therapy until your numbers are brought down. If you have type 2 diabetes, once your blood sugar has stabilized and you begin making lifestyle changes, you may be able to go off insulin and other medications.

be smarter this month!

Talk to someone. Sharing emotions with a loved one, joining a support group, or attending a class about diabetes where you can meet others with the disease can help put your feelings in perspective and make you feel less alone.

Audit your medicine cabinet.

Take a quick look in your bathroom's medicine cabinet. Are you storing any diabetes-related medication or supplies there? Because of the steamy environment, that's not the best place for those items. While rooting around in there, check labels for expired prescription and over-the-counter medications, too. Then, find a linen closet or other non-steamy place for those items.

One of the numbers your doctor will zero in on is your fasting blood-glucose level, a key test of blood sugar. While other tests also need to be considered and each case must be managed individually, you can roughly anticipate your options, depending on what your fasting blood-glucose levels are (numbers are expressed as milligrams per deciliter). As a general guideline:

▸ If fasting blood glucose is between 110 mg/dL and 125 mg/dL, you have prediabetes (also known as impaired glucose tolerance), a condition in which elevated blood-sugar levels significantly raise the risk of developing diabetes. You'll be advised to start eating a healthier diet and to get more exercise, but you're unlikely to get a prescription for drugs or insulin.

▸ If fasting blood glucose is 126 mg/dL to around 140 or 150 mg/dL, you have full-blown diabetes, but you'll probably still be able to control your blood sugar with diet and exercise, depending on your condition and results from other tests.

▸ Once fasting blood glucose exceeds 150 mg/dL and ranges to 200 mg/dL, it's likely you'll need drugs in addition to diet and exercise. You may also need occasional doses of insulin for better control at certain times of the day (after meals, for example) when blood sugar tends to be higher.

▸ When fasting blood glucose goes above 200, you may need drugs or 24-hour insulin coverage—possibly both—along with lifestyle changes.

FASTING BLOOD-SUGAR LEVELS (mg/dL) AND LIKELY TREATMENTS

110–125	Prediabetes	Diet/Exercise
126–140	Diabetes	Diet/Exercise
150–200	Diabetes	Diet/Exercise/Drugs/Occasional insulin
200 +	Diabetes	Diet/Exercise/Drugs or 24-hour insulin coverage

Master Your Medicines

Medications are an everyday fact of life for most people with diabetes—over 80 percent use insulin, pills to control blood sugar, or the newer breed of injectable drugs for type 1 and type 2 diabetes. In a perfect world these medical marvels would get the job done without causing you a moment of extra worry.

But here's a reality check: Too often it doesn't work that way. Did you know that 60 percent of people who use diabetes meds say their drugs don't keep their blood sugar under control? Or that for plenty of people (you're not alone!), diabetes drugs cause other concerns—from stubborn weight gain and other side effects to worries about safety, effectiveness, and rising costs?

Here are some of the medication issues that could crop up—and how best to manage them.

MY NEW MED IS MAKING ME FAT!

It's a frustrating fact of life that many diabetes medications can actually boost the numbers on your bathroom scale. Drugs that put more insulin into your bloodstream or make your body more insulin-sensitive help your cells absorb more glucose (blood sugar) from your bloodstream. And if that sugar isn't burned for energy, it gets stored as fat.

Oral diabetes drugs that can cause weight gain include rosiglitazone (Avandia), pioglitazone (Actos), glimepiride (Amaryl), glipizide (Glucotrol, Glucotrol XL), and glyburide (Diabeta, Micronase, Glynase). If you're taking any of these, start by asking your doctor about drugs that don't seem to increase weight. These include sitagliptin (Januvia) and metformin (Glucophage). Two new injectable drugs for type 2 diabetes, exenatide (Byetta) and pramlintide (Symlin), may even help you lose a little bit of weight.

As for insulin injections, they can also cause weight gain. Your doctor probably can't reduce your dose, but he can help you devise a diet-and-exercise plan to burn off the extra blood sugar and calories.

Don't ever let this medication side effect keep you from taking good care of your blood sugar. Stay on your meds, and battle weight gain with healthy portion-controlled eating and regular exercise. Consider joining a weight-loss program such as Weight Watchers, or work with a certified diabetes educator so you have accountability and structure—key ingredients for pounds-off success.

Losing weight is definitely worth the extra effort it takes. In one study of 5,000 people with type 2 diabetes, those who exercised and followed a portion-controlled eating plan lost nearly 9 percent of their body weight (that's 18 pounds for a person weighing 200 pounds!). As a result, their blood-sugar levels decreased, they needed less medication, and their energy levels soared.

> Keeping your drugs and supplements in your bathroom medicine cabinet or a kitchen cupboard can degrade them—*fast*.

SMARTER MEDICINE STORAGE

Store your pills in a hot, steamy rain forest? Never! New research shows that keeping your drugs and supplements in your bathroom medicine cabinet or a kitchen cupboard can degrade them fast, thanks to conditions of high temperatures and humidity. Protect your health and your investment in your medicines and supplements by storing them like this:

Pills. Cool, dry, and dark is best. Keep out of reach of children. Store in

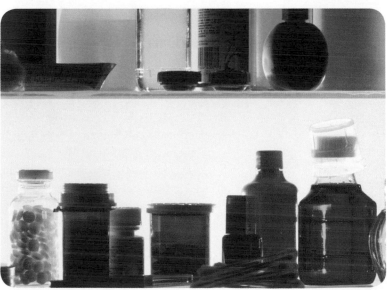

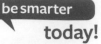

be smarter today!

Become routine.

Using your daily routine as a natural reminder can help guarantee that you take medications at the right times. Provided there are no kids or pets in the house that could get into your drugs, try leaving your morning medications beside the coffeepot, and your nighttime drugs on your bedside table. Do everything you can to make taking your medicine an unchanging daily habit.

original containers in a box high up in your bedroom closet. If you use a pill organizer or leave drug containers out so that you remember to take them, keep them up high for safety, perhaps on a dresser in your bedroom. Check your meds before you take them; toss any that are discolored or have an off taste.

Insulin. Store unused, sealed bottles in the refrigerator—never in the freezer, in direct sunlight, or in the glove compartment of your car. It's okay to store the bottle you're using at room temperature for up to one month. Always inspect your insulin before each use; toss bottles that are past their expiration date or that contain clumps, white particles, crystals or that look "frosted" on the inside. Follow label directions for storage of pre-filled insulin pens and insulin cartridges.

Byetta. Store unopened Byetta pens in the refrigerator. Once you've prepped one for first-time use, you don't need to refrigerate.

GET A MEDICINE MINDER

You may find that you're taking so many different meds that you're having a hard time remembering what to take when—and sometimes you forget whether you've taken them or not. This is a common problem, especially for people with diabetes who also are taking medications for blood pressure, cholesterol, or other health issues. A great solution is a pill dispenser. Load the compartments with the right pills (you can buy types that give you one compartment or multiple compartments per day), and you'll see at a glance whether you took them or not. Some fancy versions vibrate, flash or sound an alarm to remind you it's time for the next dose. You can also buy medication reminder watches that let you set up to 12 alarms a day (one manufacturer is Cadex).

If your pill schedule still seems way too complex, ask your doctor if she can prescribe different medications or doses so that more meds can be taken at the same time of day.

COMBO PILLS—GOOD IDEA?

The answer is maybe. Combination pills could save you hundreds of dollars per year (one co-pay instead of two!) and are more convenient than swallowing two separate pills. There are plenty of these "two drugs in one pill" products on the market these days, including Glucovance (glyburide and metformin), Actoplus Met (pioglitazone and metformin), and Janumet (sitaglipin and metformin).

Combination pills are best for people whose blood sugar has been well controlled by those same two drugs, at consistent doses. But doctors shouldn't be testing new drugs—or drug pairings—using a combination pill. So if your drugs or doses are changed frequently, or if you haven't yet found a pairing that has worked well over time, combination pills probably aren't right for you.

By the way, combo pills are also available for high blood pressure and for high cholesterol, the two other health concerns for many people with diabetes. The same upsides and downsides apply.

EASING THE WAY TO PAINLESS INJECTIONS

Check with your doctor to make sure you're using the newest and most pain-free type of needle possible. Then brush up on your injection technique:

After you sterilize your injection spot with an alcohol wipe, let the alcohol dry before you inject to avoid stinging. Next, relax your muscles and pinch up two to three inches of skin at your injection site; insert the needle and inject the medicine; then let go of the pinch and leave the needle in place for a few seconds before slowly removing it.

Finally, be sure to do an equipment check. Make sure the needle on your syringe is straight and sharp. Remove the cap by twisting and then pulling straight off to avoid bending the needle. Use each needle once; reuse can dull the end or even bend it.

THE 411 ON JANUVIA HEADACHES

Januvia (sitagliptin) can cause coldlike symptoms as well as headaches, an upset stomach, and diarrhea. These effects should diminish in a few weeks after your body begins to get used to the medicine. If they don't, tell your doctor. Watch out for allergic symptoms such as rash, hives, or trouble breathing. If any crop up, stop taking the medicine and call your doctor immediately. And if you're taking Januvia plus sulfonylurea (Glucotrol), watch out for dangerously low blood-sugar levels (you may feel dizzy or uncoordinated). Call your doctor right away if you do.

MAKE UP FOR MISSED INSULIN

You can usually make up for a missed premeal shot with a smart adjustment. Here's how it might work: If you forgot your prelunch shot but remember right after eating, a

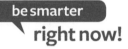

be smarter right now!

Reduce injection pain.

Take your next bottle of insulin out of the refrigerator a few hours before you need it; insulin hurts when it's cold.

Too Sweet for Our Own Good

Today nearly 20 percent of our daily calories come from sugars added to our foods or drinks at the factory. That's more than twice the amount of sugar we should be eating. A 2013 study that looked at the diabetes rates in 175 different countries determined that, for every 150 calories of sugar available per person per day, a country's rate of diabetes rose 1 percent, even after the researchers controlled for obesity. But fructose, a key component of the two most-used sweeteners in the American diet (sugar and corn syrup), may raise risk another way. Research shows it raises levels of uric acid in the bloodstream, which can interfere with your cells' ability to absorb blood sugar. High-fructose corn syrup (HFCS) and table sugar (cane or beet sugar) contain equal amounts of fructose—about 50 percent. Experts say both are metabolized in nearly identical ways in the human body.

There's nothing sweet about this story. Food manufacturers, realizing that people are naturally drawn to sweet flavors, keep adding more and more sweetening to our foods. As a result, we learn to crave sweet foods to the point that we no longer enjoy foods with more natural sweetness levels. It's a cycle that is in large part behind our obesity and diabetes crises.

How troubling is the situation? Even if you say "no thanks" to candy, desserts, and sweetened drinks like soda, iced teas, or fruit punch, you're still getting a sizeable dose of extra sugars in unlikely foods like salad dressings, ketchup, bread, yogurt, and more.

The solution is simple—and delicious. Eat farm-fresh foods, wean yourself off sweetened foods, and read food labels carefully. And ditch sugar-sweetened sodas and other drinks once and for all.

dose of insulin just one to two units smaller than your full premeal amount may be all you need. If an hour or two has passed since your last meal, a half dose may work. And if it's nearly time for your next meal, adding a few extra units to your premeal shot may be your best strategy.

These are general guidelines. Everyone's doses and injection schedules are unique, so it's wise to ask your doctor, nurse, or certified diabetes educator the best strategy for you. Ask about making up for premeal shots and what you should do if you miss a bedtime injection, too. The right solution depends on the type of insulin you use and when you realize you forgot an injection.

DEALING WITH SIDE EFFECTS: METFORMIN

About 30 percent of people who start metformin (Glucophage) have to deal with nausea, vomiting, abdominal discomfort, flatulence, diarrhea, nasty burps with a rotten-egg taste, heartburn, and even a metallic taste in the mouth. Experts say these side effects are usually temporary and subside within six weeks. To stay comfortable until they fade away, work with your doctor to be sure you're using the lowest effective dose. Taking metformin with meals can also help. If side effects don't improve after a month or so, talk to your doctor about whether another drug will work for you—without the discomfort.

INSULIN PENS VS. SYRINGES

If you're unsure whether you should use a pen or syringe to dispense your insulin, read on. Bottom line, pens can be more accurate and more convenient than filling your

Insulin pens can be more accurate and more convenient than filling your own syringes.

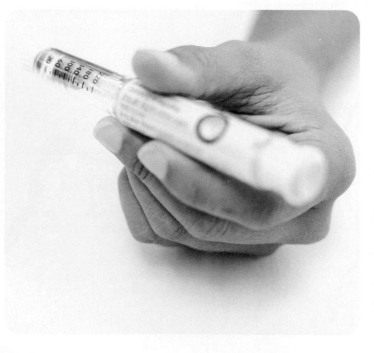

own syringes with insulin. And because you don't have to watch while you inject yourself with a pen, this nifty device could help you get over injection anxiety. To use an insulin pen, you simply insert a prefilled insulin cartridge, dial up your dose, and inject. Most contain several days' worth of insulin, and some pens come prefilled. And when you're finished, just toss the whole thing. Pens do cost more than syringes and bottled insulin, but there's a trade-off: In one study, people with type 2 diabetes who were just starting to use insulin got better results with pens, and as a result, they had fewer emergency-room visits for low blood-sugar episodes (because of too much insulin). In another study, people were more likely to use insulin regularly with a pen. So if you're new to insulin or are having trouble with bottled insulin and syringes, a pen is a wise choice.

INSULIN AND EXERCISE

Heading out to play tennis, golf, or go for a run but realize it's time for your insulin shot? Try injecting in a spot on your body that won't be getting vigorous exercise, like your thigh if you'll be swinging a racquet or golf club, or your arm if you'll be jogging, dancing, or hiking. Physical activity increases insulin absorption. Monitor yourself for blood-sugar lows, and carry a supply of "fast acting" carbohydrates with you, such as glucose tablets or glucose gel, hard candy, or a can of sweetened soda (not diet or sugar-free) or orange juice.

FEARS ABOUT ACTOS AND AVANDIA

Both these medications come with warnings, and if you're taking either of them, call your doctor and make an appointment to discuss any concerns you might have. But under no circumstances should you abruptly stop taking a prescribed medication. Doing so could be dangerous and could lead to nasty symptoms, as well as to a sharp rise in your blood sugar.

The U.S. Food and Drug Administration put restrictions on the once popular diabetes drug Avandia (rosiglitazone) in 2010 because of increased risk for heart attacks and other cardiovascular problems. Avandia is now recommended by the FDA for people newly diagnosed with type 2 diabetes only if they can't control their blood sugar with other drugs, and for those already taking it if it's working well and they have no concerns. But there's evidence both drugs raise risk for congestive heart failure in people of any age. If you have concerns about Actos (pioglitazone), talk with your doctor.

DRUGS AND PREGNANCY

Taking medication for diabetes doesn't mean you can't start a family. But you're wise to think about your blood sugar and your medications before you conceive. Talk with your gynecologist about your plans and your diabetes. You'll want to have your blood sugar under tight control for several months beforehand. Your baby's organs form during the first two months after conception, when you might not even realize you're pregnant. Oral medications for blood sugar are being studied for use during pregnancy, but until more is known, most experts recommend using just insulin to control blood sugar when you are trying to conceive, and in the early months of pregnancy.

Smart Blood-Sugar Control

This much everybody agrees on: Keeping your blood sugar under control is vital for staying healthy and warding off the complications that can accompany diabetes. But how low should you go? Doctors have long assumed that pushing patients to bring down their blood sugar as close as possible to normal with diet, exercise, and medication is the best approach. However, recent research has convinced many physicians who treat diabetes that not all patients should strive for the lowest possible blood sugar.

**be smarter
this week!**

Check ingredient lists.

During your weekly shopping trip, look for added sugars, like high-fructose corn syrup, cane or beet sugar, corn sweetener, cane crystals, or evaporated cane juice. If a sweetener is in the first four ingredients, don't buy it.

Make it a goal to lose just a little weight.

The bad news about diabetes includes many glimmers of hope. Over a decade ago the landmark Diabetes Prevention Program (DPP) study proved that losing a few pounds, exercising 30 minutes most days, and eating less saturated fat worked better than a pill for slashing risk of full-blown diabetes in people with prediabetes. The secret? You don't have to drop 50 pounds or train for a marathon to get results. Turns out, losing just 14 pounds (if you're tipping the scales at 200) and exercising a half hour most days of the week is all it takes.

A little background: The benchmark for determining success when it comes to managing blood sugar is the A1C test. By measuring certain proteins, this test gives a snapshot of your typical blood-sugar level over the past three months. A1C test results are expressed as a percent. Healthy people usually have A1C levels between 4 and 6 percent. The American Diabetes Association (ADA) has long recommended that most adults with diabetes (other than pregnant women) should try to get their A1C below 7 percent. Major studies have shown that keeping your A1C level below this threshold lowers the risk for blindness, kidney disease, nerve damage, and other diabetes complications.

However, it's also well-known that patients who strive for low A1C readings also increase their risk for hypoglycemia, or too-low blood sugar, which can cause dizziness (and in turn could lead to falls or be disastrous while driving) and even coma if untreated. Furthermore, a large 2008 study known as the ACCORD trial found that type 2 patients who were given 6 percent as their A1C goal were 22 percent more likely to suffer fatal heart attacks—which is the number one cause of death in people with diabetes—than others who had less-aggressive blood-sugar targets.

No one is sure why aiming for lower blood sugar might damage the cardiovascular system. And several other studies found no evidence that striving for near-normal blood sugar harms the heart in people with diabetes. Yet the results of ACCORD were troubling enough to persuade many doctors that low isn't always the way to go for some patients.

The ADA now advises physicians that 7 percent need not be the magic number for all diabetes patients. Experts say that less-stringent A1C goals will often be a better idea for certain patients, including the elderly, anyone at risk for heart disease, people dealing with other major illnesses, and any patient with a history of severe hypoglycemia or hypoglycemia unawareness (or the inability to feel or detect symptoms of low blood sugar). Talk to your doctor about what blood-sugar goal makes sense for you.

Deconstruct Your Diet

On the food front, it may surprise you to learn that the main issue is not the amount of sugar or other carbohydrates you eat but how many calories you get from all types of food. A dietitian can show you how to eat ample amounts of appetizing edibles (including all of your favorites, within limits, of course) yet still keep calories down so you lose weight. If you have type 1 diabetes, you'll need to balance your carbohydrate intake with your insulin injections to keep blood sugar from soaring too high or dropping too low. Whatever your diabetes type, you should put five food strategies into action right away:

1. Work up a meal plan that holds the reins on your blood sugar with tools like carbohydrate counting and food exchanges.

2. Aim to get more—not fewer—complex carbohydrates from fruits, veggies, and whole grains in your diet; these supply the greatest amount of energy with the lowest number of calories.

3. Fill up on fiber. It slows digestion and therefore controls the rise of blood sugar after a meal, keeps your appetite under control by making you feel full, and scours damaging fats from your blood.

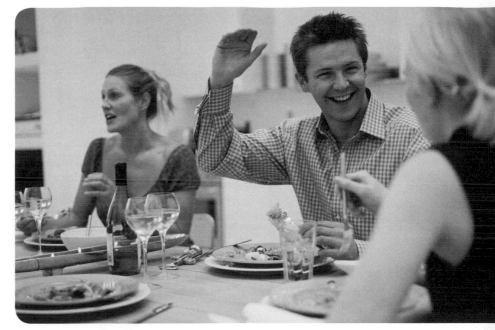

4. Cut back on saturated fat from foods like burgers and doughnuts, but allow yourself healthier monounsaturated fats in foods like peanuts, avocados, and olive oil.

5. Eat a variety of brightly colored fresh fruits and vegetables, such as apricots, berries, spinach, and tomatoes, to make sure you get enough nutrients like vitamin C and magnesium, in which people with diabetes are sometimes deficient.

Get Physical

Exercise gobbles up glucose, and this immediately brings your blood sugar down. If you do it regularly, it also enables your cells to better use glucose, even when you're not active. That can make you less dependent on insulin or medication. On top of that, exercise helps you lose weight, lowers your cholesterol and blood pressure, and makes your heart and lungs more powerful—all of which cut your risk of complications from diabetes.

Hate to exercise? Don't worry. Your workout plan doesn't have to be any more involved than making sure you pump up your heart rate and breathe a little harder several times a week, preferably for 20 minutes or more at a time. Classic aerobic exercises, like walking, running, and biking, are ideal, but ordinary chores, such as washing your car, mowing the lawn, and cleaning your house, do the trick, too. You'll know you're doing it right when your breathing becomes a little too labored to carry on a normal conversation, but not so labored that you can't talk at all.

It may surprise you to learn that the main issue is not the amount of sugar or other carbs you eat but how many calories you get from all types of food.

Beat Back Other Risks

Eating a healthy diet, getting more exercise, and losing weight are the most important things you can do to prevent complications from diabetes—but they're not the only steps you can take.

Ask about aspirin. Studies show that taking low-dose aspirin every day can cut your risk of heart attack by as much as 60 percent. Check with your doctor to see if aspirin therapy might be right for you.

Quit smoking. Besides ruining your lungs and increasing your risk of cancer, smoking narrows arteries, which raises your risk of heart attack and stroke and cuts circulation to your legs, making it harder for wounds to heal (especially on the feet). It also raises blood pressure and ratchets up your risk of kidney and nerve damage.

Take the pressure off. High blood pressure contributes to cardiovascular disease and kidney damage. If you eat plenty of fruits and vegetables, you're already bringing blood pressure down. You can bring it down further by eating less sodium (rampant in packaged foods) and more potassium from such foods as potatoes, yogurt, avocados, and bananas. Think about cutting back on caffeine, too: One cup of coffee can raise blood pressure for about two hours.

Get on a Schedule

It won't be long before dealing with diabetes will seem like old hat. Once you get used to the changes in your diet and exercise and learn to handle medications, day-to-day life may start to seem routine again. But check back with your doctor regularly to make sure everything is going according to plan. Get a physical every year, including an eye exam, cholesterol test, and a urine test to detect signs of kidney damage. Have a hemoglobin A1C test, which shows your long-term average blood sugar, every three to six months.

While there may seem to be a lot of details to deal with in the first days of a diagnosis, the steps you should take boil down to a handful of key objectives:

▸ Learn how to test your own blood sugar using lancet devices, test strips, and a blood-glucose meter.
▸ Use the results to determine your average blood-sugar levels and how they tend to fluctuate throughout the day.
▸ Make an appointment with a nutritionist or certified diabetic educator to create a diet and exercise plan you can live with.
▸ Read everything you can about diabetes—a step you're already taking.
▸ Schedule an eye exam for a month after your diagnosis. Because high blood sugar can temporarily cause blurry vision, a complete visual exam to screen for more permanent damage will be more useful after a few weeks, when you've brought blood sugar under better control.

Team Building with Your Doctor

While you probably won't be having dinner dates with your doctor, he or she can be your best friend when it comes to helping you manage your diabetes. So open your arms and be ready to embrace (figuratively speaking) that relationship, and help your doctor help you. These wise suggestions will help you forge a relationship that works for you.

Befriend the support staff. It never hurts to say a friendly word to the people who work with your physician. Office administrators, physician's assistants, and nurses can be extremely helpful when it comes to getting more face time with your doctor, answering questions about insurance coverage, or providing you a quick answer when your doctor isn't available. It's also a good idea to be considerate by arriving on time and giving at least 24 hours' notice if you need to reschedule an appointment.

Keep up with your doctor visits. Waiting too long between doctor visits and assuming everything will stay the same in the interim is like driving blindfolded and assuming that the road is straight. Most people with diabetes visit the doctor every three to four months, but that can vary depending on your health status, including your glucose levels and how stable they are. Ask your doctor how often she'd like to see you, and keep those appointments. If you go for long periods without seeing your doctor and your glucose is not under control, you could cause yourself some serious trouble.

Bring your glucose records. If you have a log book or a glucose meter that keeps track of levels, bring that information to appointments. This helps your doctor to help you pin down the food factors that seem to be influencing your blood sugar and also to point out ways to change them for the better. Unfortunately, not all general practitioners will take the time—or even have the expertise—to do this. If you're not getting enough help along these lines, you'll want to see a registered dietitian or a certified diabetes educator. Also be prepared to talk about what kind of exercise you've been doing. If you haven't been doing a lick, seeing that doctor's appointment on the calendar may spur you to lace up those sneakers.

Bring an extra set of ears. The average doctor's appointment lasts less than seven minutes. Sometimes it's hard to take everything in. If possible, bring someone with you to just listen to what the doctor says. After the appointment, compare notes. Also, if you wear hearing aids, don't forget to wear them. If you don't have anyone to bring with you, you may be able to find an advocate from a diabetes support group (look for groups at your local hospital or search www.diabetes.org) to accompany you.

> Your doctor can be your best friend when it comes to helping you manage your diabetes.

Don't dress up for the doc. Instead, wear comfortable clothing and shoes that you can remove easily. It seems like a simple suggestion, but having lots of buttons or laces can make getting undressed for examinations cumbersome. Loose pants with an elastic waist, a comfy T-shirt or sweater, and slip-on shoes are perfect.

Remove socks and shoes, even if your doctor doesn't ask you to. That'll help remind your doc to examine your feet for signs of skin breakdown, hot spots, cracked heels, or ingrown toenails.

Find out what your blood pressure is. Sometimes doctors (or their nurses) take your blood pressure and don't tell you the result—but you should know. Ideally, blood pressure for people with diabetes should be 130/80 or lower. If your pressure is higher, it means your heart is working too hard and can indicate an increased risk of heart disease, stroke, and nerve and kidney damage.

Take a few deep breaths before your blood pressure reading. This will help you get a more accurate reading, especially if you tend to get a little nervous in the doctor's office. Make sure your feet are flat on the floor.

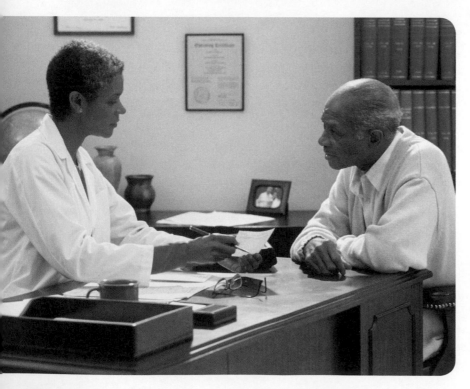

Bring a list of all your medications and supplements. Don't forget to list over-the-counter medications, vitamins, and herbs, in addition to prescription drugs. This will help your doctor quickly determine if you're taking two things that interact badly or if you're taking something you really don't need. It will also clue her in to side effects that may be related to something you're taking.

Ask when to call. Ask your doctor what blood-sugar reading is too high for you. Typically you'll need to call your doctor anytime your blood sugar is over 250mg/dL.

Learn how to get help after office hours. Is there an alternate number you should call? Who are the other doctors who will be on call when your doctor is out of town? Which emergency room should you use? Ask these questions before a crisis strikes.

Do your research if you need a new doctor. Gather word-of-mouth recommendations. Ask for referrals from friends, people you know who have diabetes, or your doctor. Do a bit of digging about why a friend is suggesting a doctor—you can turn up some interesting information by simply Googling the doc's name. Ask if she listens well. Is he experienced in working with people with diabetes? Can you get in to see her quickly? And of course, make sure any new doctor is on your insurance plan.

Look into group medical appointments. During these visits, you share a doctor and/or nurse with a group of other people who also have diabetes. Doing so can do a lot more than save you money on healthcare costs. They also can open up more time for you to ask a doctor or nurse the questions you need to get answered so you can better care for your health. A 2013 review of 93 studies found that shared medical appointments helped patients to significantly drive down blood sugar. A different study determined that these group appointments resulted in improved patient satisfaction over typical one-on-one patient visits.

Ask leading questions when doctor shopping. Does she have a large number of patients with diabetes? More diabetes patients means more experience treating people with diabetes. Does she refer diabetes patients for diabetes education? What target blood-sugar numbers does she consider acceptable? Can she tell you what her average A1C number, a long-term measure of blood-sugar control, is for her patients with diabetes? Normal is 4 to 6 percent; the goal for people with diabetes should be under 7 percent or under 6 percent, according to some sources. Does she use electronic medical records? Studies show that MDs who keep electronic records keep better track of the tests their patients need. Answers to these questions will tell you a lot about her experience with diabetes care.

Make sure your diabetes plan is a good fit for you. Speak up if for any reason you have concerns about your doctor's recommendations and expectations—for example, if your feet burn so much that you can't exercise, if you're having trouble getting rides to your doctor's appointments, if you are terrified of needles and don't think you can inject yourself with insulin, or there's nowhere to refrigerate your insulin at work. These are all problems your doctor can help you solve or work around.

What's Your Doctor's Type?

It's important to choose a primary-care doctor you feel comfortable with and whose style matches your own. You're the one ultimately in charge of your diabetes day to day, but your doctor is your trusty guide, whom you'll turn to for medications, tests, and expert advice. The better your partnership is, the better your diabetes management will be.

Some folks are most comfortable with authority figures; others, not so much. Some people like to hear about the latest scientific developments; others want just the unvarnished facts. But if your doctor resembles any of these common archetypes, you might just want to go shopping for someone new.

The Judge. Objective fact-finder; impervious; demanding of respect, maybe even fear. He's the final arbiter of your health and how to fix it.

The Scientist. Fact-driven; brilliant; often unfathomable; perhaps a bit eccentric; quite unable to communicate with the average person.

The Salesman. Has only a few minutes for you; turns on the charm; makes you feel good, then disappears; leaves you thoroughly confused, offers a prescription for a drug you never knew you needed.

The Favorite Uncle. Kindly; compassionate, but a little out of touch; hard of hearing.

Experts and patients agree that the perfect doctor is one who listens carefully, takes his or her time in both evaluating your situation and communicating what to do about it, is completely up to date on the latest medical research and methods, is deeply knowledgeable in wellness issues like nutrition and exercise, and treats you—the patient—with respect. The perfect doctor is out there, if you search carefully.

Speak your mind. If your doctor has a computer in the exam room and you find that he spends more time looking at it than at you, you need to take action. You might think this is bold, but get up and look over his shoulder to see what is so interesting. You'll make your point.

Prepare before your appointment. You probably see your doctor only a handful of times each year, so make the most of those visits with a little advance preparation. It could pay off later by eliminating the hassle of having to repeat an appointment because of a missed lab test or because you forgot to ask an important question.

Make a list of questions. Doctor visits go by so fast that it's hard to remember everything you wanted to ask or mention unless you write it down. To make sure you keep track of each question, number or bullet each item on your list, leave space to take notes, and check off each item after you've talked it over. That way, even if you get sidetracked, you'll be able to refer back to your notes to know what still needs to be discussed.

Get lab tests done in plenty of time before your visit. Your doctor may ask you to have tests done prior to your appointment, but if you wait till the last minute, you may not get your results in time and you may have to reschedule. Instead, get them done right away—you'll want your doctor to go over these with you.

Get detailed instructions for upcoming lab work. Find out if you'll need to make an appointment at the lab, or if they have walk-in times. And make sure your lab is on your insurance plan—your plan may cover some labs but not others. Will you need to refrain from eating or drinking prior to the test or wear comfortable shoes and clothes if you're going for an exercise stress test? Do you need to have lab work completed a certain number of days before your appointment? Should you avoid taking certain meds before the test?

Review your diet. Truth be told, if you're not careful, you can "out-eat" the effectiveness of most diabetes drugs. Before your next visit, take an honest look at your diet and ask yourself if you're doing everything you can to eat better foods on a better schedule. At what times of day do you generally eat? Many diabetes medications are more effective when properly timed with meals. How often do you eat out? It's much harder to keep calories under control when you eat at restaurants. What are your portion sizes—small, medium, large, or immense? Do you limit sugary or high-fat foods? Your doctor will probably ask about your food habits. If not, ask him if he would like to know what you eat and when you eat it.

Maintain your normal eating and drinking routine. That is, unless your doctor told you to fast. If you're not sure, call your doctor's office at least 24 hours before your next appointment and ask. If your eating or drinking habits were out of the ordinary in any way on the day of an appointment or lab test, be sure to tell your doctor, because that could cause altered heart rate, blood pressure, or test results.

> Getting the answers you need makes the difference between taking good care of your health and letting it slip from your control.

Ask Your Doc These Questions

Simply being in a doctor's office can be intimidating. And most doctors don't have much time to spend with patients, so it's not uncommon to feel a bit rushed. But don't stifle your questions. Getting the answers you need makes the difference between taking good care of your diabetes—and your health in general—and letting it slip from your control. Start with the tips here.

How often should I check my blood sugar? The answer will depend on several factors. At each visit, you'll want to review and discuss how you are using your monitoring results at home and whether you should increase or decrease your monitoring schedule.

How and when do I take my medications? This is critical, and the instructions for you might be different than for somebody else, so pay careful attention and take notes. Make sure you know if you should take your medication or insulin before or after meals, at night or in the morning, with or without food. Do you need to avoid alcohol? Are there potential interactions with other drugs that you should know about? This information will be in the

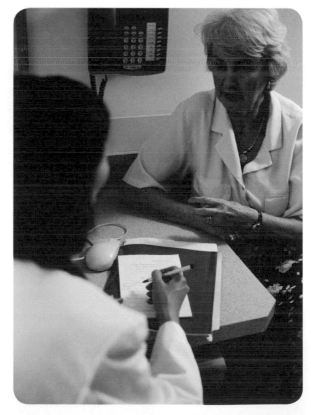

bag when you pick up your prescription, but the language can be hard to understand, so it doesn't hurt to ask while you're in the office.

Is there a generic version of my medication? If money is a concern, ask about drug alternatives. Sometimes a doctor can switch you to an older drug that's equally effective and less costly or to a generic version of the drug.

What side effects could I experience? Any prescription you receive should come with a patient pamphlet that describes possible side effects and symptoms, but it's smart to discuss these issues when the doctor first prescribes your medications. Are some side effects more likely than others? Will the medication make you drowsy or unable to drive a car? What symptoms warrant a call to the doctor? Should you stop taking a drug if you experience certain unpleasant effects? If for any reason you do stop taking a medication, call your doctor and let her know right away. Don't wait for the next appointment.

What sort of eating plan should I follow? For a real answer to this question, you'll want a referral to a registered dietitian, since most MDs are not very well trained in nutrition. In the meantime, it's still a good idea to ask your doctor for general guidelines. Most doctors' offices offer pamphlets that give healthy eating suggestions for people with diabetes. Typically this will involve not skipping meals, eating at the same time every day, eating about the same amounts of food at a given mealtime, and focusing on fresh fruits and vegetables, whole grains, low-fat dairy, and lean protein foods.

Can I drink alcohol? If you choose to drink alcohol, the general guideline is no more than one drink a day for an adult woman and a maximum of two drinks per day for an adult man. One drink is 5 ounces of wine or one 12-ounce beer. If your doctor has concerns about your kidneys or liver, he may suggest that you abstain from alcohol.

Should I avoid certain foods? Based on your blood pressure, cholesterol, and blood-sugar averages, your doctor may suggest some dietary changes. The prevailing school of thought is that you can still enjoy most of the foods you enjoyed before being diagnosed with diabetes, including sweets, though maybe not in the same amounts or prepared in the same way. Some habits, though, like drinking several cans of regular soda every day, which have the equivalent of 12 teaspoons of sugar each, will have to change.

Am I cleared for exercise? As long as you don't have serious health complications, most doctors will recommend moderate exercise such as walking, swimming, or riding a bike for 30 minutes most days a week. Still, it is a good idea to get the go-ahead from your physician if you're starting a new physical activity or exercise regimen. She may want to give you a physical or at least consider your condition (whether you have kidney disease, nerve damage, signs of heart disease, or other problems) before giving you the okay.

When can I reduce some of my meds? This is a good question to ask if you've been eating well and exercising religiously, and you've seen significant improvements in your blood sugar numbers as a result.

Get Help from a Specialist

Your regular doctor may be the one watching over your diabetes in general, but your feet, kidneys, eyes—even your diet and exercise—will need extra-special TLC because diabetes affects your whole body. In fact, it takes a team of people to properly manage diabetes, so work with your doctor to put one in place.

For stubborn blood sugar, see a specialist. If your blood sugar readings aren't showing any improvement, even after following your doctor's advice closely for at least 12 to 16 weeks, ask to see a diabetes specialist, also referred to as a diabetologist. This is a doctor who specializes in treating people with diabetes and is usually also an endocrinologist. Not all endocrinologists specialize in diabetes, though, so it is important to ask before making an appointment.

Request a referral to a certified diabetes educator. This professional, usually a registered nurse or dietitian, has specialized diabetes training and will have more time to spend with you than your doctor. He or she can help you adopt, adapt, and adhere to the better behaviors that will help improve your blood-sugar control. This person can answer questions about your medications, show you how to give yourself insulin shots, help you check blood sugar effectively, suggest better ways to keep track of your blood-sugar records, and more. Many are employed in a Diabetes Self-Management Education (DSME) program, and services from these programs are reimbursed by

Medicare. If your doctor doesn't offer DSME in his office, ask for a referral for DSME or call your local hospital to request diabetes education.

Make healthy eating habits a priority by seeing a registered dietitian (RD). What you eat and when you eat it affects your blood sugar more than any other lifestyle choice. If you have diabetes, you need an eating plan tailored just for you to help you meet your blood-sugar goals. The person who can provide that plan is a registered dietitian who specializes in helping people with diabetes. She'll help you figure out how much food you should be eating, teach you portion control, help you make healthy food choices, and plan meals that will fit your lifestyle. Not all registered dietitians specialize in diabetes; be sure to find one who does. Some RDs are also certified diabetes educators. Even if you've had diabetes for many years, a visit with a nutritionist can be very helpful. Nutrition and calorie needs change with age, and guidelines for good nutrition may also have shifted since you were diagnosed. A visit with an RD can also renew your motivation to eat better. You may even go home with some fun new recipes to try.

See an ophthalmologist at least once a year. Chronic high blood sugar can damage blood vessels in your retina (the inner layer of the eyes), which increases your chances of vision disorders and even blindness, so you'll need to make sure you have an annual comprehensive eye exam with an ophthalmologist. He will dilate your eyes to enlarge your pupils and have an extra-close look for any changes in your eyes. If you are referred to a new eye doctor, be sure to ask if he is familiar with spotting and treating diabetic eye disorders.

Go to your dentist twice a year. You learned when you were a kid that sugar causes cavities. Well, having high blood sugar can wreak havoc on your teeth, too. Bacteria that cause gum disease and cavities are more opportunistic—that is, nastier—when blood sugar is not well controlled. That's why people with diabetes are more prone to gum disease, which, believe it or not, has been linked to an increased risk of heart disease. In addition to regular dental visits, you need to brush and floss daily. It also pays to check monthly for any sores, tenderness, or redness of your gums.

Bring your feet to an expert. It's awfully hard to imagine that a simple blister or cut could lead to foot amputation, but if the injury turns into an ulcer that becomes infected, it's all too possible. That's why it's critical to take good care of your feet. A podiatrist will check for any sores, blisters, bruises, cracks, or cuts that are resistant to healing, as well as check for tingling or numbness in your feet.

Keep Your Feet Healthy

When you have diabetes, you need to direct your attention to an area of the body that usually gets little attention—your feet. That's because two common effects of diabetes are poor blood circulation and nerve damage due to high blood sugar, and those problems often affect your feet.

be smarter
this month!

Start a food diary.

Itemizing each piece of food that passes your lips might seem like a pain, but it can do you some real good. Give it a try for a month. Truly commit to jotting down everything you eat. And take that information with you on your next doctor's appointment. You'll see the payoff when you see how that lasagna dinner, or the bite of blood sugar–spiking birthday cake, affects your counts. Unconscious habits and patterns become more obvious when you see them in print. Plus, knowing that you'll be reviewing a food diary with your registered dietitian or diabetes educator might give you the willpower to pass on the cake and pick up an apple instead.

Why? Poor blood circulation makes your feet far more vulnerable to infections. Nerve damage can make it hard for you to detect any problems. That adds up to a frightening cycle: A cut or blister occurs, you don't sense it, then bad circulation hinders the healing process. The problem gets worse, but you still barely feel it, so you ignore it—and soon you're in trouble.

Foot problems are the most common cause of admission to a hospital for people with diabetes; they can even lead to amputation. And yet, all that is so easy to prevent! Treat your feet well with these tips.

Inspect 'em. Do an inspection every night or two as soon as you take off your shoes and socks. Make it automatic, just like buckling your seat belt. Start with your toes, then do the bottoms, sides, tops, and ankles. Regularity is the key. Catching a problem early will help you prevent serious complications.

Keep a mirror under your bed. It's pretty easy to see the tops and sides of your feet, but many people aren't agile enough to get a good look at the bottoms. Buy a mirror that's about the size of a sheet of notebook paper and place it mirror-side up under your bed. At bedtime, use your toes to slide the mirror out. Examine your feet in the mirror and then slide the mirror back into its hiding place.

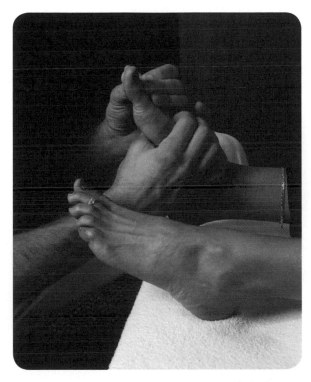

Get your spouse to play "footsie" with you. If you have a hard time checking your feet thoroughly (due to back problems, eyesight problems, or any other reason), enlist your spouse's help—and provide a kiss in return.

Watch for irritations large and small. Look for open sores, cuts, and signs of infection—swelling, redness, drainage, oozing, or warmth anywhere on your foot. Call your doctor immediately if you see any. Pay particular attention to the toes and the ball of your foot; that's where most foot ulcers develop. Smaller problems, including corns or calluses, need attention, too, but aren't an emergency.

Clean and treat minor scrapes and cuts right away. Wash your hands with soap and water. Then wash the wound with soap and water, rinse with more water, and pat it dry. Dab some antibiotic ointment onto a cotton swab and smear a thin layer of it onto the wound. (Don't apply the ointment with your finger.) Cover the wound with an adhesive bandage. If the wound doesn't look better within a day, call your doctor or podiatrist immediately.

Slather on moisturizer. When you inspect your feet each night, see if tiny white flakes are falling to the floor. Those flakes are dry skin cells, a sign that your skin is too dry.

When you have diabetes, you need to direct your attention to an area of the body that usually gets little attention— your feet.

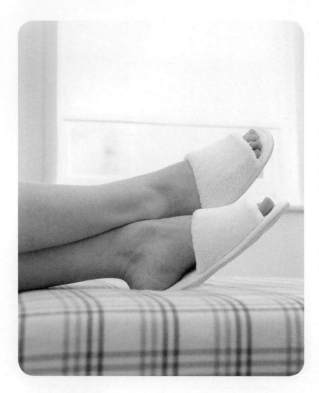

Walking
around
barefoot
is never a
good idea for
people with
diabetes.

Rub in a thick moisturizing cream or lotion thoroughly, paying particular attention to your heels and the balls of your feet. (Don't put it between your toes.) Then tuck your feet into clean socks.

Use moisturizing bar soap. Wash your feet daily in water that's warm but not hot. Avoid liquid soaps; they are more likely to leave your skin dry, which can lead to cracking. Also avoid exfoliating soaps, which can be too rough on your skin, and perfumed soaps, which cause skin reactions in some people.

Choose clippers designed for toenails. Toenail clippers are larger and have more leverage than fingernail clippers, so they can snip through thicker toenails without your applying excess pressure, which could lead to injury. Also, their blades are less rounded, making them more suitable for big ol' toes. You can purchase lever-style toenail clippers (which look like oversized fingernail clippers) or scissor-style clippers (which look like mini wire cutters). Nail files and emery boards are acceptable alternatives if used with care.

Pass on over-the-counter callus and corn treatments. When you have reduced feeling in your feet, it's easy for such treatments to damage your skin without your knowing it. The active ingredient in most callus treatments is an acid that can eat away not only dead skin, but healthy skin, too. Don't use pumice or a file, either; the risk of injury is high, and such instruments aren't sterile. Instead, for corns, calluses, or ingrown toenails, see your doctor or podiatrist.

Slip into slippers. If you've kicked off your shoes for the night, slip into a pair of slippers to protect your feet before you hit the sack. Walking around barefoot is never a good idea for people with diabetes.

Buy shoes that feel comfortable on day one. Don't tell yourself that new shoes will feel better when they're broken in or that the leather will stretch in time. All it takes is one small blister to start a cascade of trouble. Best is a shoe with ventilation that allows the shoe to "breathe."

Wear soft, sweat-wicking athletic socks. If your feet get moist, your skin will soften and blister more easily. Avoid cotton socks, which soak up sweat. Instead, wear socks made of synthetic materials like CoolMax and Dri-Fit or natural fabrics like wool and bamboo; both absorb and then release sweat into the air so your feet stay dry and free of hot spots.

Have a pair of shoes just for walking. They'll help you travel farther and faster with more comfort—and no blisters or injuries. Buy your shoe based on the terrain you'll be walking, the mileage you'll be covering, and the pattern of your foot, as revealed by the wear spots on your old shoes. For example, if the inner heel is more worn than the outer heel, your foot probably turns in excessively as you walk. In this case, you'll want some extra arch support and a shoe designed for "motion control."

Don't go barefoot. Yes, we love the feel of grass, sand, or even carpet under our feet. But we love our health even more. And nothing leads to cuts on your feet like going barefoot.

Avoid temperature extremes. Be it piping hot sand at the beach or an icy front step at home, heat extremes are hazardous to your feet. Even overheating in bed from too many blankets or a heating pad can cause real damage to your feet.

Skip the pedicures. Yes, it's a lovely luxury. But many pedicurists have a rough touch. There are countless reports of foot infections among people with diabetes caused by a pedicurist who cut away tough skin too aggressively or by instruments or foot spas that weren't completely sterile.

Tech Tools to Help Manage Diabetes

One of the side effects of having a chronic disease is that it turns you into an accountant. Numbers, numbers, so many numbers to monitor! This is particularly true for diabetes. To start, you have blood-sugar data to gather and study. Eating well for diabetes also means following the carbs, calories, and maybe even the fat levels in your diet. And if you also have high blood pressure or cholesterol issues, there are those measurements, too. Not to mention, if you're really on top of things, the calories you burn via exercise, how far you walk or jog, and other exercise-related details.

Tracking all those numbers and the other elements you need to stay on top of has become way easier these days, thanks to apps (short for applications, which are handy little programs for your computer, smartphone, or tablet device). No handheld? At least three websites offer similar support. Many systems allow you to track meals, exercise, medication, even stress levels, so you can spot patterns sooner—and see whether your lifestyle choices and diabetes drugs are providing the results you want. Some, like Agile Diabetes and Vree, even let you e-mail results to your healthcare practitioner or, like Glucose Buddy, download them to a website where your doctor or diabetes educator can review them at your next checkup.

GLUCOSE MONITORING APPS

Whether you check your blood sugar once or several times a day, monitoring the ups and downs can help you keep levels in a healthier range—and reduce your risk for serious diabetes complications. Apps that work on your iPhone or Android device make this task easy.

iPhone	Android	Blackberry
✳ Glucose Buddy	✳ eDiabetes Pro	✳ iRecordit
✳ Track3	✳ OnTrack	✳ HandyLogs Sugar
		✳ Diabetes Tracker

MEDICINE TRACKING APPS

The average person with diabetes takes four different medications—but many take eight, twelve, fourteen, or more. Keeping track of a complicated drug schedule is a big reason why 45 percent of us don't take medications as our doctor orders. These apps store info about multiple medications and buzz or beep when it's pill time. Some send reminders even when your device is locked, if you're running another app, or don't have cell phone or Internet coverage.

iPhone	Android	Blackberry
✳ Medi Reminder	✳ MediSafe	✳ MediRemind
✳ Dosecast	✳ Med Helper	
✳ MediSafe	Pill Reminder	

INSULIN MANAGEMENT APPS

Wondering how much rapid-acting insulin to take before a meal? Inject your next insulin dose with confidence by tapping a few numbers into one of these phone apps first. These insulin calculators factor in your planned carbohydrate serving intake, whether or not you plan to exercise or drink alcohol, and compute your current blood-sugar status.

iPhone		Android
✳ RapidCalc Insulin Dose Manager	✳ Structiva Insulin Dose Calculator Pro	✳ CityJams Insulin Dose Calculator

FITNESS AND HEALTH TRACKERS

A number of apps and gadgets can help you keep track of steps taken, calories burned, food consumed and even hours spent in deep sleep. Such tools can help to motivate you to get out of your chair and into your walking shoes, especially if you are using the Charity Miles app and every mile you walk helps you raise money for your favorite charity. They can also keep you honest—spitting out in undeniable numbers what you've eaten for the day and how many calories and grams of sugar it all adds up to.

You can wear some of them as a wristband (such as FitBit or Jawbone) or download others onto your phone or smart watch.

iPhone	Android	Blackberry
✳ Cyclemeter	✳ Charity Miles	✳ MyFitnessPal
✳ Lose It!	✳ Lose It!	
✳ MyFitnessPal	✳ MyFitnessPal	
✳ Pact	✳ Pact	

MANAGE YOURSELF—ONLINE!

In one study, web-based diabetes management programs helped people lower their blood-sugar levels in just three months. The easiest-to-use online programs let you transfer readings automatically from your blood-sugar meter to your computer via a cable or even a wireless connection.

Results are displayed as charts and/or graphs that can help you spot trends over time and share the info with your doctor. Programs such as DiabetEase and Lifeclinic work with a variety of meters. Others link online diabetes management software and meters from the same company—Bayer's GlucoFacts system, Johnson & Johnson's OneTouch system, and Roche's Accu-Chek system. MyGlucoHealth transmits results from a meter wirelessly via Bluetooth and your mobile phone to an online management program—then sends results directly to your doctor. What could be simpler? These sites also offer online monitoring support.

Websites	
✳ DiabetEase (diabetease.com)	✳ Lifeclinic (lifeclinic.com)

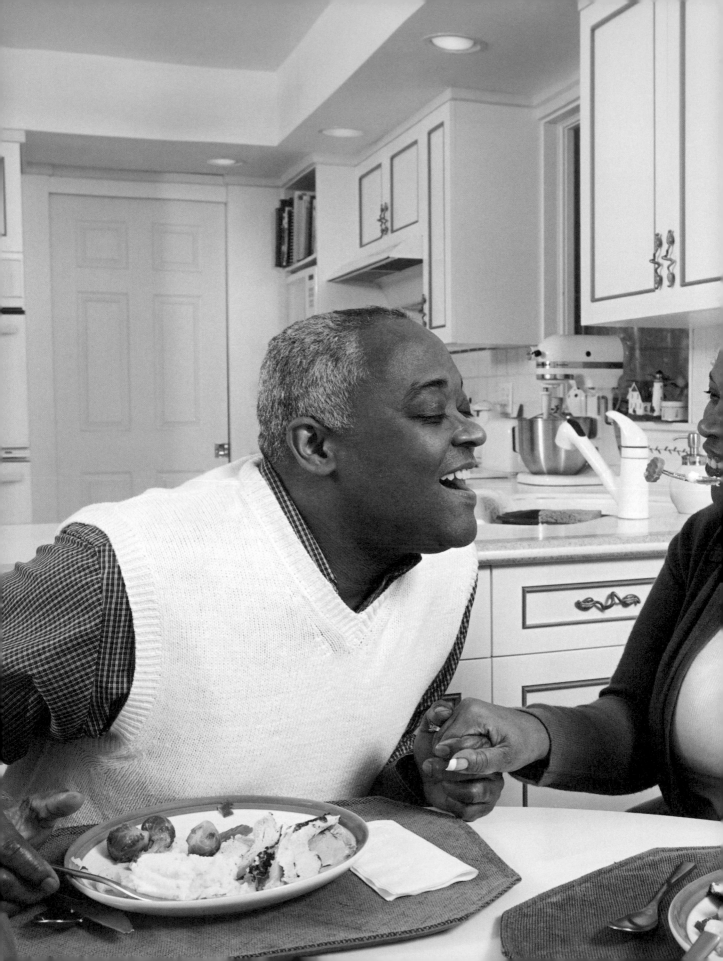

PART 2

Eat Right

Eating to beat diabetes can seem intimidating, but really, it's not. Though we'll be asking you to limit junk, processed, and fast foods, you'll be able to enjoy plenty of tasty, delectable, stick-to-the-ribs delicacies. What's more, you'll enjoy a nearly unlimited amount of brimming-with-goodness fruits and veggies, lean proteins, and satisfying complex carbs.

▼▼▼▼▼▼▼▼▼▼▼▼

Reverse Diabetes Forever with **Healthy Food**

A healthful diet for a person with diabetes isn't very different from a healthful diet for anybody else.

To a large extent, diabetes begins and ends with food, the body's glucose (read: energy) source. Improving your diet—by consuming more vegetables, fruits, and other varieties of whole foods and fewer sugar-sweetened foods—has been shown to drop risk for developing diabetes by 20 percent. Here's more: The researchers of a 2014 Harvard School of Public Health study found you have to improve your eating by only 10 percent to see a big difference! Having diabetes doesn't mean you can never enjoy your favorite dishes or desserts again. But it does mean you'll have to strike a new balance. By following the personalized meal plan we'll unveil in this chapter, you'll learn how to eat more food but consume fewer calories, control your weight, and bring down your blood sugar. And you'll learn about our tested and proven systems, including plating, food exchanges, and calorie and carbohydrate counting, which can help you make wise choices. Don't think of it as a diet but as a permanent path to better health.

The fact that diet is a key part of managing diabetes is no surprise. After all, glucose comes from food, so it makes sense that what you eat plays a role in making your blood sugar go up. But you shouldn't think of food as the problem. Instead, consider it a big part of the solution.

Food as medicine? You bet. In fact, the right diet is such powerful medicine that for people with type 2 diabetes, it could actually *reverse the course of your disease*. If you take insulin or other medication, a diet could help you reduce your dose or even eliminate your medication. For people with type 1 diabetes, the right diet can help you better manage your condition.

But if you think having diabetes means a no-fun "diabetic diet" of bland meals, with all your favorite foods forbidden, think again. The truth is, a healthful diet for a person with diabetes isn't very different from a healthful diet for anybody else. Although for many years the medical establishment recommended a restricted diet for people with diabetes—especially when it came to sugar—research has shown that sugar is not the villain it was once thought to be (with some exceptions, such as sweetened sodas). These days, the emphasis is on choices—and some choices are better than others, whether you have diabetes or not.

Eat Right > Right Now

Make the next thing you put in your mouth a piece of fruit. Think of fruit as nature's candy…but with benefits! Each piece contains an array of vitamins and minerals, and many offer a healthy dose of fiber too. Yes, some contain sugar, but because of the fiber, low calorie count, and high nutritive value, the sugar doesn't affect you the way white sugar does. Do test your blood sugar and choose the fruits that have the least impact on you. You'll soon see how easy it is to get the three servings a day you need.

Eat Right > Today

Check your watch. Now make it a point to eat at least five servings of vegetables in the next 24 hours. It's not as hard as you might think. Studies have shown that those who eat more veggies weigh less, have better blood-sugar control, and slash their risk for diabetes-related disease. Once you know that, you won't mind turning your lunch into a salad, making a snack out of baby carrots dabbed with peanut butter, or rounding out your dinner with two or three brightly colored selections from the produce aisle.

Eat Right > This Week

Weekly meal planning is essential to diet control. Not just for at-home meals but also at work and when you're dining out. If you know ahead of time what's for dinner, you'll be less tempted to turn to takeout or drive-throughs. You'll also know exactly what you need at the supermarket, so you'll be less swayed by snacks, sweets, processed foods, and other diabetes diet busters.

Eat Right > This Month

In the coming few weeks, think healthy fats. Foods such as nuts, avocados, fish, olive and canola oils, and flaxseed contain healthy sugar-controlling fats. You'll also want to limit the saturated fats found in fatty cuts of meat, poultry skin, full-fat cheese, and other dairy products. Saturated fat is not only terrible for your heart but also bad for your diabetes.

Eat Right > This Year

Closely controlling carbohydrates can take a while. But throughout the year, you can gain better control of your carb intake and how carbs affect your blood-sugar levels. Carbs make blood sugar rise—but they're also your body's main source of fuel. The answer is in choosing your carbs wisely. As you develop your sense of how carbs affect your blood sugar, you'll find after a year that you're making carb-conscious decisions without even thinking about it.

Eat Right > Forever+

When you change the way you look at food and start dividing your plate into vegetables, proteins, and carbs, you'll be able to eat at home and in restaurants, knowing that you'll be able to control your blood-sugar levels.

Eat to Beat Diabetes

How do you eat to beat diabetes? If you're like most people, you'll need plenty of additional support to stay on track. The goal is to control blood sugar while getting the right balance of nutrients for great health. But exactly what that means for you will depend on a host of factors. To plot a strategy that will work for you:

CONSULT A FOOD EXPERT

Really, aren't you worth a single, one-hour appointment with an expert who can make all the difference to your health? Your doctor can refer you to a registered dietitian, who will evaluate your current diet and make suggestions based on what, when, and how much you like to eat. Don't worry that a dietitian will only give you a list of rules and no-no's—a common fear. You may find instead that she actually provides you with more flexibility than you thought possible. For example, if you eat an ethnic diet that includes a lot of beans and rice—foods that raise blood-glucose levels—your dietitian can help make sure those staples remain a major part of your diet by, say, limiting per-meal portions or spreading your consumption out over the course of the day.

Many health-insurance and managed-care plans won't pay for ongoing consultations with a dietitian, but a diagnosis of diabetes will often allow you to schedule up to three visits. That's enough to establish a workable plan, which you, your doctor, and—perhaps occasionally—your dietitian can fine-tune as you go.

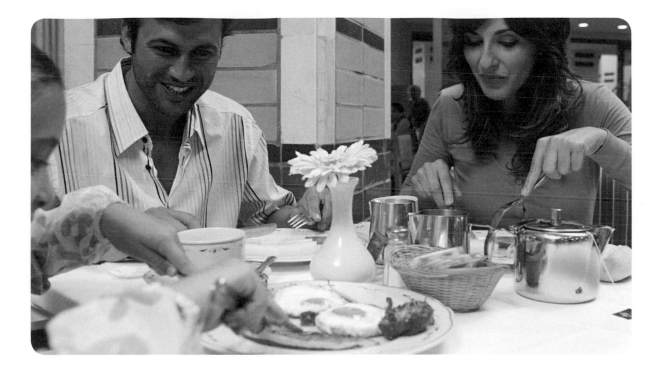

KEEP A FOOD DIARY

Before you see your dietitian for the first time, keep a log of every single morsel that you eat every day for at least a week. Also write down where you ate a particular food and what you were doing at the time. (You can use an app like My Net Daily or the food diary template on page 292 in the Healthy Tools section.) Doing this will help your dietitian find patterns that may reveal the other "w"—why you eat. If, for example, you often go out with colleagues after work, your dietitian won't want to eliminate this important social and business noshing, but she may suggest that you nibble on pretzels instead of beer nuts and switch to a white wine spritzer instead of a sugary margarita. Keeping a food diary doesn't help only your dietitian: Writing down what you eat will heighten your awareness of your eating habits, and this can help you recognize ways you can change.

For your diary, keep a small notebook handy throughout the day so you can jot down what you eat right away. Some people make notes in their smartphones. If taking notes at every sitting is inconvenient, try to reconstruct your food consumption at the end of the day; the record will be valuable even if you forget an item here and there.

FACTOR IN YOUR BLOOD SUGAR

Show your dietitian your log of daily blood-sugar readings so she can compare your glucose levels to your eating patterns. Comparing the two will indicate how much your blood sugar tends to swing in response to food and will help determine when and how much you should eat. Some people with diabetes can manage simply by eating

---

eat right
this week!

Record your eating habits.

For just one week, keep a food diary so that you can begin to understand your dietary strengths and weaknesses. You'll find the food diary template on page 292.

three balanced meals a day and cutting back on the empty calories in sweets; others need to follow a more detailed plan specifying calories, grams of carbohydrate, or number of servings from different food groups.

PUT IT ALL TOGETHER

Once you and your dietitian have a grasp of your eating and blood-sugar patterns, it's time to hammer out recommendations for specific foods you can eat at each meal or snack. This process is part negotiation and part analysis, and it involves other variables that have to be factored in, such as:

Your weight. The more excess pounds you carry, the more careful you'll need to be regarding what you eat.

Exercise habits. Exercising typically reduces your blood sugar, so how much you do—and when—will affect the number of calories you should take in at each meal.

Seven Diet Myths

Weight loss can be difficult, no thanks to popular misconceptions that have the ring of truth but can actually work against you. Among the more common myths:

1. Desserts are off the menu.
The truth is, there's room in your diet for most foods—as long as you control your total caloric intake (and grams of carbohydrate, if you tally them). Denying yourself your favorite foods can lead to binge eating and, ultimately, discouragement.

2. You have to lose lots of weight to make a difference.
The closer you can get to an ideal weight, the better—but small, sustained improvements at the beginning of a weight-loss program have the biggest impact on your health. Studies show that losing just 5 to 10 pounds can improve insulin resistance enough to allow some people with type 2 diabetes to quit medications.

3. What you eat matters more than how much.
Both matter, but recent research finds that the number of calories in your food is more important than where they come from. Example: A bagel might seem healthier than a doughnut hole, but dense bagels have the calorie content of six slices of bread. As long as you're not eating too much fat in other foods, the (just one, please) doughnut hole wins.

4. If you work out, you can eat whatever you want.
That's robbing Peter to pay Paul. You can't lose weight if you reduce calories in one way but increase them in another.

5. Skipping meals makes you lose weight faster.
Actually, studies show that people who skip breakfast tend to be heavier than people who don't. And a 2014 study of 4,116 children found that breakfast helps keep blood sugar in check, with breakfast skippers showing higher A1C readings. If you have diabetes, it's important to keep up a steady intake of small portions of food throughout the day to keep your blood-sugar levels stable and reduce the risk of hypoglycemia.

6. Starches are fattening.
If you are insulin resistant, your body may find it easier to convert carbohydrate calories to fat than to burn it as energy, but the fact remains that starches (and other carbohydrates) are less dense in calories gram for gram than other types of food. The main issue is calories, so if you load starchy foods with fat—sour cream and butter on a baked potato, for instance—or eat them in large quantities, the caloric load can add up.

7. Never eat fast food.
Never say never. Fast food can be worked into your meal plan if you choose well. Most fast-food places have healthy salads, which are great if you choose the low-cal dressing and skip crunchy or fried topping options. Some delis offer whole-wheat bread and low-fat sandwich fillings, and you can usually order a grilled chicken patty instead of burgers at many places. Whatever you do, avoid or scrape away high-fat condiments like mayonnaise, share a small-sized french fry order (better yet, choose a small side salad) to keep portion size down, and ask for water, unsweetened iced tea, or diet soda instead of sugary drinks.

Insulin use. If you're type 1, the content and timing of your meals should consistently balance the amount of insulin circulating in your blood from injections. If you're type 2 and using insulin, you'll need to factor this in on top of variables (such as weight and exercise) that affect insulin resistance.

Medication use. Which medication you take, how much, and when its action peaks may affect your dietary choices. If you have type 2 diabetes, getting off medication may be a realistic goal for your meal plan.

Special considerations. Be sure to inform your dietitian of results of tests for lipids (such as cholesterol), blood pressure, and microalbumin (for kidney function). If you already suffer such complications as poor cholesterol ratios, high blood pressure, and kidney damage, you may need to follow guidelines that specifically deal with those conditions, such as eating even less saturated fat, cutting back on salt, or avoiding excessive amounts of protein.

Consistency Is Key

Once you've developed a plan, you'll keep your blood sugar more stable if you eat about the same amount of food with the same balance of nutrients at about the same times each day. Don't figure you can be "bad" on some days as long as you're "good" on others: Eating in erratic patterns only causes blood sugar to seesaw. Instead, try to come up with a meal plan you can live with all the time.

HOW'S IT WORKING?

Self-monitoring your blood sugar will give you and your doctor a sense of how well you're able to control it with diet. From there, you can fine-tune your plan of attack by tinkering with your meal plan or changing your activity level, insulin dosage, or other variables. If you're type 2 and you're having trouble keeping your blood sugar in line through diet and exercise, that may mean you're a candidate for drug intervention. On the other hand, if you've succeeded at losing weight and controlling your blood sugar through diet and exercise, you may be able to stop taking insulin or medication.

The One Type of Fast Your Body Needs

You'll soon learn about foods that can help to stabilize blood sugar and shed pounds. But did you know that how—and when—you eat those foods is also key?

For example, you've probably heard that skipping breakfast can boost blood sugar levels, possibly by leading to cravings and overeating later in the day. But did you know that a different type of fasting—called intermittent fasting—may actually spur weight loss and help you regain control of blood sugar?

Researchers have long known that limiting calories by 50 percent helps rodents and

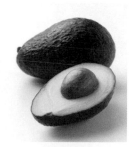

eat right
smart food
AVOCADO
Rich, creamy, and packed with beneficial monounsaturated fat, avocado slows digestion and helps keep blood sugar from spiking after a meal. When study participants consumed half an avocado at lunch, their desire to eat remained low over the following five hours, compared with when they didn't eat the avocado at lunch, found a 2014 study published in *Nutrition Journal*. A diet high in good fats may even help reverse insulin resistance, which translates to steadier blood sugar long-term. Try putting mashed avocado on sandwiches instead of mayonnaise or on bread instead of butter. To keep what's left over from turning brown, spritz the flesh with cooking spray or coat with lemon juice and wrap in plastic.

other animals live longer. But no one wants to subsist on the tiny portions these emaciated lab animals eat, so such super-low-calorie diets never quite caught on. Then, in the past few years, scientists found that intermittent fasting—eating less on some days than on others—produced the same effect but without all the hunger and suffering. A review of the available research published in a 2013 issue of the *British Journal of Diabetes and Vascular Disease* found that people with type 2 diabetes who fasted periodically lost just as much weight—and in some cases more—than those who cut calories across the board (eating the same number of calories every day). A separate study found that people who consume 600 calories twice a week—and 1,500 calories

Fasting Foods

If you'd like to try intermittent fasting as a way to stimulate weight loss and improve blood sugar control, use these suggestions for the two days a week you shrink calories to 650.

BREAKFAST	LUNCH	DINNER	SNACK
1 ounce Canadian bacon + ½ cup cooked frozen spinach + 1 cup 2% milk	Wrap: 12-inch tortilla + 5 ounces turkey breast + ½ cup sliced raw hot peppers + ¼ cup diced tomato + 2 tablespoons hummus. Side: garden salad + 1 tablespoon dressing	1 cup steamed spinach + 2 ounces grilled chicken breast + 1 cup 2% yogurt + 1½ cups air-popped popcorn	Parfait made with alternating layers of low-fat yogurt and sliced honeydew melon
½ whole-grain English muffin topped with 2 teaspons nut butter + ½ cup pineapple + 1 cup 2% milk	5 ounces sautéed chicken breast in 2 teaspoons olive oil with garlic + 1 cup prepared cannellini beans + 1 cup steamed broccoli	2 ounces pork tenderloin + ½ cup pumpkin + 1 cup fresh greens + 1 cup 2% milk	2 small plums
1 whole-grain pancake + 1 teaspoon trans-fat-free margarine	12-inch whole-grain tortilla topped with 5 ounces low-fat mozzarella	2 ounces sirloin steak + 1 cup roasted and mashed turnips + 1 cup 2% yogurt	3 prunes
1 hard-boiled egg + 1 sliced tomato + 1 cup 2% milk	1 cup mixed greens + 1 tablespoon vinegar + 1 teaspoon olive oil + 1 apple + 1 cup bouillon	2 ounces broiled salmon + 1 cup steamed green beans + 1 cup 2% milk	1 orange
1 ounce smoked salmon + ½ cup roasted asparagus + 1 cup 2% milk	2 large celery stalks + 2 tablespoon nut butter + 1 cup fresh berries + 8 ounces bouillon	Pita pizza (2 pitas topped with bell pepper, ¼ cup shredded cheese, 8 teaspoon tomato sauce and chopped onion) served with a green salad	1 cup berries

on the other days—slashed inflammation by 15 percent and insulin by 25 percent within six months.

How do you do it? Two days a week, hold your calorie intake to just 650 calories, or less than half what you normally eat. To improve satisfaction, choose low-carbohydrate and protein- and fiber-rich options (see "Fasting Foods" for meal planning suggestions). If you still feel ravenous, fill up by sipping broth made from bouillon cubes. It's nearly calorie-free—but it weighs down your stomach, making you feel full.

The other days of the week, consume reasonable portions—of up to 1,500 calories—using the good nutrition principles described in the coming pages.

What's on the Menu?

All the foods you eat, from apples to zucchini, fall into a handful of basic nutrient categories that make up the building blocks of your diet. While total calories are a major consideration, it also matters which building blocks those calories are made of. Why? Because while food raises your blood sugar within an hour or two of eating, the amount and speed of that increase depends on both how much and what types of foods you consume. In the following pages, you'll learn about the different types of foods and how that knowledge will make it easier to take control of your diabetes.

Fast Food: Inside Glycemic Load

It's human nature to want to pin the blame for our problems on a single cause. Life is simpler that way. Maybe that's why we blame all the woes of a school on the principal or all the problems with our country on the "other" political party.

And so it is with diabetes. In our quest to simplify our understanding of the disease, we often pin the blame on carbohydrates. The carbohydrates in our foods are what raises blood sugar. Therefore, they're the main cause of diabetes. Plain and simple, right?

There's a grain of truth (excuse the pun) to this thinking. Yes, carbs are the primary dietary cause of blood-sugar spikes and drops. But as with life, the truth is never that simple. As it turns out, some carb-rich foods are much healthier than others.

Thankfully, scientists have come a long way in figuring out the complexities of how carbs affect blood sugar. They also know that they need to simplify their findings if nonscientists are to understand and apply that knowledge. So they've come up with a way to make it easy to know whether a carb-rich food is a friend or a foe.

Their solution: a food ranking system called the Glycemic Load, or GL. Have you heard of it? It is quietly becoming one of the most valuable measures of the healthfulness of foods for people with diabetes. More important: Do you use it? You should. Eating foods that have low GL scores is one of the very best ways to reverse your diabetes.

What is the GL, how does it work, and how do you use it for your health? We're here to answer all your questions. Read on, and in no time you'll be an expert on carbs and how to choose the best ones for your health. Diabetes management will be so much easier as a result!

The Carb Connection

Making carbs into an enemy is a little misguided. Carbs are in *most* of the foods we eat: apples, green beans, slices of bread, a bowl of spaghetti, for instance. Even for people with diabetes, half of our calories should come from carbs.

Every food is a mix of three primary "macronutrients": protein, fat, and carbs. Beans are about one fourth protein and three fourths carbohydrate. Rice, on the other hand, is more than 90 percent carbohydrate. Whole milk contains all three macronutrients—fat, protein, and carbohydrate—because it needs to meet all the nutritional needs of a baby calf. The only foods that have no significant amounts of carbs are animal sources like beef, pork, poultry, or fish.

To understand how a food affects your blood sugar, scientists had to take into account the *quantity* of carbohydrate in foods as well as the *type* of carbohydrate in the food. This took some serious detective work. The big breakthrough came in 1981. In that year, nutrition scientist David Jenkins, MD, PhD, developed a system called the Glycemic Index (the prefix glyc means "sugar"). He had volunteers eat different foods, all containing 50 grams of carbohydrate. Then he measured the volunteers' blood sugar over the following two hours to see how high it went. As a control, he used pure glucose, the form of sugar that your body converts almost instantly to blood sugar and assigned it the number 100 on his new index.

The Glycemic Index opened a lot of eyes. In one simple number, it rated a food's impact on blood sugar based on the type of carbs it contained. A low-GI food meant that its carbs converted slowly to blood sugar; a high-GI food meant its carbs converted quickly.

The results were surprising. Most everyone had assumed that table sugar would cause the greatest increase in blood-sugar levels, much worse than the "complex carbohydrates" found in starchy staples such as rice and bread. But this didn't always prove true. Some starchy foods that contained no refined sugar, including potatoes and cornflakes, ranked very high on the index, raising blood sugar nearly as much as pure glucose.

Something else didn't make sense. Seemingly healthy foods, such as carrots and strawberries, also had super-high GI scores. And watermelon was just about off the top of the GI chart. But no one ever gained weight from eating carrots, nor do carrots, in the real world, raise blood sugar. Where did the GI go wrong?

The GI measured the effects of a standard amount of carbohydrate: 50 grams. But you'd be awfully hard-pressed to eat enough carrots—seven or eight large ones—to get 50 grams of carbohydrate. The same holds true for most vegetables and fruits. They're full of water, so there's not much room in them for carbohydrate. Bread, on the other hand, is crammed with carbohydrate. You get 50 grams by eating just one slice.

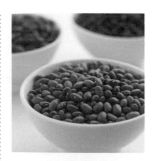

eat right
smart food
BEANS

When menu planning, think "bean cuisine" at least twice a week. The soluble fiber in all types of beans (from chickpeas to kidney beans to even edamame) puts a lid on high blood sugar. And because they're rich in protein, beans can stand in for meat in main dishes. Just watch the sodium content. Always rinse canned beans before using. To save time cooking beans, invest in a pressure cooker. Soaked beans are tender in just 10 to 15 minutes.

To solve the problem, scientists in 1997 came up with a different measurement: the Glycemic Load (GL). It takes into account not only the *type* of carbohydrate in the food but also the *amount* of carbohydrate you would eat in a standard serving. The equation is relatively simple: Multiply the GI of a food by the amount of carbs in one serving, and then divide by 100. The result is a number between 0 and 100 that accounts for both key factors: the *quality* and *quantity* of carbs in a food.

These results made much more sense. By this criterion, carrots, strawberries, and other low-calorie foods are clearly healthy to eat—they all have low GL values, since the amount of carbohydrate they contain is low. And carb-packed foods, particularly those containing fast-to-digest sugars and starches, had the highest GL scores.

The GL has become a powerful way to think about not just individual foods but also whole meals and even entire diets. When scientists looked at the GL of diets typical in different populations, they found that the higher the GL, the greater the incidence of obesity, diabetes, heart disease, and cancer. In particular, major long-term studies showed that eating meals filled with high-GL foods increased the risk of diabetes by 40 percent in middle-aged men and by a whopping 50 percent in middle-aged women. And the well-known, large-scale Nurses' Health Study found that women were twice as likely to develop heart disease over 10 years if they ate high-GL foods. The converse is also true: The lower the GL of your diet, the more likely you are to keep your weight under control and stay free of chronic disease.

When it comes to eating right, controlling weight, and preventing disease, the GL is a heavy hitter. It's a more powerful factor in keeping you healthy than the amount of carbohydrate—or even the amount of fat—you eat.

> The lower the GL of your diet, the more likely you are to keep your weight under control and stay free of chronic disease.

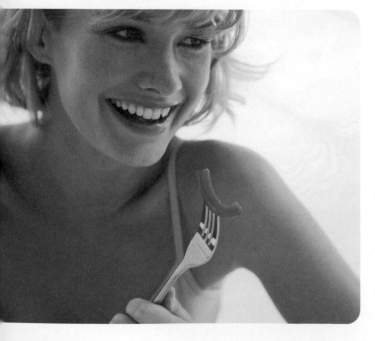

Why GLs Vary So Much

Why would one high-carb food have a different GL from another's? Why does white rice, for instance, have a higher GL than, say, honey? It has to do with the way nature constructs them.

Carbohydrates consist of starches and sugars. Starch—think of starchy foods like beans and potatoes—is made up of sugar molecules bound together in long chains. When you eat a carbohydrate-rich food, your body converts those starches and sugars into glucose, or blood sugar. Some starches, like those in white rice, are extremely easy for the body to convert, and therefore blood-sugar levels rise fast after you eat them. Others, like those in beans, take a lot more work to break down, so blood-sugar levels simmer rather than explode.

Four factors determine how fast the body breaks down carbohydrate:

1. The type of starch. Remember, starches are made of sugar molecules chained together. Some chains have straight edges, while others are branched. The straight-edged type, called amylose, is harder for your body to break down and turn into blood sugar. The branched type, called amylopectin, is much easier to break down because there are so many places for the enzymes that break down starch to get at it. Think of a tree with lots of branches—there are a lot more spots for birds to land on it compared with a simple post.

White potatoes are very high in amylopectin, the branched kind of sugar chain, which is why they raise your blood sugar in a jiffy. Peas and lentils are high in amylose, the straight kind, so they're converted to blood sugar at a snail's pace.

The more amylose a food contains, the slower it will be digested and converted into blood sugar. Take rice, for instance. Some types contain more amylose than others. In general, the softer and stickier the rice is after cooking, the lower its amylose content; this is why "sticky rice" is dastardly to your blood sugar. The firmer the rice, the higher the amylose and the harder it is for your body to turn it into blood sugar quickly. That's what makes brown rice a better choice. While some genetic variants of rice are particularly high in amylose, most of the rice we eat is low in amylose and thus has a high GL.

2. The type of sugar. Sugar is the molecule that makes up carbohydrates, but there is more than one kind. There's table sugar (sucrose) as well as the kind found in fruits and grains (fructose), the kind in milk (lactose), and the kind in malted barley (maltose). The sugars in milk and fruit tend to be absorbed more slowly than other sugars because they need to be converted into glucose by the liver first before your body can use them. That's why these foods are relatively easy on your blood sugar.

Ironically, table sugar, which is half fructose and half glucose, is turned into blood sugar more slowly than some starches, like bread or potatoes. But that doesn't make sugar—or its close cousin, high-fructose corn syrup—good for you. Why? These sweeteners aren't as sweet as you think; it takes a lot of them to turn a food into the sweet treat you've grown accustomed to. That's why one can of cola contains 40 grams of sugar. Fruit, by contrast, contains a little fructose plus plenty of water, fiber, and nutrients. A medium apple, for example, has 14 grams of fructose but lots of terrific nutrients as well.

3. Heat. All starch, whether it's made of straight or branched chains, is composed of crystals, which don't dissolve in cold water. Think of a grain of uncooked rice, a piece of raw potato, or strand of spaghetti—put it in cool water, and it stays the same. But heat breaks down those crystals so the starch can dissolve. As a result, when you cook a starchy food, it absorbs water and becomes easier to digest.

The more overcooked rice or pasta is, the faster it makes your blood sugar rise. When starch is heated and then cooled, it can return, in part, to its crystal form; that's why hot potatoes have a high GL, while potato salad's is slightly lower.

4. Processing. Have you ever noticed that some wheat breads are as smooth as white bread, while others have crunchy kernels in them? Your body takes a long time to

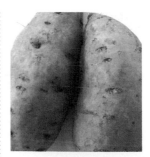

eat right
smart food
SWEET POTATOES
Choose a baked sweet potato instead of a baked white potato, and your blood sugar will rise about 30 percent less. Sweet potatoes are packed with nutrients and disease-fighting fiber, almost 40 percent of which is the soluble kind that lowers cholesterol and slows digestion. They're also extra rich in carotenoids, orange and yellow pigments that play a role in helping the body respond to insulin. Plus, they're full of the natural plant compound chlorogenic acid, which may help reduce insulin resistance.

eat right
this month!

Seek out GL data.

Sometime this month, find a book or a pocket guide on nutrition, or go online. We particularly like nutritiondata.com, which offers the most complete data on the food we eat, be it raw or processed, generic or brand name, or restaurant bought. For each food, the GL is provided in an easy-to-find box.

break down those kernels. Same for any whole, intact grains, such as wheat berries (small kernels of wheat, delicious in salads).

Modern commercial flour, on the other hand—especially white flour—has been stripped of the parts of the wheat kernel that slow its digestion; it's extremely easy for the body to turn white flour into blood sugar. That's why we continue to strongly suggest that you choose whole grains that are still intact and foods such as beans, lentils, and wheat berries instead of those made from white flour.

Until the 19th century, the main way to turn grain into flour was to grind it between stones, sometimes powered by a water wheel. Making very fine flour took a lot of work, and it was available only in small amounts to the rich. Then high-speed, high-heat steel rollers, which make very fine flour quickly and inexpensively, were invented, almost instantly transforming our diets into blood-sugar nightmares.

Modern manufacturing also turns grains into highly processed forms such as cornflakes or puffed corn snacks. These foods tend to have higher GLs than ones in which the grains are left intact, like popcorn, or those milled in an old-fashioned manner, like the coarse, stone-ground whole wheat flour used to make rustic whole-grain bread.

Swap for Zeros

When is nothing really something? When you use zero-GL foods to help manage your blood sugar. The zero tells you that a food doesn't contain any carbohydrates, the culprit behind roller-coaster blood-sugar levels. Zero-GL foods—like tomatoes, olive oil, chicken, and walnuts—aren't some exotic secret. You're likely already dishing some onto your plate on a regular basis. What you may not realize is that these foods can also help manage blood sugar by leveling out the high GLs of other foods.

However, just because they put up a GL goose egg doesn't mean that you can survive on these foods alone or eat all you want. You need to learn how to incorporate zero-GL foods into your diet.

When it comes to GL levels, foods are considered high if their GL is 20 or more; medium, 19 to 11; and low at 10 or less. Low-GL foods are often healthy options that you'll want to regularly incorporate into your diet. Finally, we have zero-GL foods.

Most zero-GL foods are nonstarchy vegetables and foods composed of protein and fat. For those with type 2 diabetes, adding more of these types of foods is good.

So good, in fact, that zero-GL foods can help tame your blood sugar by leveling out the effects of higher-GL foods. Combining a moderate- or high-GL food with a zero-GL food can result in having a blood-sugar level in the middle.

When you eat a meal, high- and low-GL foods mix in your stomach and the nutrients and glucose work their way through your system all at once. Fortunately, the high-GL foods don't convert into your blood sugar before the lower-GL foods. That means when planning a meal, you can balance the GL of foods to avoid blood-sugar spikes and crashes. However, it all comes down to portions.

For example, a high-GL food such as a heaping plate of spaghetti isn't going to be balanced by just a small serving of broccoli. There's no formula to achieve this balance, but think of any high-GL food as a side dish–size serving and zero- or low-GL foods as the main course. Finding the right balance can be a little tricky. Some people do better glycemic-wise with slightly more protein and a moderate amount of fat as they cut back on carbohydrate intake.

One way to add some zero-GL foods is to mix pinto beans into high-GL foods like rice. Or squeeze lemon juice over foods, because acidity decreases the GL. And when combining zero-GL foods with others to manage your blood sugar, frequently check your blood sugar. That way, you can tell if the combinations are actually achieving the desired result.

Remember, though, that zero-GL foods aren't magic. Eating them exclusively will leave you with an empty fuel tank. It's like gas for your car. Carbohydrates in higher-GL foods provide energy and act as your body's main fuel source. Even people with diabetes need carbohydrates for energy. The point is not to stop eating high-GL foods but to control the amount and make healthier choices. Another reason not to skip those higher-GL foods is that they often have other important nutrients that you need.

And just because a food has a zero GL doesn't automatically make it a health food. It may be high in fat, calories, and cholesterol. For example, zero-GL olive oil and nuts have healthy fat but are loaded with calories. As you look for zero-GL foods, stick with more heart-healthy protein foods.

To help balance your blood sugar, here's a guide to some common zero-GL foods.

A Taste of GL

Experts say a food has a low Glycemic Load if it scores zero to 10; a medium-GL food is 11 to 19; and a high-GL food is 20 or higher. Here are the GLs for a sampling of common foods in typical portion sizes:

Food	GL
Butter (1 tablespoon)	0
Sirloin steak (12 ounces)	0
Chicken breast (roasted)	0
Cucumber (½-cup slices)	1
Egg (1 large)	2
Carrot (1 medium, raw)	2
Strawberries (1 cup)	3
Peach (1 medium)	5
Whole-wheat bread (1 slice)	5
Dark chocolate (1 ounce)	7
Graham cracker (1 rectangle)	7
White bread (1 slice)	9
Milk (8 ounces, skim)	9
Orange juice (8 ounces)	9
Honey (1 tablespoon)	10
Corn (1 medium ear, boiled)	10
Banana (1 medium)	10
Lentil soup (1 cup)	12
Cheerios (1 cup)	12
Doughnut (3-inch, glazed)	13
Pretzels (1 ounce)	15
Pancake (6-inch)	15
Cornflakes (1 cup)	17
Chocolate cake (1 slice)	19
Raisins (1 small box)	20
White pita bread (6½-inch)	21
French fries (McDonald's, medium)	22
Garbanzo beans (1 cup, canned)	23
Spaghetti (1 cup, cooked)	23
White rice (1 cup)	24
Bagel (4-inch, seeded)	26
Baked potato (1 large)	29

When eaten with high-GL foods, nonstarchy vegetables such as asparagus can help to balance blood sugar.

CHEESE

These four cheeses may have a GL of zero, but they are still high in fat and saturated fat, meaning a zero-GL cheese may not be the overall healthiest choice.

▸ Cheddar (full-fat), 1 ounce
▸ Provolone, 1 ounce
▸ Monterey Jack, 1 ounce
▸ Colby, 1 ounce

MEAT, POULTRY, FISH & EGGS

The GL of meat, poultry, and fish is zero because they have no carbs. When choosing protein, look for lean meats and trim any visible fat. Remove skin from chicken and turkey and eat only egg whites to cut cholesterol. Tuna packed in water and tuna packed in oil both have a GL of zero, but go for the healthier version packed in water, well drained. Also, just because bacon has a GL of zero doesn't make it healthy for you.

▸ Bacon, ½ ounce or 2 strips cooked
▸ Beef, 3 ounces cooked
▸ Pork, 3 ounces cooked
▸ Chicken, 3 ounces cooked
▸ Turkey, 3 ounces cooked
▸ Tuna, 3 ounces cooked
▸ Salmon, 3 ounces cooked

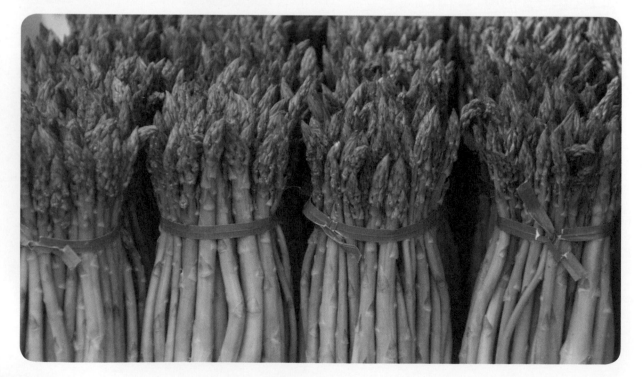

OIL, BUTTER & MARGARINE

Here's a category of zero-GL foods where you can find better selections within the bunch. For example, olive oil leads the pack for a heart-healthy choice. Butter contains saturated fat, and margarine contains hydrogenated oil, or trans fat, neither of which is recommended as part of a heart-healthy diet—even though the GL of each is zero.

- Canola oil, 1 tablespoon
- Vegetable oil, 1 tablespoon
- Olive oil, 1 tablespoon
- Butter, one pat
- Margarine, 1 tablespoon

NUTS & SEEDS

Nuts and seeds in small amounts can also provide a good source of fat. But keep the portion small because nuts do contain some carbs and lots of calories per serving.

- Almonds, 1 ounce
- Walnuts, 1 ounce
- Pecans, 1 ounce
- Sunflower seeds, 1 ounce

NONSTARCHY VEGETABLES

Here's one group of food in which more is better. Pile on your vegetables and mix them with high-GL foods to help balance out your blood sugar. In addition to being zero GL, these foods are packed with fiber and diabetes-friendly nutrients. But, remember, not all veggies fit into this category. Starchy vegetables such as corn, peas, legumes, and potatoes won't help balance other higher GL foods. But these will:

- Asparagus, five spears
- Broccoli, ½ cup
- Celery, one rib
- Eggplant, ½ cup
- Lettuce, 1 cup
- Peppers, ½ cup
- Spinach, 1 cup
- Tomato, 1 whole
- Zucchini, ½ cup

ARTIFICIALLY SWEETENED OR UNSWEETENED DRINKS

Sipping zero-GL drinks will help you avoid a spike in your blood sugar. The following beverages contain no carbs and are good choices for people with diabetes.

- Black coffee, 1 cup
- Black tea, 1 cup
- Diet beverages with artificial sweeteners, 8 ounces

Healthy Carbs

America is in love with carbohydrates. The spud is our favorite "vegetable." Bread and butter is our...bread and butter. Soda is our national beverage. For people with diabetes, this is bad news indeed. That said, if you think having the disease means never eating another potato or plate of pasta, think again. Many of the foods that are supposedly off-limits because they raise blood sugar can be easily adapted to help you manage your diabetes while still enjoying your food. Best of all, by swapping simple or fast-digesting carbohydrates for "slower-burning" foods, you'll find your cravings diminished and your once-spunky energy levels restored.

Most of the food we eat contains carbohydrates. There's no way to avoid them, and frankly, you shouldn't. Carbs are the body's main fuel source. What's more, eating whole-grain carbohydrates actually lowers your risk for disease. But not all carbs are alike. Some of them convert quickly to glucose after you eat them, raising your blood sugar and increasing the demand for insulin. The faster and higher a food raises glucose levels in the blood, the higher its "glycemic load" or GL.

Swapping high-GL foods for ones with a lower GL is a critical step in keeping your weight and blood sugar under control. Bonus: Cutting back on high-GL foods will also protect your arteries and slash your risk of heart attack and stroke.

ALL ABOUT BREAD

If you're eating white bread, you might as well be eating pure sugar, since the effect on blood sugar is similar. Take a look at the ingredients label on the brand you're eating now. What's listed first? If the word "whole" is missing, don't buy it again, even if the front of the package makes it sound miraculously healthful—and even if the bread looks "brown." Without the word "whole" in front of "wheat," you're looking at processed flour to which some brown coloring may have been added. Multigrain bread? It doesn't matter how many grains it contains if none of them is whole.

"Enriched wheat flour" is another common marketing ploy. At the very least, all flour must be enriched with folic acid as mandated by federal law. (Folic acid helps protect against birth defects.) Manufacturers will often add back some of the nutrients stripped away by processing, but much of the fiber is usually still missing, and without it, your bread is veering into doughnut land. Even if bread is made from whole grain, check to be sure that sugar in any form isn't listed among the top four ingredients. If it is, don't buy it.

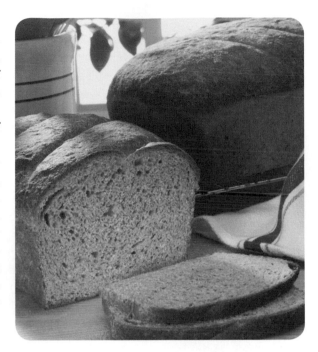

Here are four ways to improve your bread:
- ▸ Buy whole-grain bread with the word "whole" as the first ingredient.
- ▸ Look for at least 4 grams of fiber per serving—more is better.
- ▸ The coarser the bread, the better. A coarse texture indicates the best parts of the bread have been preserved—including the flavor. If the bread contains nuts and seeds, better still. They will slow down digestion of the bread, making for a slower glucose spike.
- ▸ If you see sugar in any form in the first four ingredients, just say no.

CEREAL—IT'S WHAT'S FOR BREAKFAST

When it comes to choosing diabetic-friendly cereals, there's no surprise: Sugar is the big concern. In fact, you'd be better off buying an unsweetened brand and spooning on the white stuff yourself, because you'd have a hard time adding as much sugar as manufacturers add to a typical serving.

But sugar isn't the only problem to watch for. If you favor cornflakes or rice cereal for breakfast, their lack of fiber can send your blood sugar soaring. (Corn and rice both convert to glucose very quickly in the body.)

Finally, even if you choose the healthiest cereal on earth—let's say a low-sugar bran cereal—there's still room for error. The GL is tied to portion size, and many people seriously overestimate the proper portion size for cereal. Double it and you've just doubled the GL.

Here are four tips for healthier cereal:
- ▸ Multiply the grams of sugar per serving by four (sugar has 4 calories per gram);

---

eat right this week!

Shop smart for bread.

Not all white bread is bad for you. The glycemic load of sourdough is actually on par with some whole wheat brands and 40 percent lower than standard white. Look for a crusty artisanal loaf. It will most likely use fermented sourdough yeast, which contains acids that slow the bread's digestion. Ordinary supermarket sourdough isn't the same; its sourness may result from added flavoring.

eat right
this week!

Switch to hot cereal.

One answer to the cereal problem is to switch to hot cereal in the morning. Oatmeal (old-fashioned, not instant) has a much lower GL than most cold cereals. It's also loaded with soluble fiber, which blunts the rise of blood sugar—and lowers your cholesterol to boot. It's also stick-to-your-ribs filling. In one study, people who ate oatmeal for breakfast consumed one-third fewer calories at lunch than those who ate a sugary, flaked cereal.

the result should be no more than one fourth of the total calories per serving.

▸ Look for whole-grain cereal that provides at least 4 grams of fiber per serving. Most cereals high in fiber are made with whole grains, but manufacturers also have sneaky ways of adding "fake" fiber, so check to make sure.

▸ Be wary of corn and rice cereals, even if they're low in sugar. Because they're made from refined grains, they can still raise blood sugar. Bran cereal is a much better choice.

▸ Don't pour more than one and a half times the serving size listed on the box. Fill the rest of your bowl with high-fiber berries and/or nut pieces to slow digestion.

USE YOUR NOODLES

Noodle lovers will be pleased with this news: The GL of pasta is fairly low—provided you prepare it al dente, or just a little chewy. If you favor angel hair or thin spaghetti though, you may want to rethink your selection. The thinner the pasta, the higher the GL. Couscous, which is essentially granules of pasta, has the highest GL.

The main problem with pasta is that many of us tend to overcook it. We also serve ourselves large platefuls, often topped with butter or cheese. Then we enjoy a piece of French or Italian bread on the side, ratcheting up our carb total for the meal even higher—without adding much fiber.

Here are five smart ways to choose noodles:

▸ Choose thick noodles over thin. Farfalle, penne, fettuccine, and lasagna noodles are good choices.

▸ Cook noodles al dente, not well-done.

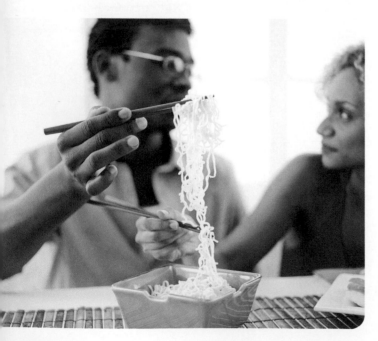

▸ Your best bet? Whole wheat pasta and other new choices. The pasta aisle in your supermarket is loaded with new products that offer more fiber than plain white pasta. Some pastas contain veggies, for even more benefits. All these cook and taste like traditional white pasta but deliver more fiber and nutrients.

▸ Add vegetables such as zucchini, broccoli, peas, bell peppers, or onions to your pasta dish to lower the calories and GL per serving.

▸ For an even lower-glycemic choice, consider pasta made with Jerusalem artichoke flour. This type of starch is not readily digested. And Jerusalem artichokes contain inulin, which may help smooth out blood sugar and insulin levels after a meal.

RICE, REALLY?

White rice may look like a grain, but as with white bread, in your body it acts more like sugar. Rice doesn't start out white. Only a rigorous milling and polishing produces those familiar milky grains. This processing strips away fiber and nutrients. White rice loses up to 90 percent of its heart-healthy vitamin B, half its manganese (which helps convert protein and carbohydrates into energy), 60 percent of its iron, and all its fiber and essential fatty acids. That's a high price to pay for rice that cooks a little faster.

Substituting brown rice will ensure you get all these nutrients (brown rice has six times the fiber of white!), and you'll eat less because it's more filling. Unfortunately, even brown has a relatively high GL.

To make rice more blood-sugar friendly:
- ▸ Choose brown rice over white. When brown won't do, wild rice is a good side-dish option. Wild-rice blends include seeds and other grains that substantially lower the GL.
- ▸ When you must serve white rice, use the "converted" kind. It's steamed under pressure before the husk is removed, which forces some of the husk's nutrients into the grain, preserving it for when you cook. As a result, converted rice offers a slight nutritional advantage over other types of white rice. Although it's still missing all the fiber and essential fats of brown rice, it has a lower GL than other white rice.
- ▸ Keep barley on hand as a tasty rice substitute with a much lower GL.
- ▸ Look for red and black rice, which are more nutritious than white rice, in gourmet shops and natural food stores.
- ▸ Convenience isn't everything, especially when your health pays the price. Instant rice is practically predigested, meaning it will turn into glucose almost as soon as it hits your stomach. Avoid it at all costs.

SCRATCH THE SODA

Some experts consider soda, aka liquid candy, the biggest single contributor to the obesity epidemic. In countries where soft drinks are popular, they're the number one source of added sugar in the diet. The worst part is that hunger sensors in the gut and brain don't register these liquid calories. In other words, you could drink hundreds of calories and still feel just as hungry as when you started. Diet sodas are no better and may be even worse. When rats are given artificial sweeteners, they eat more food and gain more weight than those fed real sugar. Here's another reason to kick soda out of your life once and for all: Its extreme sweetness dulls the flavor of other foods—the subtle yet rich taste of fruits, grains, and vegetables all pale by comparison. What's more, if you're drinking a lot of soda, you're probably not drinking good-for-you beverages such as milk and tea.

To make over your sipping habits:
- ▸ Get rid of the soda. You don't need it, and soon enough, you won't miss it.
- ▸ Instead of soda, try seltzer flavored with lemon, lime, or fruit juice. Consider getting a home soda maker so you can spritz up a bottle of seltzer whenever you want it (good for the environment, too—you reuse the plastic bottles!).
- ▸ If you drink soda for the caffeine, substitute more-healthful coffee or tea.

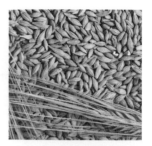

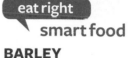

BARLEY

Choosing this grain instead of white rice can reduce the rise in blood sugar after a meal by almost 70 percent—and keep your blood sugar lower and steadier for hours. That's because the soluble fiber and other compounds in barley dramatically slow the digestion and absorption of the carbohydrate. Even brown rice can't compare. Add barley to soups, serve it as a side dish, or make it the basis for a stir-fry or casserole. Pearled, hulled, and quick-cooking varieties are all crackling good choices.

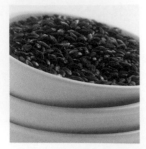

FLAXSEED

No, this is not something you fill the bird feeders with come winter. Rather, these shiny brown seeds hit the diabetes trifecta: They're rich in protein, fiber, and good fats similar to the kind found in fish. They're also a source of magnesium, a mineral that's key to blood-sugar control because it helps cells use insulin. Ground flaxseed spoils quickly, so buy whole seeds in bulk, keep in the fridge, and grind as needed. Sprinkle on cereal, yogurt, or ice cream or blend into meat loaf, meatballs, burgers, pancakes, and breads. It works in just about anything—including bird feeders.

DON'T GET JUICED

Fruit juice? Dangerous? That's right. Compared with the fruit itself, a cup of juice can have as much as twice the calories but none of the fiber. That's a problem because it's the fiber in fruit that prevents the fruit's natural sugars from causing a glucose spike. Drink a cup of orange juice, and you'll get 100 calories and less than ½ gram of fiber. Eat an orange, and you'll get seven times the fiber (3.5 grams) and only 65 calories. Which one do you think will fill you up more? The same is true of apple juice. It contains practically zero fiber, while an apple has four grams and about half the calories. And like the calories in soda, the ones in juice don't satisfy hunger very well.

To **squeeze the most health from juice:**
- When you can, have a piece of fruit instead of a glass of juice.
- When you want juice, buy 100% juice (not some juice "drink" with added sugar or high fructose corn syrup) and limit yourself to four ounces (a small juice glass) at a time.
- Want more juice? Pour yourself four ounces and fill the rest of your glass with no-calorie seltzer.

Cut Back on Carbohydrates?

That would seem to make sense. After all, the major types of carbohydrate—sugars and starches—both break down into glucose and are the main source of blood sugar, making them an important target of dietary control. But carbohydrates are also the body's primary source of energy, so they play a critical part of any healthy diet. According to the American Diabetes Association, carbohydrates should account for up to 60 percent of your total diet.

Why so much? One gram of carbohydrate contains only 4 calories, while a gram of fat contains 9 calories. That means, gram for gram, you can eat more than twice as much carbohydrate as fat for the same number of calories. A carb-based diet allows you to eat larger quantities of food and therefore a greater variety of foods (both nutritionally and taste-wise) even if you're restricting your total calories.

But shouldn't sugars be avoided? The answer is yes, but only because they often come in packages that are high in fat and low in vitamins and minerals: desserts, candies, and baked goods, for instance. Otherwise, there's nothing inherently wrong with sugars (sometimes called simple carbohydrates because their chemical structure consists of only a few molecules that are easily broken down during digestion). Milk contains sugar (called lactose), and so does fruit (fructose), and there's no reason to ban these foods. There's even room for sucrose (table sugar) and sweets in your diet, as long as you eat them in small amounts.

That makes starches, or complex carbohydrates, the main staple of your diet. Starches lack the sweetness of sugars but are found in some of the most nutritious foods you can eat, including beans, potatoes, pasta, rice, whole-grain breads and cereals, and vegetables like broccoli, carrots, corn, and peas. Starches not only are energy powerhouses, but they're also rich in vital nutrients, such as vitamins and minerals.

Counting Carbs: An Easy Solution

One of the most useful tools for controlling your caloric intake and blood sugar at the same time is carbohydrate counting. This method is a favorite of dietitians since researchers discovered that all types of carbohydrates, whether sugars or starches, are converted into glucose and released into the blood at about the same rate—within an hour or so of eating. (Fat and protein are eventually broken down into glucose, too, only at a much slower rate.) So the level of glucose in the blood after a meal is determined primarily by the amount (not the type) of carbohydrate consumed.

This makes following a meal plan relatively easy because you can control the amount of glucose entering your body by simply counting the grams of carbohydrate you ingest—information that's printed on every package of food you buy. This approach is particularly useful to people with type 1 diabetes or those with type 2 who must take insulin because it allows more precise matching of insulin doses to glucose intake.

To start you out on a carbohydrate-counting plan, your dietitian will first come up with the number of carbohydrates that you should eat at every meal and snack, based on your individual calorie needs. Ideally, carbohydrate should make up 50 to 60 percent of your daily calorie intake. You then have flexibility in choosing the foods you like in order to hit your target. A similar program of fat-gram counting can be helpful for people with type 2 diabetes who are trying to lose weight.

Your dietitian can provide carb-counting food lists, or you can find more extensive lists in books. But a general rule of thumb is that one serving of starch, fruit, or

Crave That? Eat This

When a carb craving hits, satisfy it with the foods on the right instead of the ones on the left. In most cases, the substitute foods offer more fiber, fewer calories, less sugar, and/or a lower GL. The dark chocolate contains antioxidants that are powerful weapons against diabetes complications.

CRAVE THIS?	EAT THIS
Mashed potato	Baked potato with the skin
A dinner roll	Real (bakery) sourdough bread
French fries	Sweet potato fries
White rice	Pearled barley
Bagels	Whole-wheat English muffin
Raisins or dried bananas	Dried apricots
Potato chips	Corn chips
Candy bar	A single piece of dark chocolate
Pretzels	Air-popped popcorn
Glazed donut	Plain donut
White crackers	Whole-grain crackers or pita chips

Cooking with Whole Grains

If these whole grains are missing from your cupboard—and they probably are—pick some up next time you shop. These are among the healthiest grains on the planet, each high in fiber and nutrients. Here's how to cook with them.

Barley. Use this nutty grain as an alternative to pasta or rice, or sauté it with vegetables for a side dish. Or chill it and make a barley salad with herbs, dressing and a sprinkling of Parmesan cheese.

Bran. Use it to replace half the flour in muffin recipes. Mix into meat loaf or sprinkle bran flakes on casseroles.

Bulgur (also known as kasha). Make bulgur pilaf as a side dish or use the grain cold to make a salad, such as tabbouleh. Or cook hot bulgur cereal in salted water as you would oatmeal.

Quinoa: Use it as a side dish for an alternative to white rice or pasta. It's rich in protein and fiber.

milk contains about 15 grams of carbohydrate; vegetables, five grams; and meat and fats, none. Unfortunately, that doesn't mean you can load up on meat or eat the same three carbohydrates at every meal; you still need to aim for variety and balance. Try to spread your carbohydrate intake evenly throughout the day so the amount of glucose released into your blood is fairly consistent from meal to meal.

Solve Your Carb Crisis

Lots of us have the same problem: We're eating too many unhealthy carbs—and it shows on your blood-sugar tests and your waistline. The solution is simple enough: Cut back on empty carbs and choose ones that help keep blood sugar under control.

But first, let's talk about refined carbohydrates and other so-called high-glycemic foods that may be standing between you and better diabetes control. They are blood-sugar boosters and excess-weight creators. And, if you're like most Americans, you're eating way too many of them.

What makes these foods so problematic? Simple: the extraordinary ease and speed at which they break down into glucose during digestion. This sudden surge of available glucose quickly enters your bloodstream, sending blood-sugar levels into orbit—the very problem that causes diabetes. Even worse, these high-glycemic carbs tend to be empty calories that do little more than pad your waistline.

Which foods are the main offenders? Sweetened soft drinks, candy, and baked goods, as well as three ubiquitous "white" foods: potatoes, white rice, and white bread. By upgrading your carb intake, you can lower your blood sugar as much as some diabetes drugs do. Follow these three simple steps to slash your consumption of refined carbs by 50 percent or more, and replace them with whole grains, fruits, vegetables, and other super-nutritious foods.

1. START SWAPPING CARBS

Simply cutting back on, or cutting out, a few specific foods can give you a serious edge in controlling diabetes. A major study of middle-aged women found that the worst offenders by far when it came to raising blood sugar were the following:

- ▸ Potatoes
- ▸ Sugary breakfast cereal
- ▸ White bread
- ▸ Muffins
- ▸ White rice
- ▸ Sugary drinks

Here's how to blunt the impact of these sugar-raisers:

Cut your pasta in half. Pasta isn't as big a blood-sugar booster as you might think. Because its starch molecules are interwoven with protein molecules, it converts to glucose slowly as you digest a meal. That means pasta is fairly friendly to your blood sugar, as far as grain foods go. (Cook it al dente instead of well-done, and it will have even less impact on your blood sugar.) The issue is portion size: Most people eat a huge bowl of pasta when it's the main course. Limit yourself to half a cup of pasta instead.

Make sandwich wraps out of lettuce. A 13-inch tortilla can contain as many as 330 calories, not to mention 55 grams of carbs. Instead, make your sandwich wraps out of lettuce, using broad-leaf choices like romaine or red leaf. For a tasty lunch, fill a large lettuce leaf with canned tuna or salmon, shredded carrots, diced celery, and pepper slices.

Skip the dinner rolls. Bread isn't bad for you, especially if it's whole grain. But if you had a sandwich at lunch or toast with your eggs at breakfast, that's probably all the bread you need for the day.

Eat less rice. Limit yourself to one serving, or ½ cup. Avoid jasmine rice, arborio rice (the kind used to make risotto), sticky rice, and long-grain quick-cooking rice; these varieties raise blood sugar the most. Choose brown and wild rice instead.

Indulge in vegetable "fries." Say good-bye to French fries made from potatoes, and say hello to fries made from vegetables with a lower glycemic load. Cut parsnips, turnips, sweet potatoes or carrots lengthwise into thin vegetable strips. Place on a baking sheet, drizzle with olive oil, sprinkle with salt and pepper, and roast in a 400°F oven for about 40 minutes. Truly delicious!

Say so long to soda. We're sprinkling this warning throughout this book because we consider it so important. If the FBI had a most-wanted list for the foods that are hurting your health, Public Enemy Number One would certainly be sweetened drinks. Experts report that sugary drinks—not just soda but also many supposedly healthy fruit drinks—have rapidly become the biggest single source of calories in the American diet, comprising 7 to 10 percent of our total caloric intake. Pretty much all those calories come from refined sugar or corn syrup: One 12-ounce serving of regular soda has the equivalent of nine packets of sugar! Banishing colas and other sweetened beverages from your life is the fastest, easiest way to gain better blood-sugar control and cut empty calories. Need we say more? Make a commitment to get zero calories from your mealtime drinks, by choosing water, sparkling water, iced tea, or lemonade made from fresh lemon juice and a sugar substitute.

eat right this week!

Review your eating patterns.

At the end of the week, look over your diary for patterns. You may find that you consume more calories than you've ever imagined in the form of midday or late-night snacks or beverages such as juice, soda, lattes, and beer. Also look critically at your diary to see how well your eating habits match up with the Eat Right goals, and figure out where they fall short. Are your breakfasts full of carbs but no protein? Are you getting anywhere near five servings of veggies a day? It's amazing what you'll learn when you look at your diet in black and white.

2. EAT MORE WHOLE GRAINS

Why all the fuss over whole grains? Here are three good reasons to make them part of your daily menu.

- ▸ Women who eat the most whole grains are about 50 percent more likely to maintain a healthy weight.
- ▸ Eating more whole grains may cut your risk for heart disease—the number one killer in people with diabetes—by up to 25 percent.
- ▸ A diet rich in whole grains helps keep blood sugar steady.

Adding more fiber is easier when you follow these tips:

Start your day with a high-fiber cereal. Look for a brand with the word "whole" in the first ingredient and at least three grams of fiber per serving. Avoid sugary cereals; try to keep the sugar grams per serving in the single digits. That way, you'll control calories and stay off the blood-sugar roller coaster that leads to midmorning hunger pangs and food cravings. Top your cereal with berries to squeeze in a fruit serving. For protein, pour on some fat-free milk and maybe some ground flaxseeds.

Buy bread and rolls with the word "whole" first on the ingredients list. Don't be fooled if the label says "made with wheat flour;" that could be true of both whole wheat bread and angel food cake. If a product is truly whole grain, the label will list whole wheat, whole oats, or some other whole grain as the first ingredient.

Switch pastas. Try whole wheat pasta, especially the new high-fiber, high-protein varieties; they're even friendlier to your blood sugar. Some are made from grains such as oats, spelt, and barley in addition to durum wheat, which means they're higher in soluble fiber. And yet their taste and texture are surprisingly close to regular pasta choices.

Bake with the whole stuff. Give a boost to homemade baked goods by replacing one-third of the white flour with whole-wheat flour.

Use fibrous fixings. Bran cereal, oat bran, and wheat germ make good toppings when sprinkled over oatmeal, applesauce, cottage cheese, and yogurt. In recipes that call for bread crumbs, try oatmeal or whole-grain bread—toasted, then reduced to crumbs in your food processor.

Choose brown rice. Eat brown rice instead of white, and you'll get six times more fiber and far more vitamins, minerals, and other healthy plant compounds. Just keep in mind that even brown rice bumps up blood sugar quite a bit, so limit yourself to ½ cup per serving. Remember that brown rice takes about 45 minutes to cook, so start early—or make a big batch and freeze meal-size portions.

3. MAKE FIBER A PRIORITY

Fiber, an indigestible complex carbohydrate found in plant foods such as bran, broccoli, oatmeal, and whole grains, should be part of your diet for a number of reasons—primarily because it slows the rise of blood sugar after a meal.

eat right **this month!**

Start by adding more fiber slowly.

Foods like beans and broccoli are notorious for producing gas in the intestines, but the effect is temporary, and your body will adjust as you eat more fiber. You may feel more comfortable if you add fiber gradually over a period of weeks to give your system a chance to get used to it. Start by adding about 5 grams a day (about the amount in half a cup of kidney beans) until you reach the 25- to 30-gram daily target. Your body will also handle added fiber more effectively if you drink more water.

There are two types of fiber: soluble and insoluble. Both are good for you, but only soluble fiber, found in oats, barley, beans, and some fruits and vegetables, lowers your blood sugar in a big way. Here's why: Most whole grains are rich in insoluble fiber, which passes through you undigested. Soluble fiber dissolves in water, causing it to form a gum in your digestive system. This gum creates a barrier between the digestive enzymes in your stomach and the starch molecules in food. That slows down the conversion of starchy carbs in a meal into glucose. And that means lower blood sugar for you.

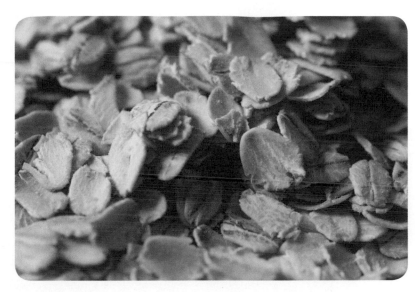

In one study, people with type 2 diabetes who got 50 grams of fiber in their diet every day for six weeks (after starting with six weeks of 25 grams, the amount recommended for the general population) brought their blood-sugar levels down by about 10 percent. In addition to lowering blood sugar, soluble fiber helps lower cholesterol, reducing your risk of cardiovascular disease. Insoluble fiber (the other type) improves overall digestive function by helping waste move through your system. What's more, fiber adds bulk to food, which makes you feel full without adding a single calorie.

While food labels list grams of fiber for processed and packaged products, don't worry about "counting fiber" to get the recommended 25 to 30 grams per day. It's much better (and easier) to simply work as many grains, beans, and fresh fruits and vegetables into your diet as you can. Here are some smart strategies:

Bump up beans. Whether dried or canned, beans and other legumes are among the best fiber sources you can find. For example, half a cup of black beans provides about a quarter of your recommended daily fiber intake.

Hail the whole. Whole-grain foods contain far more fiber than more processed foods, in which such fiber-containing grain parts as the bran are thrown out. For example, whole-grain bread contains about twice the fiber as bread made with refined flour.

Preserve the peel. Routinely thrown away, the peel is often the most fiber-filled part of a fruit or vegetable. You're better off eating apples, carrots, and potatoes with the peel still on (be sure to wash them first if you eat them raw).

Savor stems. We also often toss out the stalky stems of vegetables like asparagus and broccoli, but that's where the plant's fiber is most densely concentrated. To make them less tough, chop the stalks into small pieces and cook them a bit longer, adding the florets slightly later.

> Soluble fiber, found in oats, barley, beans, and some fruits and vegetables, lowers your blood sugar in a big way.

Use fibrous fixings. Products like bran cereal, oat bran, and wheat germ make good condiments when sprinkled over oatmeal (which is high in fiber itself), applesauce, cottage cheese, and salads. In recipes that call for bread crumbs, try substituting oats.

The Skinny on Sugar Substitutes

You'd think sugar-free foods like candy and soft drinks would have less impact on blood-glucose levels than regular candy or soft drinks. But you can't eat sugar-free foods with impunity.

Here's why: Common sweeteners, such as maltodextrin, sorbitol, and xylitol, may not be sucrose (the technical name for regular sugar), but they do contain carbohydrate, each gram of which can raise blood glucose just as much as sugar does. Nonnutritive sweeteners like aspartame contain no carbohydrate or calories, but products that contain these sweeteners (such as yogurt and soft drinks) might.

The best advice: Pay no attention to "sugar-free" claims on the packaging. Look instead at a product's total carbohydrate count.

ARE FAKE SUGARS SAFE?

For people trying to reduce their calorie and carbohydrate intake, artificial, nonnutritive sweeteners have been a godsend, allowing a wide variety of foods and drinks to taste more delectable without sugar or added calories. But two of the most popular artificial sweeteners, saccharin and aspartame, have been battered by storms of controversy regarding their safety. Should you worry?

Saccharin. Back in the 1970s, the Food and Drug Administration banned saccharin (marketed as Sweet'N Low) after studies indicated that high doses of it caused cancer in rats. Since then, studies have suggested that differences between rat and human anatomy make the rats' risk inapplicable to people, and in 2000, saccharin was taken off the official list of cancer-causing compounds. Some consumer-advocate groups and nutrition researchers are uneasy about the change and claim the evidence of a cancer risk still warrants caution. Still, even they admit that if a risk exists, it's very small.

Aspartame. Heated debate preceded aspartame's FDA approval in 1981, partly because investigators found research by the manufacturer to be riddled with inconsistencies and errors. An outside advisory board recommended withholding approval but was overruled by the FDA, which felt (after an audit) that the evidence proved aspartame (sold as NutraSweet) to be safe. Even after the approval, skeptics charged that aspartame interfered with normal brain chemistry, triggering headaches, seizures, and (it was feared) brain cancer. However, numerous studies over the past 15 years have found these concerns to be groundless, and even strong advocacy groups, such as the Center for Science in the Public Interest, no longer sound alarms about aspartame.

Diabetes and Dessert

Want some cake or a few cookies after dinner? Yes, you can still have sweet desserts when you have diabetes. The secrets? Use less refined sugar, cut back on the fat, include whole grains or wheat, add nuts, and keep portion sizes reasonable. These two cookie recipes show that delicious diabetes-friendly desserts are yours to enjoy, if you follow these secrets.

CHOCOLATE WALNUT MELT-IN-YOUR-MOUTH COOKIES

A wonderful treat or reward awaits you at the end of a busy day: A delightful hit of sweetness, with just the right crisp texture and rich chocolatey goodness.

Makes: 30

Prep Time: 25 minutes
Cook Time: 12–15 minutes

6 ounces semisweet chocolate chips

2 large egg whites, at room temperature

1/8 teaspoon cream of tartar

1/2 teaspoon vanilla extract

1/2 cup packed light brown sugar

1/3 cup finely chopped walnuts

1/4 cup all-purpose flour

30 walnut pieces

1. Preheat the oven to 350°F. Coat two baking sheets with nonstick cooking spray.

2. Melt the chocolate chips in a small glass bowl in the microwave, 1 to 1½ minutes. Cool slightly.

3. In a medium bowl, with an electric mixer, beat the egg whites together with the cream of tartar and vanilla until soft peaks form. Gradually beat in the brown sugar, 1 tablespoon at a time, to make stiff peaks.

4. Drizzle the chocolate on top of the egg whites, and gently fold until thoroughly incorporated.

5. In a small bowl, stir the chopped walnuts and flour until blended. Sprinkle over the egg whites and gently fold until blended (batter will deflate slightly). Immediately drop the batter by rounded teaspoons onto baking sheets. Place a walnut piece in the center of each.

6. Bake, turning pans halfway through baking time to ensure even baking, until firm around the edges, 12 to 15 minutes. Remove the cookies from the pans and cool on wire racks.

Per cookie: 70 cal, 4 g fat (1g sat), 9 g carbs, 1 g protein, 1 g fiber, 0 mg chol, 5 mg sodium, 9 mg calcium

CHOCOLATE CHIP OATMEAL COOKIES

Look what has happened to the traditional chocolate chip cookie! This one has only half the fat of the original plus old-fashioned oats add fiber. Yet none of these changes have slimmed down the flavor.

Makes: 36

Prep time: 15 minutes
Cook time: 20 minutes

1 cup all-purpose flour

1½ teaspoon baking soda

Salt to taste

1 cup old-fashioned oats

4 tablespoons margarine

2/3 cup packed light brown sugar

1/2 cup granulated sugar

1 large egg

1½ teaspoons vanilla

1/3 cup reduced-fat sour cream

3/4 cup semisweet chocolate chips

1. Preheat oven to 375°F. Line two large baking sheets with parchment paper. Whisk flour, baking soda, and salt in medium bowl. Stir in oats.

2. Cream margarine, brown sugar, and granulated sugar in large bowl with electric mixer at high speed until well blended. Add egg and vanilla, and beat until light yellow and creamy, about 3 minutes. Blend in sour cream with wooden spoon, then flour mixture all at once, just until combined (don't overmix or the cookies may become tough). Stir in chocolate chips.

3. Drop dough by heaping teaspoonfuls 2 inches apart onto baking sheets. Bake cookies until golden, about 10 minutes. Cool on baking sheets 2 minutes, then transfer to wire racks and cool completely. Store in airtight container for up to 2 weeks or freeze for up to 3 months.

Per cookie: 91 cal, 3 g fat (1 g sat), 14 g carbs, 1 g protein, 0.2 g fiber, 7 mg chol, 34 mg sodium, 8 mg calcium

Sucralose. Marketed as Splenda, sucralose is one of the newest artificial sweetener on the market. Studies have shown it to be safe. In a 2003 study, 128 people with type 2 diabetes were given sucralose capsules or a placebo for 13 weeks. At the study's end, blood tests showed that sucralose had no effect on the fasting blood glucose or HbA1C levels of people with type 2 diabetes. However, some recent animal studies have raised concerns about sucralose's effect on absorption of prescription medications and its effects on reducing the amount of good bacteria in the gut. Because sucralose is found in so many food products and can be used in cooking, you could unknowingly consume as much as a cup or more of the stuff every day—and we simply don't know what the long-term effects of that might be.

THE BOTTOM LINE

It's fine to drink an artificially sweetened beverage now and then or to eat a serving or two of a food product containing artificial sweeteners. But the point of the Reverse Diabetes diet is to acquaint you with naturally delicious foods and to show you that even a little real sugar won't affect your blood-sugar levels. When it comes to food, keeping it real (and in moderation) is your best defense against blood-sugar problems.

Factoring in Fat

Fat is usually seen as a dietary evil, mainly because it's so dense in calories and a known contributor to heart disease. But fat also has important roles to play in the body, such as helping to form cell membranes, distributing fat-soluble vitamins, and insulating the body against heat loss. And there's an upside to fat for diabetics: It slows the digestion process, which means that glucose enters the blood more gradually. As a result, fat should play a bigger role in your diet than you might assume, making up as much as 25 to 30 percent of total calories.

But watch out—there's a caveat. The type of fat you eat makes a difference. According to the American Diabetes Association's dietary recommendations, less than 10 percent of your diet should consist of the kind of fat we're likely to eat most: saturated fat. For most of us, this works out to about 20 grams of saturated fat per day, a pretty tiny amount when you consider that just 1 ounce—about four dice-size pieces—of cheese can have 8 grams of saturated fat.

Found in animal-based foods like meat and eggs and in dairy products like butter, saturated fat tends to raise levels of LDL ("bad") cholesterol and is associated with an increased risk of cardiovascular disease, thus magnifying the metabolic problems that worsen diabetes. What's more, experts have discovered that saturated fat actually increases insulin resistance, making blood-sugar control more difficult. Even worse than saturated fat: trans fat. Found in margarine and processed foods, it raises LDL cholesterol and lowers the healthy HDL kind. No amount of

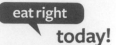

eat right today!

Have a serving of peanut butter.

A daily serving of peanut butter could cut the risk for type 2 diabetes by 21 percent. Meanwhile, studies have shown that munching on nuts every day may lower the threat of heart attack.

trans fat is good for you. It's so bad that experts advise you to eliminate it entirely.

But if you eat only small amounts of saturated fat (easily recognized because it usually stays solid at room temperature) and no trans fat, where should the rest of your fat calories come from?

The answer is monounsaturated and polyunsaturated fats, neither of which raises your levels of bad cholesterol. Monounsaturated fat is especially recommended because it actually raises levels of good cholesterol, making it the best source of fat in your diet. (Polyunsaturated fat, found in such foods as corn oil, safflower oil, and mayonnaise, ranks second because it's been shown to lower levels of bad cholesterol.)

According to the ADA, monounsaturated fat may also reduce insulin resistance.

These fats are so good for you that the ADA says either monounsaturated fat or carbohydrates can be eaten in place of saturated fat. In fact, either one can make up as much as 60 to 70 percent of your total calories. This allows you even more latitude when planning your meals, especially if you eat an ethnic diet. For example, a person who eats an Asian diet may prefer a diet high in carbohydrates like rice, while someone who eats a Mediterranean diet may want more calories from foods like olive oil. Both are allowed. But remember: Even monounsaturated fat is rich in calories, so don't go overboard, especially if you're trying to lose weight.

Unsaturated Fats

These types of fats have fewer hydrogen atoms than saturated fats (so named because the carbon atoms aren't saturated with hydrogen atoms). They are often derived from plants, but seafood is also rich in healthy unsaturated fats. Unsaturated fats come in two categories:

POLYUNSATURATED FAT

There are two main types of polyunsaturated fats, or PUFAs: omega-3 fatty acids and omega-6 fatty acids. You probably get plenty of the latter, since they're found in vegetable oils like safflower, sesame, corn and sunflower-seed oils, as well as nuts and seeds. However, omega-3s are one of the heart-healthiest foods available and they may be largely missing from your diet. They are found mostly in seafood, particularly cold-water ocean fish like salmon.

MONOUNSATURATED FAT

Often called MUFAs, these fats are liquid at room temperature but start to solidify in the refrigerator. They include olive, canola, and peanut oils, as well as the fat in avocados. Swapping saturated fat for monounsaturated fat helps reverse insulin resistance and improves cholesterol levels. Olive oil is the best-known source of this nourishing fat, but there are plenty of other ways to slip MUFAs into your menu.

Good Fats for Breakfast

Traditional breakfast foods are often loaded with saturated fat (think bacon) and trans fats (such as doughnuts). On the other hand, many sources of good fats, such as olive oil, fish, and avocados, are rarely associated with morning foods. However, there are plenty of ways to slip good fats into breakfast.

Go nuts. If your cereal doesn't contain nuts, add some chopped almonds, walnuts, or pecans yourself. If you're enjoying a piece of toast or a whole wheat English muffin, peanut butter is the perfect spread. You can also add chopped nuts to waffle, pancake, and muffin batter.

Find flax. Flaxseeds are loaded with ALA, a form of fat that resembles omega-3 fatty acids. And they have a pleasant, slightly nutty taste. Buy whole flaxseeds, store them in the fridge, and grind them as needed. Don't eat whole flaxseeds, or they'll come out the way they went in.

Spread smart margarine. If you have high cholesterol, consider buttering your whole-grain toast with a margarine such as Benecol, which is enhanced with plant compounds called stanols. Stanols prevent the intestines from absorbing cholesterol in food. Eat several servings of stanol-rich margarine a day, and you can lower total and LDL cholesterol by 10 percent and 15 percent, respectively. New research shows that these margarines also reduce triglycerides, another unhealthy blood fat. But beware: If a margarine's ingredients list contains the words "partially hydrogenated," don't buy it—that's a tip-off that it contains trans fats, the unhealthy stuff that's to be avoided at any cost.

Eat eggs. They're nature's best source of protein, and here's a little-known fact: One large egg contains two grams of MUFAs, the good fats also found in nuts and olive oil.

Serve smoked salmon. A few slices with your eggs or toast will provide you with the omega-3s you need, plus a wonderfully rich and bold flavor. But don't create monster bagel sandwiches filled with cream cheese.

▸ MAKING THE SWITCH AT BREAKFAST

INSTEAD OF	TRY
Bacon and sausage	Whole-grain cereal sprinkled with chopped nuts
Doughnuts	Whole wheat English muffin with 1 tablespoon peanut butter
Pastries	Scrambled eggs with smoked salmon
Waffles and pancakes	Low-fat or nonfat yogurt topped with fresh fruit and low-fat granola

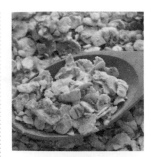

eat right
smart food

OATMEAL

Ever wonder why oatmeal is so good for you? It's because it's loaded with soluble fiber, which forms a paste when mixed with water. Just as it sticks to your bowl, it also forms a gummy barrier between the digestive enzymes in your stomach and the starch molecules in your meal. So it takes longer for your body to convert the carbs you've eaten into blood sugar. Don't like oatmeal in the morning? Buy oat flour and use it as a thickener in autumn stews, casseroles, and soups. Or add ground oatmeal (not the instant kind) to muffin, pancake, or waffle batters. You won't even know it's there.

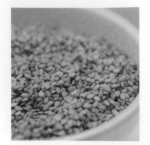

SEEDS

Like nuts, seeds of all types—pumpkin, sunflower, sesame—are filled with good fats, protein, and fiber that work together to keep blood sugar low and stave off heart disease. They're also a natural source of cholesterol-lowering sterols—the same compounds added to cholesterol-lowering margarines. Fill an empty Altoids mint tin with your favorite unsalted seeds and stash it in your purse or pocket in case of snack emergencies. Or tell the waiter to hold the croutons on your Caesar and substitute pumpkin or sunflower seeds instead.

Good Fats for Lunch

Skipping takeout burgers in favor of green salads for the midday meal will spare you lots of saturated fat. But that plan backfires if your stomach is groaning by 2:00 p.m. and you give in to cravings for high-calorie, tide-you-over snacks. Adding good fats to your lunch, either on the side or right on top of that salad, will give your midday meal a first-class upgrade and keep you satiated longer.

A is for avocados. Replace the cheese in your sandwich or salad with avocado slices. Or mash some avocado and use it as a spread in place of mayonnaise. Avocado slices are also great additions to black bean soup.

Butter nutter. Talk about an easy lunch: Start with a slice of whole-grain bread (preferably one with lots of visible nuts and seeds) and slather on a tablespoon of peanut butter, and you've got a belly-filling companion for that lonely green salad.

Other ideas for peanut butter and nuts at lunch:
▸ Spread peanut butter on a banana or some apple slices.
▸ Top whole wheat noodles with spicy Asian peanut sauce.
▸ For a change of pace, try almond butter.

Try tahini. Like nuts, seeds are full of good fats. Try seed spreads, such as tahini, an essential food in Middle-Eastern cuisine that's made from sesame paste. Tahini is delicious on its own (spread it on bread or whole-grain crackers), but it's also the key ingredient in easy-to-make healthy dishes such as hummus and baba ghanoush.

▸ MAKING THE SWITCH AT LUNCH

INSTEAD OF	TRY
A fast-food burger	Tomato stuffed with tuna salad made with low-fat mayonnaise or plain yogurt, hard-cooked egg, chopped apples, celery, and onions
A breaded fish sandwich	Tuna or salmon sandwich with lettuce and onions on whole-grain bread
A deli sandwich topped with mayonnaise	Green salad topped with dried cranberries, chopped nuts, and an olive-oil-based dressing
A burrito	Mixed-greens salad with peanut butter–smeared apple slices on the side

10 Ways to Trim the Fat

Fat is a beloved dietary staple because it's both tasty and versatile: It can be creamy, crunchy—and sometimes both at once (think fried ice cream). But while no one needs to forgo all of fat's pleasures, a lot of the fat in our diet comes hidden (and unbidden) in cooking or eating habits that can easily be changed without sacrificing taste.

1. Choose leaner loins
Oddly enough, meats labeled "prime" are the ones you should avoid; they're loaded with saturated fat. Lean cuts include flank steak, top round, and pork tenderloin.

2. Chill out
Trimming obvious fat from meat quickly carves off lots of saturated fat. To do it better, put meat in the freezer for 20 minutes first; this will firm up the meat for closer cutting and make marbled fat more visible. When preparing soups or stocks, chill broth overnight and skim congealed fat from the surface.

3. Forgo fried snacks for baked snacks
Salty, fried snacks like potato and tortilla chips can have as much saturated fat content as beef. Better options: low-fat chips, pretzels, or—best yet—fresh-cut veggies with salsa.

4. Switch to skim
Whole milk gets almost half its calories from fat, while fat-free milk has almost no fat and fewer calories. If you don't like the taste of skim, blend varieties to start, progressively adding fat-free milk as you get more used to it. Or, try ultra-pasteurized varieties. Always use fat-free in recipes.

5. Use butter-besting spreads
Instead of butter, switch to a margarine-like spread. Look for one that does not contain hydrogenated oils or trans fat.

6. Skin your chicken
About half the fat in poultry is concentrated in the skin, which you can leave on while cooking to keep the meat moist but remove before eating—especially if you like drumsticks, which contain more than twice the fat of chicken breast, even with the skin off.

7. Take advantage of nonstick
Why use butter or margarine to keep food from adhering to frying pans when nonstick pans eliminate the need? If you still want to coat the pan, use a cooking spray.

8. Retire the fryer
Even with healthier oils, frying adds fat calories you can do without. Better bets are baking and broiling, which add little fat and bring out the flavor of beef, poultry, fish, and hearty vegetables like peppers and eggplant.

9. Mix your meats
When recipes call for ground beef, cut the amount in half and bulk up the meat by substituting lower-fat ground turkey, soy crumbles, or shredded vegetables such as onions, carrots, and green peppers.

10. Repair the recipe
When baking foods like breads, cakes, muffins, and brownies, try using only half the amount of fatty ingredients like butter and oil and substituting an equal amount of applesauce or pureed fruit, such as prunes.

eat right this month!

Choose a variety of proteins.

So meals don't get boring with the same protein over and over again (how much chicken can we eat?), include eggs, fish, beans, and lean cuts of beef. How important is this protein? Protein makes you feel full, so be sure lean proteins are part of every meal. They help keep blood sugar low, cut between-meal cravings, and even help preserve calorie-burning muscle while you're losing weight. We'll show you easy ways to work protein into every meal.

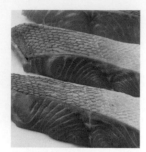

smart food

FISH

The single deadliest complication of diabetes is heart disease, and eating fish just once a week can reduce your risk by 40 percent, according to a Harvard School of Public Health study. The fatty acids in fish reduce inflammation in the body—a major contributor to coronary disease—as well as insulin resistance and diabetes. And unless you're pregnant, don't worry too much about potential chemical contaminants. An exhaustive review of the scientific literature on fish and human health by Harvard researchers led to the conclusion that eating it far outweighs any accompanying risks.

Good Fats for Dinner

If you have a busy schedule—and who doesn't?—dinner is the only meal where you might have time to strap on an apron and do some real cooking. That makes the evening repast a prime opportunity for fitting in more good fats, since some of the best sources are cooking oils (tops for MUFAs) and seafood (unparalleled for omega-3 fatty acids).

Opt for olive oil. In fact, feel free to drizzle it over cooked vegetables to make them more appealing. And if you're serving a crusty whole-grain or sourdough bread with dinner, put out a small bowl of olive oil for dipping rather than butter. Other cooking oils are good for you, too, in moderation.

Cook fish. Many people avoid fish because they think it's just too hard to make a great-tasting fish dinner. But simple techniques such as steaming, baking in foil, and grilling (thick, firm-textured fish only) can produce delectable results. Or, for a quick dinner, try albacore tuna with cannellini beans, sliced red peppers, chopped cilantro or parsley, cucumbers, and onions, tossed with an olive-oil-based dressing.

Swap nuts for meat. Nuts, especially peanuts and cashews, are tasty, filling stand-ins for meat in veggie-heavy stir-fry dishes. (Remember to serve the stir-fry over brown rice and use low-sodium soy sauce.)

Sprinkle some sesame seeds. They liven up broccoli, and they're another great addition to Asian-inspired stir-fries and beef and chicken dishes.

▶ MAKING THE SWITCH AT DINNER

INSTEAD OF	TRY
Lasagna and other cheesy pasta dishes	Fish (4 ounces) that's baked, steamed, grilled, or cooked in foil
Porterhouse steaks and other fatty cuts of meat	Whole wheat pasta tossed with olive oil, basil, pine nuts, and sun-dried tomatoes
Chicken or turkey with the skin on, swimming in gravy	Lean beef (such as sirloin) marinated in oil and vinegar, grilled or broiled
Vegetable side dishes cooked in butter	Steamed vegetables dressed with extra-virgin olive oil

Good Fats for Snacks

Aside from giving you a moment to pause and relax in the middle of a busy day, having a healthy snack serves an important purpose: It staves off hunger between meals and helps keep your blood sugar from spiraling downward. Choose well, and snack time can also be an opportunity to fit in some good fats.

Go nuts. Nuts are high in protein and good fats—and you can't do much better for a snack. Have a handful, or try some peanut butter on whole wheat crackers or spread on apple slices or celery sticks.

Sweeten the deal. If you need to spark your blood sugar at snack time, pair nuts with a small amount of raisins or other dried fruit.

Get creative. Don't limit yourself to traditional snacks. For example, avocado slices or hard-cooked eggs make great between-meal treats.

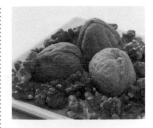

eat right
smart food

NUTS

Because of their high fiber and protein content, nuts are "slow burning" foods that are friendly to blood sugar. And even though they contain a lot of fat, it's that healthful monounsaturated kind again. Roasting really brings out the flavor of nuts and makes them a great addition to fall soups and entrées. Just spread shelled nuts on a cooking sheet and bake at 300°F for 7 to 10 minutes.

▸ **MAKING THE SWITCH AT SNACK TIME**

INSTEAD OF	TRY
Candy	Tapenade (olive spread) on toasted whole-wheat pita triangles
Cookies	Spiced almonds (1 ounce)
Energy bars	½ avocado drizzled with lemon juice or avocado slices on whole wheat crackers
Potato chips	A handful of pumpkin or sunflower seeds
Granola bars that contain tropical oils (such as palm oil)	1 tablespoon all-natural peanut butter on whole wheat crackers

Get Creative with Avocado

This rich, creamy fruit is loaded with fat—a whopping 25 to 30 grams each—but most of it is "good" monounsaturated fat, the same fat you get in nuts and olive oil. Research suggests that diets rich in this type of fat may help keep blood sugar in check by slowing digestion after a meal. And unlike the saturated fats in butter and meat, monounsaturated fat won't increase insulin resistance. There's even some suggestion that eating more of it could help insulin-producing cells in your pancreas stay healthier. That means avocados are great additions to your diet if you eat them in moderation.

1. Start with a ripe avocado. Hold the avocado in your hand and press it gently, then roll it to the other side and press again. If it gives just a bit but pressure doesn't leave a permanent dent (an indication that it's too ripe), it's ready to eat.

2. Eat it as a snack. Instead of a handful of pretzels—practically all carbs—or cheese, cut an avocado into five pieces and eat two of them, drizzled with lemon juice, for a satisfying 110-calorie snack.

3. Use avocado in place of cheese. Rich in sterols, compounds shown to lower cholesterol, avocado is also a calorie bargain when eaten the smart way. Have one of those slices you cut in the tip above on your sandwich for 55 calories—half the 100 or so calories in an ounce of cheese. Or mash some avocado and spread it on in place of mayonnaise.

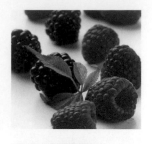

BERRIES

Think of them as nature's M&M's: sweet, convenient, colorful, and satisfying. Berries are full of fiber and antioxidants. The red and blue varieties also contain natural plant compounds called anthocyanins. Scientists believe these may help lower blood sugar by boosting insulin production. Put some in an easy-to-grab location or freeze a handful to suck on or use as ice cubes.

Good Fats for Dessert

It's OK to enjoy dessert now and then, though you'll need to exercise some restraint with many popular sweet treats to spare yourself a heavy dose of bad fats. It's probably no surprise that candy and cookies are loaded with sugar, saturated fat, trans fat, and calories, so avoid them. Another surprise may be that healthy-seeming granola bars, energy bars, and trail mix can contain surprising amounts of bad fat, so read ingredients lists. When you pick up your favorite snacks, check for trans fats, including crackers.

On the other hand, you'll be surprised by how easy it is to use healthy fats to make desserts that taste absolutely decadent.

Go Greek. Greek yogurt is thick, rich, and nearly as satisfying as whipped cream on berries, especially when you add a drizzle of really good honey. And a 2014 study published in *Diabetologia* found that yogurt consumption dropped risk of developing diabetes by 28 percent. Part of yogurt's goodness stems from the healthy bacteria used to ferment it. Look for a variety that is either plain (no sugar) or has natural fruit and sugars. Stay away from yogurt sweetened with artificial sugar, as new research shows that these sugars may spur the growth of unhealthy bacteria in the gut, counteracting the healing properties of the yogurt.

Dark chocolate. A square of the best, darkest chocolate you can find is immensely rewarding—just savor it in tiny bites.

▸ MAKING THE SWITCH AT DESSERT

INSTEAD OF	TRY
Cake	Dark-chocolate-covered almonds
Pie	Half an apple baked with cinnamon, walnuts, and maple syrup
Ice cream	Half a fresh peach baked with honey and cardamom and topped with toasted ground almonds

The Power of Protein

Getting the right amount of protein isn't difficult if you're already controlling your fat and carbohydrate balance—protein will account for the rest of your calories. You need protein to build and repair tissues and ensure the proper functioning of hormones, immune-system cells, and hardworking enzymes throughout the body.

Almost none of the protein you eat is converted to blood sugar, making low-fat protein foods a good choice for people with diabetes. Protein may have another advantage: Recent studies have shown that high-protein foods, as well as high-fiber foods, keep you full longer than high-fat foods. And getting enough protein is important when you're trying to lose weight because it helps your body hold on to calorie-burning muscle tissue. If you need to shed pounds, as many people with type 2 diabetes do, it's a good idea to eat some protein at every meal.

Meat, chicken, and fish aren't your only protein possibilities. Dairy foods such as low-fat milk and yogurt and plant foods like beans, nuts (including peanut butter), and soy foods also offer plenty of protein. (Beans are about one-third protein and two-thirds carbohydrate.) Eggs are another good source.

Doctors once advised people with diabetes to cut back on protein. They feared that eating too much protein would strain the kidneys, which excrete excess protein. But studies have laid these fears to rest. Only people with significant kidney problems, such as renal insufficiency, need to worry about consuming too much protein.

Just how important protein is for blood-sugar control emerged from a fascinating study. Researchers at the University of Minnesota tested two diets, one high in protein and one with only half as much. The fat content was the same in both diets, but the carbohydrate content varied—volunteers ate fewer carbs on the high-protein diet, more carbs on the low-protein program. In the group that followed the high-protein diet, blood-sugar levels were reduced by as much as if the participants had taken pills prescribed to lower blood sugar.

Does that mean that you should sit down to a 12-ounce T-bone steak or fried chicken tonight? No. Fatty cuts of beef, poultry with skin, and some cuts of pork, as well as bacon and some lunch meats, pack lots of heart-threatening saturated fat, which raises levels of bad cholesterol. This bad fat has also been linked to increased insulin resistance, which contributes to higher blood-sugar levels.

It's important to focus on lean protein foods so that you get the blood-sugar and weight-loss benefits of this important macronutrient without the health risks. By cutting back on saturated fat in fatty protein foods like hamburgers and fried chicken, you'll leave room in your diet for eating more blood-sugar-friendly "good fats."

Here's a look at some delicious protein choices.

Take Another Look at Pork

Pork loin is a very lean and affordable cut of meat that's flavorful and satisfying, like beef. Among its charms: It cooks quickly in the oven or on the grill and tastes great with a wide variety of marinades and spices (we love garlic and oregano or low-sodium soy sauce and grated fresh ginger). Pork loin is perfect when company is coming for dinner. Or throw a couple of chops on the grill (try garlic-lime marinade or a rub made of chili and garlic powders).

> Lean beef not only tastes good but is also great for helping you achieve and maintain a healthy weight, thanks to its protein.

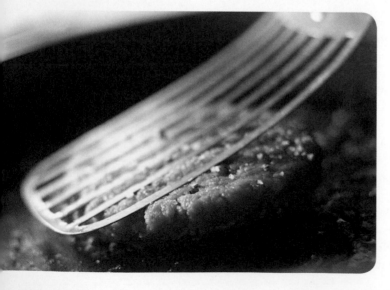

Turn to Chicken

Chicken and turkey can be high-fat disasters or perfect Reverse Diabetes fare. It all depends on the cut and how it's prepared. Breast meat is lower in fat than dark meat such as thighs and drumsticks. And in fact, a 3-ounce serving of skinless chicken breast has 95 percent less saturated fat—the stuff that clogs arteries and blunts insulin sensitivity—than an equal serving of beef tenderloin. It also has 40 percent fewer calories, making it a practically perfect protein food. Just remember that even breast meat loses its health appeal when it's fried (especially in the oils used at many fast-food joints, which essentially turn chicken into a heart attack in a bucket). The skin, meanwhile, with all its saturated fat, is just about the worst thing you can eat. Be sure to remove it either before or after cooking.

Here are six easy ways to add poultry (and a healthy amount of protein) to your diet:

Enjoy a fast dinner of supermarket rotisserie chicken. Instead of the fast-food drive-through tonight, run into the supermarket for a bag of salad greens and a rotisserie chicken. At home, enjoy a big salad and a slice of breast meat. To keep it lean, skip the skin and don't eat the greasy drippings.

Order turkey or chicken breast at the deli counter. Roll up a few slices and add to salads to pump up their protein content, or eat them in sandwiches on whole wheat bread topped with mustard, tomato, and plenty of lettuce or even baby spinach. Have two slices or 1.5 ounces per sandwich.

Roast some turkey even when it's not Thanksgiving. Turkey breast is actually lower in fat and cholesterol and higher in protein than chicken breast. You can now buy just the turkey breast in many grocery stores.

Try this instead of fried chicken. Brush boneless, skinless chicken thighs with olive oil and sprinkle with rosemary, salt, and pepper. Bake or grill until juices run clear, about 45 minutes. Chill overnight—this is great lunch or picnic fare. For another option that's just as finger-lickin' messy as the real thing, mix the juice of one lemon with 1 tablespoon Dijon mustard, ½ cup honey, a pinch of curry powder, and a pinch of salt. Roll skinless chicken drumsticks in the mixture to coat well and bake until done, 45 to 60 minutes.

Use ground chicken or turkey breast in place of ground beef. Make sure it's ground breast meat; if it includes dark meat it will be much higher in fat. This lean meat makes good burgers and tastes great in meat loaf, meatballs, chili, tacos, and lasagna.

Keep chicken tenderloins in the freezer for fast meals. Two tenderloins are about three ounces, a perfect portion. These skinless, boneless cuts thaw quickly in the fridge overnight or in a bowl of cold water (seal in a ziplock bag first).

No Beef with Beef

Yes, beef can still be for dinner—or, more accurately, part of dinner. Lean beef doesn't just taste good—it's great for helping you achieve and maintain a healthy weight, thanks to its protein. That doesn't mean that sitting down to a giant T-bone or eating mega-cheeseburgers with enough calories and fat for breakfast, lunch, and dinner combined is suddenly OK. It isn't. But it's more than OK to fill one-quarter of your plate with a lean choice like tenderloin. Here's how to get the leanest, most flavorful red meats on your plate.

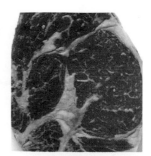

eat right
smart food

BEEF

Yes, beef can be "what's for dinner," as long as you choose the leanest cuts and keep portions to one-fourth your plate. Getting enough protein at mealtime keeps you feeling full and satisfied. Plus, it helps maintain muscle mass when you're losing weight, so your metabolism stays high. The skinniest beef cuts are eye of round, top round, ground round, tenderloin, sirloin, flank steak, and filet mignon. To lean up other cuts, put them in the freezer for 20 minutes. This hardens the meat so it's easier to slice off the fat. Lean cuts can be tenderized and made more flavorful by marinating in any mixture that contains an acid such as vinegar, wine, or citrus juice.

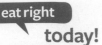

eat right today!

Trimming the fat made easy.

Put meat and poultry in the freezer for 20 minutes before you get to work trimming away excess fat. This firms it up for easier cutting (the meat will become harder than the fat, making a closer "shave" possible) and make marbled fat more visible so you can locate and remove it.

To add beef in a healthy way, check out these five tips:

Pair beef strips with veggies. Stir-fry strips of beef with lots of veggies for an easy way to have your beef and get your vegetables too. Or throw together fajitas made with flank steak and generous amounts of bell peppers and onions for a quick weeknight meal. Or for a refreshingly delicious Asian-inspired salad, toss hot grilled beef with crisp lettuce, lime juice, and chopped onion.

Remake meat loaf. Create healthier meat loaf by combining finely chopped spinach and onions and grated carrots with extra-lean ground beef. Use oats as a binder instead of bread crumbs.

When company comes, serve up roast beef tenderloin. This delicious, but expensive, roast is impressive enough for a dinner party but lean enough to enjoy guilt-free. Serve a nicely garnished salad as a first course and at least one veggie side dish.

Try a little tenderness. Make any cut of beef a standout by marinating it in balsamic vinegar, olive oil, basil, Dijon mustard, and garlic. Or use any marinade that contains vinegar, wine, or citrus juice. The acid softens the tissues of the meat, making it more tender.

Use half the beef; get all the flavor. In chili, tacos, spaghetti sauce, and casseroles that call for ground beef, use half extra-lean ground beef and half ground, skinless turkey or chicken breast. You'll cut the fat content but still get the assertive, satisfying flavor of beef.

Go for Fish

The fattiest protein on your plate should be oily cold-water fish like salmon and mackerel (and to a lesser extent, tuna and other fish). These fish contain diabetes-fighting, heart-protecting omega-3 fatty acids—a fat you almost certainly need to get more of into your diet. A study at the Harvard School of Public Health found that women with diabetes who ate fish just once a week had a 40 percent lower risk of dying from heart disease than did women with diabetes who ate fish less than once a month.

The fats in fish do even more than guard against heart disease. They also cool chronic inflammation in the body, a major contributor to numerous chronic diseases, including insulin resistance and diabetes. Inflammation may even play a role in brain diseases such as Alzheimer's as well as certain cancers.

Any fish is a great source of protein, and we encourage you to eat it twice a week when you might otherwise have chicken or beef. Shellfish counts, too, so go ahead and indulge in grilled shrimp, lobster, and mussels. They don't contain as much omega-3 as salmon, but they're still low in saturated fat and calories and rich in protein. Worried about your cholesterol? You don't need to avoid shrimp. It does contain cholesterol, but for most of us, shrimp should still get the green light. In a definitive

Rockefeller University study, eating large servings of shrimp every single day raised bad LDL cholesterol by 7 percent, but it also boosted good HDL cholesterol 12 percent—a net benefit.

Here's how to fit in two servings of fish or seafood a week:

Keep frozen fish fillets in the freezer. Vacuum-packed sole, cod, and salmon fillets are the next best thing to fresh. You'll have dinner on the table in a flash—even if you have to spend a few minutes defrosting it first—because fish is done before you know it, making it a perfect weeknight meal.

Fire up the grill. Almost any type of fish tastes fabulous grilled, especially salmon. Brush it with a little olive oil to keep it from sticking. Throw some zucchini strips on the grill, too, and you'll have a blood-sugar-friendly meal. Or, try wrapping trout in foil with lemon slices, dill, thyme, salt, and pepper and bake. Serve over quinoa.

Don't overlook salmon in cans and pouches. This is usually wild salmon—same as the pricey, sometimes hard-to-find stuff from the fish counter. Use it to make salmon salad or salmon croquettes and use in quiches and pasta dishes.

Stuff a tomato with tuna or salmon salad. Make the tuna or salmon salad with low-fat mayonnaise or plain yogurt, hard-boiled eggs, chopped apples, celery, and onion. Serve with whole wheat crackers.

Think sushi for supermarket takeout. Many larger supermarkets have their very own sushi chefs on staff. If you need a quick, prepackaged meal, this is the place to stop. Sushi delivers protein and is generally low in calories. But nix the bluefin tuna sushi—it's being fished to extinction and is contaminated with mercury, to boot. Instead, choose yellowfin or albacore tuna, bonito, black cod, crab (kani), squid, salmon and salmon roe. And ask for brown rice instead of white.

Order grilled salmon when you dine out. You'll avoid temptations packed with saturated fat (like cream sauces and deep-fried goodies) and ensure that you get a serving of healthy omega-3 fatty acids.

Keep a bag of frozen shrimp in the freezer. Thaw them according to the package directions, and you'll have the makings of a fast, high-protein meal or appetizer. Serve boiled shrimp with shrimp sauce as a party hors d'oeuvre. Leftovers? Chop some cooked shrimp and sprinkle over your salad to add low-fat protein. Use a lemony dressing. Or place a shrimp, small chunks of avocado and tomato, and a bit of salsa onto a lettuce leaf. Roll it up and eat! In stir-fries, use shrimp instead of chicken or beef. Add in the last five minutes to avoid overcooking. Also try shrimp in your tacos instead of beef.

> Oily cold-water fish contain diabetes-fighting, omega-3 fatty acids—a fat you almost certainly need more of in your diet.

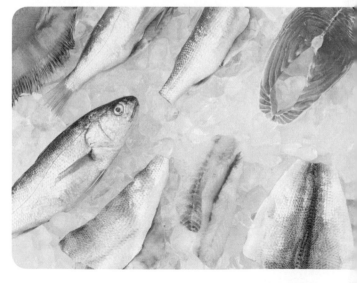

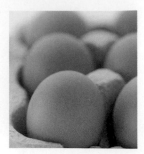

eat right
smart food

EGGS

Eggs are another excellent, inexpensive source of high-quality protein—so high, in fact, that egg protein is the gold standard nutritionists use to rank all other proteins. An egg or two won't raise your cholesterol and will keep you feeling full and satisfied for hours afterward. Such a magic food deserves a little sleight of hand in its preparation. To flip an egg, spritz the skillet with cooking spray, wait for the egg white to bubble, and in one continuous motion, slide the pan quickly toward you and then forward with a slight upward flick of the wrist. Bow to your guests.

Have lobster for lower blood sugar. Indulge in this fancy feast—without the melted butter. The upper crust of the crustacean kingdom happens to be a particularly rich source of a little-known mineral called vanadium, which studies suggest enhances insulin's effect in the body, helping to keep an anchor on blood sugar.

Foil some fillets. Baking fish in foil packets makes a perfect fish meal surprisingly easy to pull off. Just coat a couple of fish fillets with olive oil, lemon juice, salt and pepper, and a fresh herb of your choice, and bake at 400°F for 15 to 20 minutes. For a complete meal, throw cut-up vegetables, such as zucchini, summer squash, red peppers, and scallions, into the foil packet too.

Don't Forget Eggs

Eggs have been much maligned in recent years, but the fact is, they're an excellent and inexpensive source of protein and the most nutritionally complete of all protein sources. One large hard-boiled egg has seven grams of protein, to keep you full, and just two grams of saturated fat. In studies, people who ate eggs and toast for breakfast stayed fuller longer and consumed significantly fewer calories for the rest of the day than people who started the day with a bagel and cream cheese. Because they're all protein and fat, eggs have virtually no impact on your blood sugar, making them a much better breakfast choice than, say, a stack of white-flour pancakes.

Eggs do contain cholesterol, but dozens of studies show that saturated fat, not dietary cholesterol, raises people's cholesterol the most. For people with elevated cholesterol or those who are especially sensitive to the cholesterol in foods (for some people, cholesterol levels do rise after eating a cholesterol-rich meal), experts recommend eating no more than three or four egg yolks a week. Egg whites, which contain no cholesterol, don't count.

If you have an egg tray in your refrigerator door, ignore it. Eggs stay fresh best if you keep them in their original container, pointed ends down.

And here are three ways to incorporate eggs into your diet:

Keep hard-boiled eggs in the fridge. It's hard to find snack foods rich in protein, but a hard-boiled egg is the perfect solution. It's portable, too—but you do have to keep it cold.

Serve a frittata for dinner. Think of it as Italian egg pie. You can add almost anything to your frittata, such as lean ham, diced tomato, spinach, and goat cheese. Use one to two cups of filling for every four or five eggs.

Dress up egg salad sandwiches. Add veggies such as grated carrots, chopped leeks, finely chopped shallots, red onion, pea shoots, or plain old lettuce. Mix with a combination of low-fat mayo and plain yogurt. Sprinkle in a classic "egg salad" herb such as tarragon or dill. Or throw in some canned tuna to up your fish quotient for the day.

Make It Milk

Within the subject of protein, dairy deserves special mention. Foods such as fat-free milk and yogurt and low-fat cheese are high in both protein and calcium. Why is calcium important? Studies find that making sure you get adequate amounts can help you lose weight. The reason: A lack of adequate calcium triggers the release of a hormone called calcitriol, which prompts the body to store fat. Eating two or three servings of calcium-rich dairy foods per day helps keep calcitriol levels low so your body burns more fat and stores less. Taking calcium supplements doesn't seem to produce the same effect, which leads researchers to conclude that dairy foods may have some other, as-yet-undiscovered weight-loss advantage as well.

But there's more. A mysterious factor in milk seems to help directly protect against insulin resistance. Two Harvard studies found that people who made dairy foods part of their daily diets were 21 percent less likely to develop insulin resistance and 9 percent less likely to develop type 2 diabetes for each daily serving of dairy they had. Pretty impressive!

Not everyone tolerates the lactose in milk well, but if you're bothered by symptoms such as bloating and gas, you can ease dairy into your diet by having small amounts with meals, which slows the rate at which lactose enters your system. You can also forgo milk in favor of dairy foods that are naturally lower in lactose, such as low-fat cheese and yogurt. Thanks to the healthy bacteria used to ferment it, yogurt may further help to control diabetes by improving your gut health. In one study, people who consumed yogurt and other fermented foods (such as sauerkraut) dropped their risk for diabetes by 28 percent.

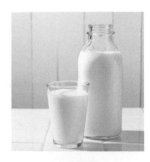

eat right
smart food

MILK AND YOGURT

Both are rich in protein and calcium, which studies show may help people lose weight. And diets that include plenty of dairy may fight insulin resistance, a core problem behind diabetes. Go low-fat or fat-free, though. If you don't like the taste of nonfat milk, try a brand that's ultra-pasteurized. It's thicker and creamier than regular skim. Likewise, reduced-fat Greek-style yogurt tends to taste richer than its American counterparts because of how it's made. Drizzle with honey and imagine you're on the Mediterranean.

Perfect Produce

Five. Yes, five servings of vegetables a day. That's the number, and the key, for being able to reverse diabetes through diet. So many wonderful, healthy results spring from crunching on crudités. Right about now, you're probably thinking, "That's a lot of vegetables." If you're not used to eating vegetables, yes, bumping up to five servings a day may seem overwhelming. So if you're not used to eating veggies at all, start with three servings a day. Then, with tips in this section, you'll be easily able to boost your intake. If you're already eating five servings of vegetables a day, there's no harm in bumping that up to seven. There's new evidence that getting seven vegetable servings a day is even better for your health.

Because vegetables are low in fat and calories and packed with fiber, vitamins, minerals, and other powerful nutrients, they help fight disease, pamper your blood sugar, and help you maintain a healthy weight. And let's face it, if you're eating more vegetables, you're eating less of everything else, including fatty meat, carbohydrate foods, and junk food.

Over the past few decades, researchers have found that eating more vegetables is a key strategy for losing weight and keeping it off. Vegetables make you feel full and satisfied, for very few calories. The simple truth: The more vegetables you eat, the less you'll weigh. In one study at Pennsylvania State University, women who started a meal with a low-calorie salad and then ate a pasta dish consumed about 12 percent

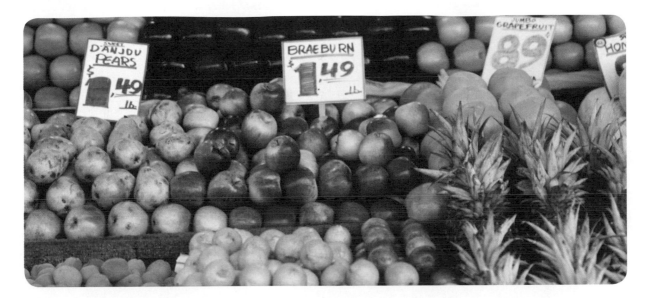

fewer calories in total than women who skipped the salad and started right in on the pasta. In another study, adding about six ounces of vegetables (in this case, carrots and spinach) to dinner helped people feel fuller on fewer calories.

Making sure you get your daily five (or more) servings doesn't have to be tricky. All it takes is a little planning ahead. If you don't have any veggies handy, the default is often to eat a dinner that's virtually veggie-free or go for chips, cookies, candy, cheese, or whatever else is on hand when you're hungry and need a snack. Remember this: Make sure vegetables are ready and waiting and as handy as possible.

Easy Does It

Here's a case where we go against our advice to avoid prepared foods. They're more expensive and often high in artificial flavorings, sugars, and sodium. But when it comes to prepared veggies—bagged salads, prewashed spinach, peeled and diced butternut squash, washed and chopped kale—we're all for it. Numerous consumer studies find that we're more likely to use bagged salads and other produce than produce that requires more preparation.

To make sure you've always got veggie items handy, stock your pantry and freezer with canned and frozen vegetables. These can be as nutritious as fresh veggies because they're picked at their peak, when they are the most nutrient-rich. Frozen vegetables are flash-frozen, which seals in the nutrients until the veggies are thawed. Don't worry about losing nutrients that leach into water in cans: The amounts are small, and you lose nothing if you use the water in dishes such as soup. Just be sure to choose naked veggies—those without sauce or cheese.

Ready to munch and crunch? Read on.

> Making sure you get your daily five (or more) servings doesn't have to be tricky. All it takes is a little planning.

Look! There's a Veggie Serving!

Part of what seems so daunting about eating five servings of vegetables a day is actually knowing what a such a serving looks like. To help, here's the definition of a serving from the National Cancer Institute. All varieties of fruits and vegetables—fresh, frozen, canned, dried, and 100 percent juice—count. Measure out some of these in your kitchen so you can see how reasonable a serving size is.

▸ ½ cup raw, cooked, canned, or frozen vegetables
▸ ¾ cup (6 ounces) 100 percent vegetable juice
▸ ½ cup cooked or canned legumes (beans and peas)
▸ 1 cup raw, leafy vegetables such as lettuce and spinach

Choose All-Star Veggies

Vivid colors—dark greens and bright reds, oranges, yellows, and purples—signal that a vegetable is packed with vitamins, minerals, and other vital nutrients. Often, these nutrients are especially helpful for people with diabetes. We highly recommend these five versatile superstars:

Broccoli. Big on volume and small on calories, broccoli is a great way to bulk up carbohydrate-rich dishes (think pasta, casseroles, and baked potatoes) to blunt their effect on your blood sugar and your waistline. This classic is one of the best food sources of chromium, a mineral required for insulin to function normally (remember, insulin helps the body use up blood sugar so there's less in the bloodstream). One cup of broccoli provides almost half of your daily chromium requirement. Fiber, at a hearty four grams per stalk, is also part of broccoli's "benefits package."

Carrots. Don't believe the hype that carrots raise your blood sugar rapidly. Chalk up that myth to a problem with the Glycemic Index, a system that preceded the more accurate Glycemic Load. While the type of sugar carrots contain is transformed into blood sugar very rapidly, the amount of sugar in carrots is extremely low. Thank goodness, because they're one of the richest sources of beta-carotene, which is linked to a lower risk of diabetes. Like most vegetables, carrots are also a good source of beneficial fiber. By the way, carrots won't help you throw away your reading glasses, but they will help protect against two sight-robbing conditions: macular degeneration and cataracts.

Spinach, kale, and other dark, leafy greens. Thanks to rich stores of carotenoids (including beta-carotene and other "carotenes"), these yummy greens are among the most antioxidant-rich vegetables on Earth. Antioxidants are powerful weapons against diabetes-related complications, including heart disease and nerve damage, not to mention cancer. They're also loaded with potassium and magnesium, which help keep blood pressure in check.

Sweet potatoes. Eat a baked sweet potato instead of a baked white potato, and your blood sugar will rise about 30 percent less! A sweet deal indeed, especially because these potatoes are packed with nutrients and disease-fighting fiber, almost 40 percent of which is soluble fiber, the kind that helps lower blood sugar and cholesterol.

Sweet potatoes are extraordinarily rich in carotenoids, orange and yellow pigments that play a role in helping the body respond to insulin. They're also full of the natural plant compound chlorogenic acid, which may help reduce insulin resistance.

New Rule: Veggies Always on the Side

When planning and making meals, this needs to become automatic. Fortunately, it can be as easy as tossing baby carrots or cherry tomatoes into a ziplock bag. These strategies can help make the most of the great flavors and textures in these amazing foods.

Here are four ways to make that side really, really simple:

Give veggies a roast. Here's one of the great side dishes—easy to make, delicious to eat, and amazingly healthy. Plus, it tastes surprisingly sweet and lasts well as a leftover, meaning you can make large batches and serve throughout the week. Cut hearty root vegetables like parsnips, turnips, rutabagas, carrots, and onions into inch-thick chunks and arrange in a single layer on a cookie sheet. Other good candidates include Brussels sprouts, whole if small or halved if large, as well as broccoli and cauliflower cut into two-inch chunks. Drizzle with olive oil and sprinkle with kosher or sea salt, freshly ground pepper, and fresh or dried herbs. Roast in a 450°F oven until soft, about 15 to 45 minutes, turning once, until tender (some veggies cook more quickly than others). That's it!

Throw 'em on the grill. If you use your grill for meats only, you've been missing out! Peppers, zucchini, asparagus, onions, eggplant—even tomatoes—all taste amazingly good when grilled. Generally, all you need to do is coat them with olive oil and throw them on. Turn every few minutes and remove when they start to soften. Or skewer chunks of veggies on a bamboo or metal skewer and turn frequently. You can also buy grilling baskets that keep the veggies from falling through the slats in the grill.

Buy a vegetable steamer. It's one of the healthiest ways to cook vegetables because nutrients aren't lost in the water. Choose a metal or bamboo steamer basket, fill it with veggies, place over a saucepan of rapidly simmering water, cover, and cook for five to 10 minutes. It's that simple.

Season to taste. Think beyond butter when it comes to seasoning vegetables. For example, asparagus tastes great with lemon, garlic, and oregano. When serving broccoli, don't ruin it with a pat of butter—instead mix it with garlic, mustard, or dark sesame oil. And add a little zing to carrots with lemon, orange, curry powder, ginger, or dill. Experiment, be creative. You'll likely find a new taste that the whole family will enjoy.

> If you use your grill for meats only, you've been missing out! Peppers, zucchini, asparagus, onions, eggplant—even tomatoes—all taste amazingly good when grilled.

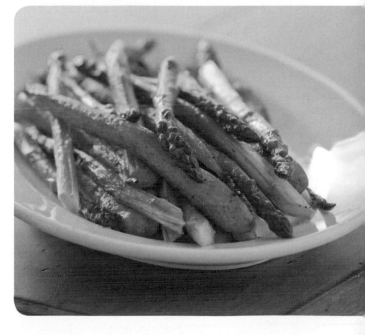

The High-Protein, Low-Carb Controversy

Not everyone agrees with the generally accepted recommendations about what your diet should look like. In fact, proponents of a number of popular diets argue that the picture is upside down for people with diabetes. If carbohydrates produce the largest and fastest increases in blood sugar, the argument goes, it doesn't make sense to eat more of them than of anything else. What's more, critics note, eating a lot of carbohydrates can contribute to obesity (as can eating too much of anything).

But if you take this message to heart and cut back on carbs, what should replace them? The answer, inevitably, is protein or fat, particularly monounsaturated fat. Proponents of alternative eating plans say that, contrary to popular opinion, people with diabetes can lose weight on such diets and keep blood sugar more stable. The popularity of the low-carb approach suggests that it works for some people—or at least appeals to their desire to eat more bacon, eggs, meat, and other favorites. But the consensus in the medical community is that you should view low-carbohydrate diets cautiously, with an eye to your unique needs.

Who should go low carb?

The American Diabetes Association acknowledges that some people may legitimately need to lower their carbohydrate intake. For example, certain people who have type 2 diabetes and are insulin resistant may find that eating a diet rich in carbs raises triglyceride levels and brings down levels of HDL cholesterol. It's another reason the ADA's latest recommendations allow 60 to 70 percent of total calories to be distributed between carbohydrates and monounsaturated fat. If your main concern is keeping your blood sugar in check after meals and improving your triglyceride levels, eating more monounsaturated fats may be the way to go. If losing weight is your main concern, then, according to the ADA, favoring carbs over fats (which contain more calories gram for gram) may be preferable.

Something to keep in mind: According to a recent U.S. Department of Agriculture report that evaluated a variety of popular diets, how much weight you lose depends more on how many calories you eat than on where they come from.

Lunch and Snacks

One reason we don't get enough vegetables is that many of us consider them merely a side dish to dinner. Here are some scrumptious ways to boost your veggie quota:

Build a sandwich with more lettuce and tomato than meat. Stack the meat filler in the sandwich to no higher than the thickness of a standard slice of bread. Then pile on lettuce (choose darkest green and red varieties for best nutrition) and tomatoes to the combined height of both slices of bread.

Have a veggie burger for lunch once a week. Top it with a sliced tomato and lettuce for even more veggie power. Honestly, it will taste better than you imagine.

Open a can of low-sodium soup and add veggies. Toss in a bag of precut broccoli and carrots, either fresh or frozen, and voilà! You have a superfast and easy lunch or dinner entrée, ready to be flavored with your preferred spices, herbs, or hot sauce. As the soup simmers, it will simultaneously cook the veggies, boosting the nutritional value and fiber.

Eat vegetables as if they were fruit. Half a cucumber, a whole tomato, a stalk of celery, or a long, fresh carrot are as pleasant to munch on as an apple. It may not seem typical, but who cares? A whole vegetable makes a terrific snack.

Dinner and Dessert

Start each dinner with a mixed-greens salad before you serve the main course. Not only will doing so help you eat more veggies, but by filling your stomach first with a nutrient-rich, low-calorie salad, you'll be less hungry for the higher-calorie items that follow. For an instant, perfectly dressed salad, open a bag of prewashed, precut romaine lettuce or mixed greens, add a tablespoon of olive oil and a splash of lemon juice or balsamic vinegar, and shake.

And another great suggestion: Put a plate of raw vegetables in the center of the table. Nearly everyone likes carrot sticks, celery sticks, cucumber slices, string beans, cherry tomatoes, and/or green pepper strips. They're healthy, they have virtually no calories, they have a satisfying crunch, and they can substantially cut your consumption of the more calorie-dense main course.

Some other veggie-licious ideas:

Once a week, have an entrée salad. A salade niçoise is a good example: mixed greens, steamed green beans, boiled potatoes, sliced hard-boiled egg, and tuna drizzled with vinaigrette. Serve with crusty whole-grain bread. Bon appétit!

Fill your spaghetti sauce with vegetables. Then replace half the pasta you normally eat with more vegetables. Take a jar of low-sodium prepared sauce and add in string beans, peas, corn, bell peppers, mushrooms, tomatoes and more. Like it chunky? Cut them in big pieces. Don't want to know they're there? Shred or puree them with a bit of sauce in the blender, then add. And don't stop there. Steamed broccoli or green beans, or baked spaghetti squash (use a fork to remove the spaghetti-like strands), are filling and delicious replacements for the mounds of pasta that often find their way onto our plates.

Order your pizza with extra veggies. Instead of the same old pepperoni and onions, do your blood sugar and digestion a favor and ask for half the cheese, double the sauce and add toppings like artichoke hearts, broccoli, hot peppers, and other exotic vegetables many pizza joints stock these days for their gourmet pies.

Puree cooked veggies into soup. Carrots, winter squash, parsnips, cauliflower, and broccoli—just about any cooked (or leftover) vegetable can be made into a creamy, comforting soup. Here's a simple recipe: In a medium saucepan, sauté 1 cup finely chopped onion in 1 tablespoon vegetable oil until tender. Combine the onion in a blender or food processor with cooked vegetables and puree until smooth. Return puree to saucepan and thin with broth or low-fat milk. Simmer and season to taste.

Make Mondays meatless. Simply substitute the meat serving with a vegetable serving (suggestion: make it a crunchy, strong-flavored vegetable like broccoli). Or you can dabble in the world of vegetarian cooking, in which recipes are developed specifically to make a filling, robust meal out of vegetables and whole grains. For those times, get yourself a good vegetarian cookbook.

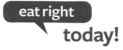

eat right today!

Make asparagus pop.

Roast whole spears in the oven with a little olive oil, salt, and pepper. For an extra pop of flavor, grate on some lemon zest right before serving. Delicious! Or make instant asparagus soup by pureeing cooked asparagus, heating it with a little milk, and adding chopped parsley or tarragon.

Get Enough Vitamins and Minerals

As a rule, if you eat a wide variety of foods, you'll have no trouble getting all the nutrients you need. However, people with diabetes appear more likely to be deficient in certain micronutrients—something your dietitian can evaluate. Nutrients you may need more of include:

Vitamin C. Evidence for diabetes-related deficiencies is most clear for vitamin C, which, like glucose, requires insulin to help it enter cells. It's not hard to add more vitamin C to your diet. Just one cup of steamed broccoli contains 123 milligrams—a whole day's supply.

Vitamin D. Deficiencies of the sunshine vitamin are linked to poor diabetes control, according to a 2010 study—and in that same year, the Institutes of Medicine upped the RDA for vitamin D to 600 IU a day; people 71 and older should get 800 IU. Since your body synthesizes vitamin D from sunlight, getting enough is difficult, especially during the winter, and even in the summer, since wearing sunscreen blocks vitamin D formation.

Magnesium. The most common mineral deficiency, especially in people with type 1 diabetes, is of magnesium. Getting too little of it may promote eye damage, a common complication of diabetes.

Vitamin E. An antioxidant, vitamin E may protect against such complications as eye, nerve, and kidney damage. But amounts in food tend to be small, so you may want to take a supplement. Check with your doctor first.

Vitamin B$_{12}$. Some diabetes medications, such as metformin, may interfere with the body's absorption of B$_{12}$ from food, potentially leading to deficiencies.

Before taking any dietary supplements, check with your doctor. As a rule, if you suffer from deficiencies, you'll want to correct them by eating more foods containing the nutrients you need. Supplements are generally considered less desirable because some vitamins and minerals can be harmful in high amounts; in addition, supplements lack other nutrients or elements, such as fiber, that may make it easier for the body to absorb and use what it ingests.

Is Alcohol Off-Limits?

There are plenty of reasons to avoid drinking alcohol, starting with the obvious: inebriation and addiction. But assuming you're a responsible drinker, is there room for alcohol in your diet if you have diabetes? Most experts agree that the answer is a qualified yes. Alcohol may even have some benefits in terms of preventing cardiovascular problems associated with diabetes.

A 2015 study published in *Diabetes & Metabolism* found that people who have one alcoholic drink a day are 53 percent less likely to develop diabetes than people who don't drink at all. Other studies in both men and women have shown that alcohol raises HDL ("good") cholesterol and thins the blood slightly, protecting against the formation of clots that can cause a heart attack or stroke.

Drawbacks of drinking

There are a number of caveats. In a recent Harvard study, women who had more than about 1½ drinks a day had a 30 percent higher risk of elevated blood pressure than nondrinkers did. Furthermore, alcohol affects people with diabetes more significantly than non-diabetics. The main threat is hypoglycemia. Alcohol is processed in the liver, which also stores and releases glucose. Result: Wine, beer, and spirits hinder the liver's ability to release glucose, which can lead to hypoglycemia as much as a day after you drink. Moreover, symptoms of hypoglycemia mimic those of inebriation, making the danger harder to spot.

Another consideration is that alcoholic drinks have seven calories per gram—almost as much as fat—but provide no nutrition, making them a poor choice if you're trying to lose weight. And if you're taking medication, alcohol may be out of the question.

Should you drink? Talk it over with your doctor or dietitian. If you get the OK to imbibe, here are some basic guidelines to keep in mind.

Keep it to one. Most studies find few risks and possible benefits from one drink a day or less. "One drink" is defined as a 12-ounce beer, 5 ounces of wine (about a half cup), or a 1½-ounce shot of distilled spirits, such as scotch, whiskey, or vodka (mix only with sugar-free soda or water).

Eat something. Food slows the absorption of alcohol into the bloodstream, allowing the liver to better process glucose while handling the alcohol. Also try to nurse your drink over a couple of hours to further ease the burden on your liver.

Sidestep the sweet stuff. In addition to their calories from alcohol, sweet wines and liqueurs pack extra amounts of carbohydrate. Likewise, sugary sodas and other sweet mixers added to distilled spirits can boost the calorie quotient.

Exchange cautiously. As a rule, doctors and dietitians would prefer that you not drop a nutritious item from your meal plan to make room for alcohol. But for the record, alcoholic drinks (except for beer) count as two fat exchanges, which may be consistent with your dietary goals. Beer counts as one and a half fat exchanges and one starch exchange.

Finally, there's one mineral you may need less of: sodium. High blood pressure is common among people with diabetes, and studies suggest that consuming less sodium can help bring blood pressure down. Use table salt sparingly, and avoid canned or packaged foods, which tend to pack a wallop of sodium. Rely more on herbs and spices when cooking.

WHERE THE NUTRIENTS ARE

Vitamin C: Citrus fruits, tomatoes, spinach, bell peppers, broccoli, and strawberries

Magnesium: Leafy green vegetables (like spinach), whole grains, dairy products, brown rice, apricots, and bananas

Vitamin E: Many nuts, such as almonds, Brazil nuts, and peanuts, as well as whole wheat flour

Vitamin B$_{12}$: Poultry and a variety of seafood, including clams, crabs, scallops, and shrimp

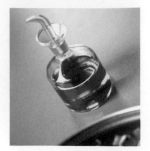

eat right
smart food

OLIVE OIL

This stuff is liquid gold. In fact, it contains an anti-inflammatory component so strong that researchers liken it to aspirin. This may be one reason that people who follow a Mediterranean diet—a traditional way of eating that emphasizes olive oil along with produce, whole grains, and lean meat—have such low rates of heart disease and diabetes, both of which are linked to inflammation. Unlike butter, the good fat in olive oil won't increase insulin resistance and may even help reverse it. A touch of olive oil also slows digestion, so your meal is less likely to spike your glucose. Dribble it on salads, baked potatoes, pasta... just about anything.

Food Swap System

Another tool your dietitian may bring into play is the food-exchange system, which looks beyond carbohydrates at the diet as a whole, organizing foods into several groups—generally breads and starches, fruits, vegetables, milk, meat and protein-based substitutes, fats, and other carbohydrates like sweets. While food exchanges are designed for people with diabetes, many nutritionists find them valuable for anyone trying to control calories, reduce fat, and eat a balanced diet.

The idea behind the exchange system is that every item within a given category is nutritionally equivalent to every other item on that same list—providing roughly the same amount of carbohydrate, fat, protein, and calories. Using the portion sizes laid out on the lists is important for making the system work. But the big advantage is that—as with carbohydrate counting—you have a lot of flexibility in choosing foods within each category, as long as they add up to the nutritional budget allowed in your meal plan. Fortunately, portion sizes for many of the groups tend to be similar, which helps give you an intuitive grasp of how much you should eat. One bread/starch exchange, for example, is usually measured in slices or half cups (as are many vegetable exchanges). One meat exchange is about one ounce—much smaller, by the way, than the two to three ounces that typically constitute a serving.

The exchange system strives to give you a range of nutrients from a variety of foods, but it does so with greater precision. Still, using the exchange system requires

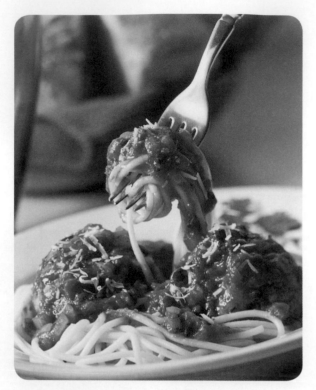

guidance. Your dietitian can help you figure out how many exchanges from each group you should eat.

The groupings themselves may take some getting used to because they're organized by calorie and nutrient content rather than source. Cheeses, for instance, are listed with meats rather than milk because their protein and fat makeup are more similar. Corn, green peas, and potatoes appear with starches rather than vegetables because of their high carbohydrate content. Once you're familiar with the system, however, its combination of flexibility and consistency can help you keep blood sugar down while providing enough nutrients.

Ranges of Exchanges

Some exchange lists are subdivided into groups that specify exchanges of, say, very lean meats and substitutes (separate from high-fat meats), or nonfat-milk products (separate from whole-milk products). Foods within each category are nutritionally equivalent in the exchange system.

> The big advantage of a food swap system is that you have a lot of flexibility in choosing foods within each category, as long as they add up to the nutritional budget.

▶ **Starches**
One slice white bread, ½ cup cooked lentils, ½ cup cooked pasta, ½ cup corn, one small potato

▶ **Vegetables**
½ cup cooked carrots, ½ cup cooked green beans, 1 cup raw radishes, 1 cup raw salad greens, 1 large tomato

▶ **Fruits**
One small banana, 1 large pear, seven small grapes, 2 tablespoons raisins, ½ cup fruit cocktail

▶ **Very lean meats and substitutes**
1 ounce skinless chicken breast, 1 ounce canned tuna (in water), 1 ounce fat-free cheese, ¼ cup low-fat cottage cheese, two egg whites

▶ **Nonfat and very-low-fat milks**
1 cup skim milk, 1 cup plain nonfat yogurt, ½ cup nonfat fruit-flavored yogurt (containing nonnutritive sweetener), ½ cup evaporated nonfat milk, 1 cup nonfat buttermilk

▶ **Other carbohydrates**
One 2-inch-square brownie, two small cookies, 1 tablespoon 100 percent fruit spread, ½ cup gelatin, five vanilla wafers

Making It Work

Knowing what your ideal diet should be is one thing. Putting it into practice—especially if you're trying to cut calories—is quite another. Anyone who has tried to lose weight can attest to the fact that it's easy for the best-laid dietary plans to go awry—at least temporarily. Not to worry. This is a long-term project, and occasional lapses are to be expected. In the meantime, a few smart strategies can help you peel off those unwanted pounds.

Control the Calorie Crunch

Researchers have recently noticed what seems to be a curious trend: According to a number of national surveys, the proportion of fat in the average American diet has actually gone down, even as rates of obesity have gone up. This has come to be called the American paradox. Does this mean fat isn't the villain we've been led to believe it is? No. The explanation: While the percentage of fat in the diet may be dropping, the sheer amount of fat we consume as a nation is going up because we're eating larger portions of everything.

Controlling your calorie intake is the bedrock of all weight-loss plans. But how can you stay the course when food is abundant and the temptation to overindulge is strong? Start by making a few small adjustments to your dining and snacking habits. For instance:

Keep food off the table. If you portion out servings on plates at the stove or kitchen counter and don't set food out on serving platters, you'll be less tempted to take more once your plate is empty.

Don't eat from packages. It's all too easy to lose track of how much food you've gobbled if you're nibbling straight from the box. Instead, portion out crackers, pretzels, and other snacks on a plate to give yourself a visible sense of what you're consuming.

Downsize your dishes. Smaller plates and bowls make portions appear larger.

Take it slow. It takes about 20 minutes for the brain's appetite-control center to register that there's food in the stomach. To wait it out, put down your fork between each bite and take small sips from your drink.

Work for your food. Eating foods that require some effort—peeling an orange, cracking open crabs, or cutting open a baked potato, for example—slows you down even more, giving food a chance to make you feel full.

Socialize outside the kitchen. People seem to congregate in the kitchen, but you'll be less tempted to nosh if you move the action to the living room.

Shop Smarter in 13 Easy Steps

You came, you saw, you shopped. But then you got home from the supermarket and started unloading fatty snack items and deli meats. What went wrong? You fell back into the habit of shopping like an average American rather than a person with a dietary purpose. In an enticing palace of eating designed to lead you astray, here's how to stay on track:

Make a list. The meal plan you develop with your dietitian will help you figure out which foods you should be buying. Before you shop, write down what you need to reduce the chances of buying what you don't.

Limit your trips. Make your shopping list long so you have to make only one or two trips to the store per week. Besides being more efficient, doing this will provide less opportunity to make impulse purchases.

Avoid shopping on an empty stomach. When you're hungry, you're more likely to grab high-fat snacks and desserts.

Follow the walls. Limit browsing to the perimeter of the store, where you'll find the freshest, most healthful foods: raw produce, low-fat dairy products, fresh lean meats and fish. Venture into the interior aisles only when you're after specific foods, such as pasta and dried beans, to avoid picking up extra items not included in your diet plan.

Pay attention to portions. Those cookies look great—and hey, eating them costs you only 12 grams of carbohydrate. But check the serving size: one cookie. Eating

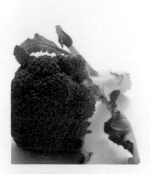

eat right
smart food
BROCCOLI
Broccoli is filling, fibrous, and full of antioxidants (including a day's worth of vitamin C in one serving). It's also rich in chromium, which plays an important role in long-term blood-sugar control. If you don't already love it, sneak it into soups, pasta dishes, and casseroles, or sauté it with garlic, soy sauce, ginger, and mustard or dark sesame oil (or any combination thereof) for a taste you'll fall for.

"them"—say, three cookies—brings your total carb count up to 36 grams, more than the flesh of a baked potato.

Ignore the pictures. Golden sunshine glows on heaps of freshly harvested grains—an image of good health that signifies nothing. Look at the side of the box instead for the facts, and choose foods that are high in fiber and low in fat and calories. Which also means you should…

Read the back of the package, not the front. Some manufacturers add polydextrose, maltodextrin, and inulin to their foods so they can boast they're high in fiber. But there's no proof that these purified powders or "faux fibers" stabilize blood sugar or lower cholesterol the way real fiber does. In general, ignore the front of the package and focus on the ingredients. They should be few and recognizable.

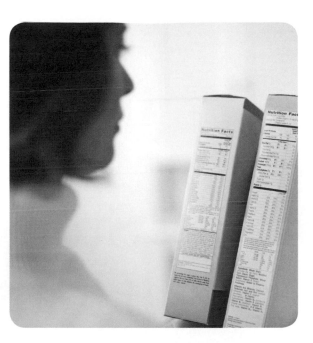

Grade your grains. Want high-fiber bread? Look for the words "whole grain," "100 percent whole wheat," or "stone-ground" on the label. Breads labeled simply "wheat"—even if they are brown in color—may not contain whole grains. True whole-grain bread contains at least two grams of fiber per serving—but you're much better off selecting breads that contain four or five grams per serving.

Choose prepared foods with short ingredients lists. The shorter and more natural-sounding the ingredients are, the healthier the food usually is. Of course, if the top ingredients are sugar and butter, put the item back on the shelf. And watch the sodium content: Even otherwise healthy processed foods can contain a day's worth of sodium. Avoid products that have more than 500 milligrams of sodium per serving.

Leave the ice cream coupons behind. No matter how much you're saving, it's not a deal if it isn't healthful.

> In general, ignore the front of the package and focus on the ingredients. They should be few and recognizable.

Watch the language. Beware of foods labeled "no sugar added"—the wording is carefully chosen because the product may be loaded with natural sugar. You'll find the real story on the label, under "Sugars."

Add some spice to your life. Instead of creamy condiments, load up on such spices as basil, chives, cinnamon, cumin, curry, garlic, ginger, horseradish, nutmeg, oregano, paprika, parsley, and Tabasco sauce. They're so low in carbohydrates, fat, protein, and calories that they're considered "free" items in meal planning.

Keep your eye on the cashier. You're waiting in line, nothing to do—a captive audience. It's no accident that supermarkets pile their impulse items next to the registers. Keep a couple of items from your basket in your hands: It'll stop you from reaching for the candy bars.

Stock a Healthy Pantry

Having a shopping list is a huge help in making your grocery choices smarter and healthier, and we hope this pantry guide helps you organize your needs. To help, here are tips for knowing what to do when standing in the grocery aisle, staring at a bewildering array of seemingly similar products.

Purge the Bad

All the diabetic-friendly advice in the world won't help if your pantry is packed with unhealthy food. Say it out loud: Sugary treats, processed snacks, candy, and similar products are no longer welcome here! Then grab an empty box for food to be given away and a garbage can for open packages to be tossed, and start sorting, using the following tips:

Lose the bad sugars. Sugar comes in many forms, but no matter what it's called, factory-sweetened foods should be eaten as little as possible. Though it's fine to occasionally use products that contain a little honey, maple syrup, or even white sugar, for that matter, toss anything that contains corn syrup or high-fructose corn syrup within the first four ingredients. These calorie-dense, nutritionally empty sweeteners may be much worse for you than white sugar.

Toss the toxic fats. Get rid of anything in your pantry that lists "partially hydrogenated oil" on the label, and don't buy any products with labels listing anything partially hydrogenated. Eating these fats, called trans fats, is like putting cement in your arteries—there's no such thing as a "healthy amount" of them. These fats raise your bad (LDL) cholesterol and lower your good (HDL) cholesterol. Eating foods containing trans fats increases your risk for developing heart disease, stroke, and type 2 diabetes.

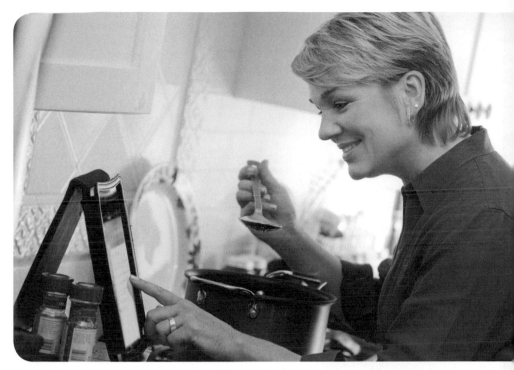

Dump products with chemical ingredients. A laundry list of chemicals means that a food product has been processed beyond recognition. Products that contain more ingredients than you can count, especially those with lots of unpronounceable chemicals, should be purged from the pantry.

Sack the loser cereals. Here's what a serving of nutritious cereal (about 1 cup) looks like. Get rid of those that fall short of these recommendations:

- 120 calories or less
- 2 grams or more protein
- 5 grams fiber (more is better)
- 8 grams (or less) sugar, unless it's an otherwise healthy cereal containing dried fruit
- 3 grams or less fat; no trans fat. If an otherwise healthy cereal contains nuts, it's fine if the fat content is a little higher.
- 10 to 25 percent of the daily value for key vitamins and minerals (e.g., iron, folate, B_6, and B_{12}).

Check for expiration dates. Though not all outdated pantry items are unhealthy, there's a good chance they've lost their nutritional value and should be discarded.

Get wise to "natural." Some food marketers list terms like "natural" and "healthy" on product labels. That's meaningless, because there are no standards governing the use of the words. If you're interested in "natural" products, skip the promotional messages and read the nutrition label to make sure the product is free of chemical ingredients.

For a truly healthy pantry, you should stock many of the items listed on page 118.

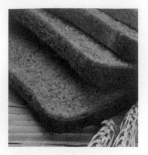

WHOLE-GRAIN BREAD

Eating white bread is practically like eating table sugar when it comes to raising blood sugar. So if you eat a lot of it (and this includes bagels), simply switching to whole grain may improve your sensitivity to insulin. In one study of nearly 1,000 men and women, the higher their intake of whole grains, the greater their insulin sensitivity and blood-sugar stability. Don't mistake any old brown bread, or even multigrain, for whole grain. If it doesn't have the word "whole" in the first ingredient, don't buy it. And look for the coarsest bread you can find; the coarseness will slow digestion.

Keep the Good

Once you've gone through the pantry and tossed out the stuff that's not so good for you and your family, check to see which of these items you already have on your shelves. Then shop as needed for the staples you'll want to have on hand to make home remedies—and healthful meals—for your family. For a truly healthy pantry, you should have many of the following ingredients:

Canned or dry legumes and fresh or frozen vegetables

Beans: cannellini, kidney, chickpeas (garbanzos), pinto, black, and other varieties

Carrots

Corn

Leafy greens such as spinach and collards

Lentils

Sauerkraut

Split peas

Tomatoes, whole, crushed, pureed

Healthy cereals (high-fiber, low-sugar) and whole grains

Bulgur

Barley, regular and quick-cooking

Oat bran

Oats, rolled and steel-cut

Whole-wheat couscous, flour, and pasta

Condiments

Capers

Horseradish

Hot pepper sauce

Mustard

Sea salt

Salsa

Tamari or soy sauce

Fish (canned)

Anchovies

Chunk light tuna

Herring

Sardines, packed in sardine oil

Wild Alaskan salmon

Mackerel

Groceries

Broth, low-sodium, preferably organic (available in cans and cartons): chicken, vegetable, and beef

Brown sugar

Chocolate, dark (65 percent cacao or higher)

Coffee

Cocoa powder

Lemons

Limes

Mushrooms, dried

Onions

Oils

Canola oil

Extra-virgin olive oil (look for the words "cold-pressed" on the label for the best quality; use for dressings)

Toasted sesame oil

Walnut oil (nice for salads)

Nuts and seeds

Almonds

Brazil nuts

Flaxseeds

Pecans

Pistachios

Sesame seeds

Sunflower seeds

Walnuts

Vinegar

Apple cider vinegar

Distilled white vinegar

Wine vinegar

Build a Healthy Plate

Now, after hearing about what goes into a healthy diet, it's time to tie it all together on your plate—literally. The plate method of dividing your meal by types of food can help you trim portion sizes, curb carbs, and maintain blood sugar.

Such thinking is spreading. The USDA recently scrapped its tricky-to-fathom food pyramid—a graphic guide designed to help you design a healthy daily diet—for the My Plate graphic. We applaud the switch! The My Plate illustration is a colorful dinner plate divided into four equal triangles, one each for fruits, vegetables, grains/starchy foods, and protein, with a small circle representing a fat-free or low-fat dairy serving. What's even better: This approach is effective *and* easy to follow.

So now you're ready to get down to the nitty-gritty—putting the healthy, tasty foods on your plate today, this week, and forever. Your assignment: Get a plate and set yourself a place at the table. Learning to fill it with perfect portions of fruit and vegetables, grain and starch-based carbs, and protein is the key to successful blood-sugar control, successful weight loss, and success at lowering your risk for diabetes complications.

The good news: Using the plate approach can make weighing and measuring food for portion control obsolete.

The plate method rebalances your meals to give you the ideal proportions of vegetables, protein, and carbohydrates. Dividing the types of food on the plate automatically

**eat right
today!**

Swap fruit for veggies at breakfast.

We're not going to ask you to fill half your plate with vegetables at this meal, since most of us don't eat vegetables in the morning (although if you're making an omelet, go ahead and pack it with as much produce as possible). Instead, substitute fruit, such as blueberries, strawberries, or bananas. A 2013 study published in *Nutrition Journal* found that people who included two servings of fruit a day, as part of a healthy eating plan, lost more weight than did people who ate a serving or less of fruit a day.

cuts your calorie intake—the real goal of any weight-loss plan. It also ensures that you won't get too many carbohydrates at one sitting, with no need for you to keep a tally. Best of all, your plate will contain plenty of food, so you'll never feel deprived.

Complicated eating plans, such as the food exchange system that dietitians sometimes recommend for people with diabetes, are supposed to be effective because they make you track everything you eat, theoretically leaving less to chance. But many people find the exchange system too confusing. This approach accomplishes the same objective (controlling portions and calories) in a simpler way—and it works.

In one study at Emory University School of Medicine in Atlanta, people who used a basic visual guide to make healthy choices lowered their blood sugar, cut calories, and lost weight just as successfully as those who took the trouble to follow a plan that used food exchanges. And in a Canadian study, people with diabetes who followed a similar plate approach lost more weight than those who got conventional weight-loss advice. And they kept using their plate approach even after the study ended.

The biggest change you'll likely see on your plate? That humble helping of vegetables in the typical American meat-and-potatoes diner will become a hearty helping, shrinking the space left over for fatty meat and carbs—the major sources of calories, fat, and blood-sugar-raising starches and sugars.

Use the three main elements of a typical meal—meat, carbs, and vegetables, and add fruits—as your starting point. When you dish them out, your plate in effect becomes divided into four sections. Of course, it's the size of the sections that matters. To picture how your plate should look, mentally divide it into quarters. Whenever you eat a meal, keep these sections in mind and fill them in the following way.

TAMES CARBS

The plate approach automatically controls carbs and so helps regulate blood sugar. However, if you use insulin or you're having trouble controlling your blood sugar, you may need a stricter approach, such as carbohydrate counting, a system that helps you keep tight control on carb levels at every meal. You can combine carb counting with the plate approach to achieve better blood-sugar control and to reach a healthy weight.

CURBS STARCHES

Using the plate approach, the number of calories you save by eating more vegetables and fewer fatty foods can be significant. When you incorporate this method of meal planning, the result is fewer starches, which means much less impact on your blood sugar.

½ PLATE = VEGETABLES AND FRUITS

With the plate approach, one-half of your entire plate should be reserved for produce. This is where you'll put all your vegetables as well as fruit. Choose anything you like except potatoes and corn, which belong in the grains and starchy foods section. For some meals, you can eat fruit instead of (or in addition to) vegetables.

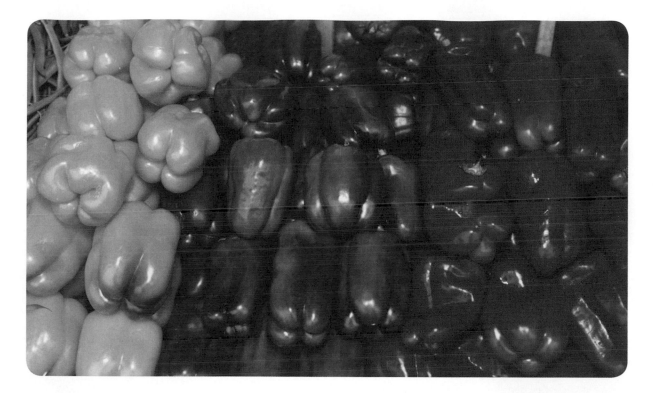

There's no escaping it: To lose weight, you need to take in fewer calories than you burn. The plate approach's solution to cutting calories is remarkably simple: Eat more produce and less of everything else. In the plate approach, half the real estate on your plate is taken up by vegetables and fruit, which are naturally very low in calories, so there's less room for starches and calorie-dense meats.

Vegetables are low in calories yet high in volume because a lot of their weight comes from water. Such "high-volume" foods have the advantage of looking big, so they make your brain expect that you'll be satisfied by eating them. They also take up more room in your stomach, so they trigger a signal in your brain that makes you stop eating sooner. It's small wonder that researchers in weight-loss programs such as the one at the University of Alabama in Birmingham find that when people eat lots of vegetables, their calorie consumption goes down—and they lose weight.

As an example, half a medium head of iceberg lettuce weighs around 10 ounces, and is about 40 calories. By comparison, one Oreo cookie, which weighs less than 1 ounce, is about 55 calories.

At the same time, vegetables are the most nutrient-dense foods around, filled with vitamins, minerals, and other micronutrients that you can't get in other foods but that are crucial to good health and healing.

This two-pack of benefits is huge. It means that if you avoid using lots of oil, butter, or creamy sauce in the cooking process, you can eat as many vegetables as you want without jeopardizing your health or blood sugar.

> Vegetables are low in calories yet high in volume because a lot of their weight comes from water.

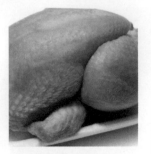

CHICKEN OR TURKEY

These meats can be high-fat disasters or perfect Reverse Diabetes fare. It all depends on the cut and how it's prepared. Breast meat, whether ground or whole, is always lower in fat than dark meat such as thighs and drumsticks. Never eat the skin, because of its high saturated fat content, and when buying ground turkey, make sure the package says ground turkey breast. Otherwise, you may as well be eating hamburger. And need we remind you, the Colonel is not your friend. (Why are you eating anything that comes in a bucket, anyway?) If you stick to these rules, you'll enjoy a nice, low-calorie dose of sustaining protein. No time to cook? Pick up a rotisserie chicken.

Still hungry? You can fill the vegetable section again and again. That's right, there's no limit on the amount of food you can eat from this part of the plate as long as you stop when you feel satisfied. On the rest of the plate, however, stick with one helping of grains/starchy foods and one helping of protein.

Almost all vegetables are inherently good for you, but beware of transforming low-calorie vegetables into high-calorie ones by frying them in oil or smothering them with toppings such as cheese sauces, full-fat salad dressings, or butter. By adding just one teaspoon of butter, you more than double or triple the calories in a serving of vegetables.

Another great thing about vegetables: There are so many terrific choices! Don't limit yourself to the same ones over and over (can you say broccoli, green beans, or cucumbers—again?). Serious chefs will tell you that vegetables are one of the most interesting, delightful, and tasty foods to experiment with. Consider cooking greens (collards, chard, and kale), Asian choices (bok choy, napa cabbage, long beans, and snow peas), and any of the many varieties of eggplant, squash, peppers, and tomatoes that are available.

And if you haven't tried roasting your veggies, you're in for a treat! As a cooking technique, it couldn't be easier. Preheat your oven to 450°F. Cut into pieces roughly two inches around, and toss in olive oil seasoned with salt and pepper. Spread out on rimmed baking sheet and roast until browned and tender, turning to brown on both sides. Especially yummy for Brussels sprouts (cut larger ones in half; leave smaller ones whole), cauliflower, and broccoli.

¼ PLATE = WHOLE GRAINS

Grain-based carbohydrates and starchy veggies such as potatoes belong in the upper right-hand side of your plate. This area is reserved for whole-grain pasta, brown rice, barley, noodles, potatoes (white or preferably sweet), or corn. If you're serving starchy beans (legumes such as black beans, pinto beans, kidney beans, or chickpeas) as a side dish, put them here too.

The benefit? When starches are limited to one-fourth of your plate, you've got automatic carb control, which translates into better blood-sugar control. With the plate approach, you'll enjoy a generous yet safe and controlled amount of carbs—no more worries, no more guilt.

You already know that carbs aren't dietary disasters and that having three servings of whole grains a day will enhance your health and your blood sugar if you have diabetes. But limiting portions is important with both starchy and grain-based carbs. First, they raise blood sugar. Second, some researchers now believe that eating too many carbohydrates makes weight control especially hard for people who are already heavy. The reason: Carbs break down easily into glucose, and with enough glucose on hand, the body never has to burn its fat stores for energy.

Bottom line: With the plate approach you'll enjoy a generous yet safe and controlled amount of carbs. Stick with it, and you can enjoy rice and mashed potatoes, without worrying that your blood sugar could be in peril.

¼ PLATE = LEAN PROTEIN

Reserve one-fourth of your plate for satisfying, sugar-controlling protein foods. These include lean red meat, eggs, fish, and chicken and turkey. If legumes, such as lentils, are part of your entrée, put them here.

You've already learned that making sure you get protein at every meal is critical. Protein makes you feel full longer than carbohydrates do, and it doesn't raise blood sugar. So why not eat more of it? We're glad you asked. The first reason, of course, is calories. Just about any protein food you eat has more calories than veggies do. The second reason is fat. As you know now, saturated fats directly impair the body's ability to react to insulin, the hormone that keeps blood sugar in check, and many protein foods contain these fats. Finally, if you fill up on protein at the expense of vegetables or whole grains, your body will be deprived of nutrients that are essential for good health.

ON THE SIDE: DAIRY

The USDA My Plate program recognizes that a serving of nonfat or low-fat dairy should be part of every meal, so add a glass of milk or other dairy products such as yogurt and cheese.

eat right
today!

Serve your meal on just one plate.

That means no bread plate or separate salad bowl. How come? Having multiple plates at a meal makes it hard to keep track of how much food you are eating. Plus, they double up your portions; having a scoop of corn on your plate and a roll on a bread plate means you are having two courses of carbs, not one. And that separate salad bowl can trick you into thinking that you have covered your vegetable needs, giving you permission to put more carbs and protein on your main plate.

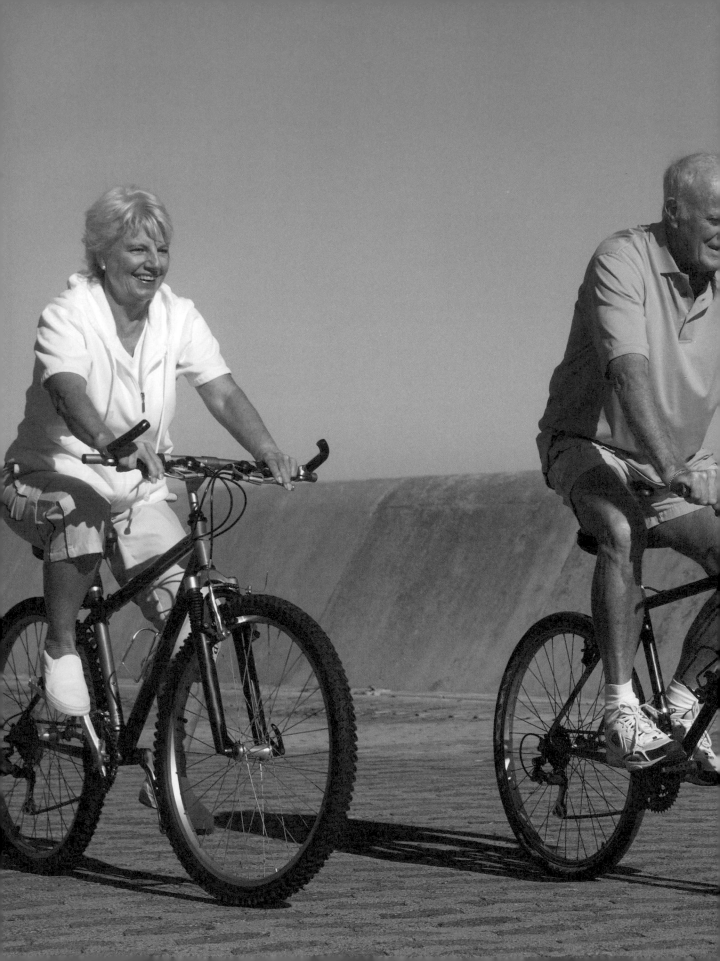

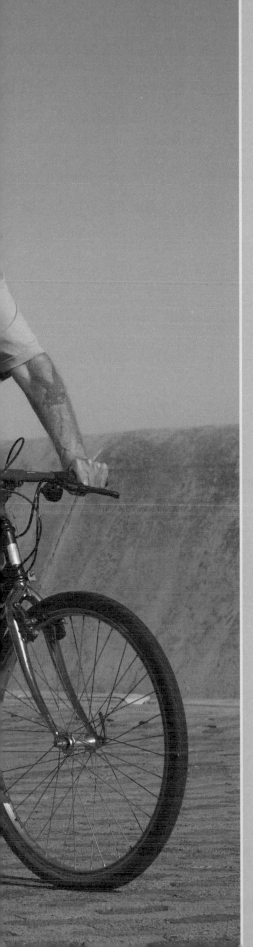

 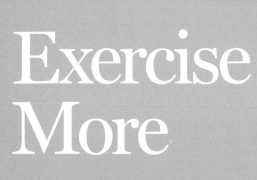

PART 3

Exercise More

Here's something amazing about exercise: It can naturally help you manage blood sugar and functions just like some diabetes drugs. Exercise sensitizes cells to insulin so they soak up more glucose. In fact, when you start exercising more, chances are you'll see your blood-sugar levels drop—maybe even enough to reduce some of your medications. In addition, your body will burn more calories all day long, making it easier for you to lose extra weight. Let's get up and move!

Reverse Diabetes Forever with **Active Living**

Getting active trims fat from your body and helps you tip the scales in the right direction.

If a dramatic treatment hit the market that could drop your blood sugar from 386 to 106 mg/dL, help you lose 100 pounds in 14 months, and guarantee that you'd never have to use insulin, you'd jump on it, right? Well, that's exactly what you should do: jump, walk, jog—anything that moves you in the right direction when it comes to reversing your diabetes.

It takes just 30 minutes a day—the time spent watching a mindless sitcom—to put you on the path to better blood sugar today and for months and years to come. At the same time, you'll ease stress, boost your brain's feel-good chemicals, and give your weight-loss efforts a big nudge in the right direction.

Studies show that making active choices, from doing lawn work to going bowling, is a no-sweat way to lose weight and reduce your risk for diabetes and other health problems. We'll show you how to energize your life and burn hundreds of extra calories each day.

Maybe you're interested in exercise but tend to put other commitments—and other people's expectations—first. Now's the time to renew your commitment to yourself and your health. It's not hard. Just start by fitting in small bouts of exercise all day long (like taking the stairs instead of the elevator) and setting aside time for fun physical activity, like shooting some hoops or taking the grandkids to the park. Yes, these count as calorie-burning exercise—and they'll get you into the mindset for moving every day.

Take a look through these pages to find exercise plans that are right for you. There are low-impact exercise options, walking plans, yoga workouts, bicycling fitness tips, and lots of other options to exercise more. Find one that appeals to you and that you know you'll stick with.

Just remember, it doesn't matter whether you walk, dance, or bicycle your way to better fitness and blood-sugar control. It all comes down to this: Getting active trims fat from your body and helps you tip the scales in the right direction—two key ways to reverse diabetes forever.

Exercise More >
Right Now

Put this book down and take a 10-minute walk. You'll immediately find that you do have time for exercise. It doesn't take a major time commitment to reap the rewards of physical activity, exercise feels good—and fits into any schedule. Remind yourself of the benefits: better blood-sugar control, a healthier weight, lower stress, and less risk for serious diabetes complications.

Exercise More >
Today

During the course of your usual day, look for opportunities to exercise. Perhaps you can commute to work by bike once or twice a week. At the very least, you can take more stairs or make the long circuit to the bathroom. Then take note of how your time is spent in the evenings. Try to swap TV or web-browsing time with exercise. Being aware of these "movable moments" today can help your plan for long-term fitness.

Exercise More >
This Week

Make time to walk at least five days a week. Being more physically active could be a walk in the park...or around the neighborhood...or on a treadmill. Putting one foot in front of the other is a simple yet powerful way to lower blood sugar and lose weight. Start with just 10 minutes a day and build up to 45-minute walks— energizing, calorie-, and fat-burning workouts that feel great.

Exercise More >
This Month

Exercise can make or break your efforts to lose weight and control your blood sugar—but when you have diabetes, you need to make sure you're exercising smartly and safely. It's important to guard against hypoglycemia (blood sugar that dips too low), protect your feet, and time your workouts, especially if you take insulin.

Exercise More >
This Year

Muscle mass is the secret to blood-sugar control and to maintaining a healthy weight with ease. Find some sort of comparison so you'll be able to gauge your progress after a year. Perhaps it's the amount you can lift or the muscle defini- tion in your arms and legs. Or it could be how much of that spare tire melts off your midsection. Whatever your measure, have something you can use to check your progress after a year.

Exercise More >
Forever+

When you begin an exercise program, you often feel dread. But if you make it through the initial weeks and months, you'll discover something amazing: You miss it when you don't exercise. Your body will become accustomed to the new, invigorated you. You'll also likely find new friends and activities as you continue to enjoy a more active lifestyle. Reversing diabetes forever with exercise is sort of like that law of physics: Bodies in motion tend to stay in motion. Keep moving!

Why Exercise Works

You've heard for years that exercise is good for you. But it has specific benefits for people with diabetes—a fact that healers from ancient cultures in India and China recognized centuries ago. Since then, scientists have discovered exactly how exercise works its magic. Here's what exercising more can do for your diabetes.

LOWERS BLOOD SUGAR

Putting your muscles into action is like hitting your car's accelerator: It instantly boosts the demand for fuel—namely, glucose. Once your muscles exhaust their own supply of glucose, they clean out the stores in your liver, then draw glucose straight from the bloodstream, lowering your blood sugar. When you're done exercising, your body gives top priority to replenishing glucose stores in the liver and muscles rather than the blood, which means that your blood sugar will stay lower for hours—perhaps for as long as a couple of days, depending on how hard you worked out.

BEATS "SITTING DISEASE"

Believe it or not, sitting can kill you—especially if you're a woman. Turns out, a recent study by researchers from the American Cancer Society's Epidemiology Research Program—which looked at over 100,000 healthy men and women ages 50 to 74—

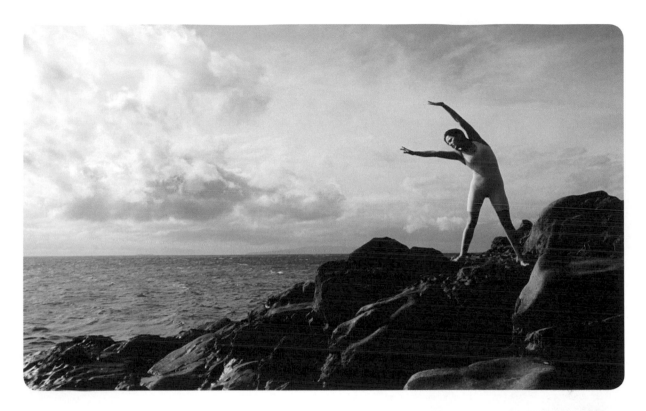

revealed that if you're a woman who spends more than six hours a day sitting down, your risk of dying from any cause is 40 percent higher than women who sit for three hours or less. The researchers noted that it was prolonged sitting—sitting for hours at a stretch—that were lethal, so if you've got a desk job, take frequent walk breaks, even if it's just to the watercooler and back.

BOOSTS INSULIN SENSITIVITY

If you exercise regularly, you can actually lower your level of insulin resistance. That's because exercise forces muscles to use glucose more efficiently by making cells more receptive to insulin. It's as if getting physical gives your cells a kick in the pants: If they absolutely must have more glucose, they'll work harder to get it. Exercise also boosts the number of insulin receptors. Do it regularly and you'll perpetuate good blood-sugar control. In fact, the effect won't entirely fade away unless you go for about 72 hours without a workout. Even if you've been a die-hard couch potato for years, you can ratchet up your insulin sensitivity with exercise in as little as one week.

BURNS FAT

What happens when muscles use up the glucose in the liver and blood? After about 30 minutes of continuous exercise, the body turns to fatty acids both in flabby storage sites throughout the body and in the blood. Using fat for energy helps clear the blood of harmful fats, such as LDL cholesterol and triglycerides. It also boosts "good" HDL

exercise more today!

Celebrate your good choices.

Every time you make an active choice instead of an inactive choice during your day, give yourself a pat on the back by writing it down. That includes small stuff, like taking the stairs instead of the elevator, or bigger stuff, like mowing the lawn or playing a game of softball in the backyard. Recording these choices will motivate you to get up and move even more often.

> As you lose fat, build muscle, and gain energy, you'll feel livelier, more capable, and maybe even younger!

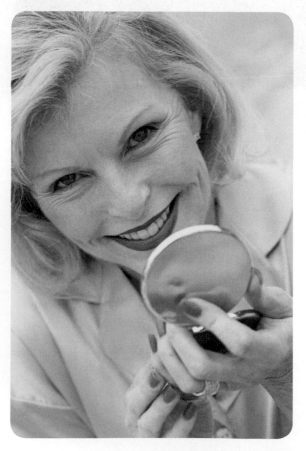

cholesterol and helps trim abdominal fat, which is linked to a higher risk of diabetes and complications.

SHAVES POUNDS

The more active you are, the more energy you use, and if you control your diet as well, you'll end up with a calorie deficit that eventually tips the scales in a favorable direction. A bonus: Exercise also builds up your muscle mass, and since muscle burns energy faster than other types of tissue (especially fat), that means you'll burn more calories all the time—even when you're not exercising.

PROTECTS YOUR HEART

Exercise cuts your chances of having a heart attack, stroke, or other cardiovascular problem linked with diabetes by helping to improve your risk profile. In one study, type 2 patients who took part in an aerobic-exercise program lasting only three months saw their triglyceride and HDL cholesterol levels improve by about 20 percent, along with a significant drop in blood pressure. And the benefits aren't limited to those with type 2 diabetes. Researchers at the University of Pittsburgh found the risk of dying from cardiovascular illnesses to be three times higher among sedentary people with type 1 diabetes than among those who regularly burn about 2,000 calories a week through exercise.

MAKES YOU FEEL GOOD

This isn't a minor point. Dealing with a chronic disease day after day can sometimes feel discouraging, stressful, or even depressing. Exercise helps by producing feel-good chemicals in the brain that can boost your mood, relieve stress, and alleviate the blues. It also does wonders for your sense of confidence and self-esteem. When you finish a workout, you're justified in feeling that you've accomplished something important. You might feel that if you can do this, maybe you really can get your health under control. And you'd be right.

MAKES YOU LOOK BETTER

It's not the most important health benefit, but it sure is a strong motivator. Without a doubt, if your fitness improves, your appearance does, too. You lose flab and gain muscle, strength, and energy, which make you seem livelier, more capable, and maybe even younger. Is that sweat on your brow? Then you look fabulous!

100 Calories—Burned!

One of the wonderful things about exercise is that there are plenty of ways to get your heart pumping and those calories burning. That's what we're showing you in this chapter: It doesn't matter how you get more exercise, just that you do. Even little everyday activities can make a big difference. For instance, if you burn an extra 100 calories a day, even if you don't change your eating habits at all, you'll lose about 10.5 pounds over the course of a year. What does it take to burn 100 calories? Not much. Below are 15 activities that burn 100 calories, based on a 150-pound, 42-year-old woman. How many have you done today, this week, or this month?

1. Go roller-skating. In just 12 minutes you burn off 100 calories.

2. Go grocery shopping. A 38-minute grocery shopping trip burns 100 calories; you'll burn another 100 calories carrying the groceries to your car and then into your house.

3. Play Frisbee. Half an hour is all it takes—and that's assuming you're not doing a lot of running after wild throws.

4. Put up your Christmas tree. Forty minutes of stringing lights and hanging ornaments is all that's needed to burn 100 calories and decorate for the holidays.

5. Usher for your church or synagogue. After 45 minutes you'll have not only greeted all the attendees but will have burned 100 calories as well.

6. Make dinner. Pick one that requires chopping. If it takes you 35 minutes to prepare dinner, you've burned your 100.

7. Jump rope. Even slow jumping burns 100 calories in 11 minutes; jump faster and it takes only about 7.

8. Clean out your garage. Put in half an hour of sorting. By then, you'll have cleared at least one small space and burned 100 calories.

9. Jog in place. Do it for 11 minutes during the commercials of a 30-minute TV show.

10. Dance the flamenco. Just 15 minutes of fast ballroom dancing will do it.

11. Walk your dog. In a half hour, you'll have burned 100 calories, and he'll have stretched all fours and sniffed to his heart's content.

12. Iron your clothes. And your partner's and your kids'. Do it for 40 minutes.

13. Hit the driving range. You'll improve your golf game and burn 100 calories in 30 minutes.

14. Play golf. Carry your clubs and walk the course, and you'll burn 100 calories every 20 minutes.

15. Go fishing. It's peaceful and stress-free, and 30 minutes of it burns about 100 calories.

HAS FRINGE BENEFITS

Exercise helps control diabetes and reduce the risk of heart attack and stroke. As if that weren't enough, it also:

▸ Helps prevent certain malignancies, such as colon cancer.
▸ Improves or maintains blood flow to sex organs, potentially enhancing sexual function and enjoyment.
▸ Preserves cognitive functions, such as memory.
▸ Retards bone loss that can lead to osteoporosis.
▸ Boosts the ability of immune-system cells to fight invaders.
▸ Slows physical decline that accounts for most impairments associated with aging.
▸ Eases arthritis pain by strengthening and stretching the muscles, tendons, and ligaments that support joints.
▸ Guards against back pain by strengthening muscles that support the spine.
▸ Aids digestion and helps prevent such ailments as irritable bowel syndrome.
▸ Promotes good sleep.

Personalize Your Exercise

Exercise is so powerful it's almost like taking medicine.
But a prescription that works for you won't be ideal for everybody with diabetes. That's why it's important to work with your doctor to customize your exercise plan to fit your circumstances, starting with which kind of diabetes you have and how you're treating it now.

Whichever strategy you choose, you'll want to bring blood sugar down—but not too far. To keep close tabs on it, test an hour before your workout, then again a half hour later to find out if your levels are rising or falling. If they're falling and on the low side, you may want to eat about 15 grams of carbohydrate before you start exercising. If your blood sugar is high and rising, you may need more insulin. Once your blood sugar becomes more stable, your doctor may allow you to monitor less often, but self-testing following a workout is always a good idea.

The readings you get will help clarify how exercise should work into your overall diabetes-management plan, which will vary from one situation to the next.

If You Have Type 1

People with type 1 diabetes need to approach exercise with extra caution. If you work out too soon after taking insulin, the glucose-lowering tag team of insulin plus exer-

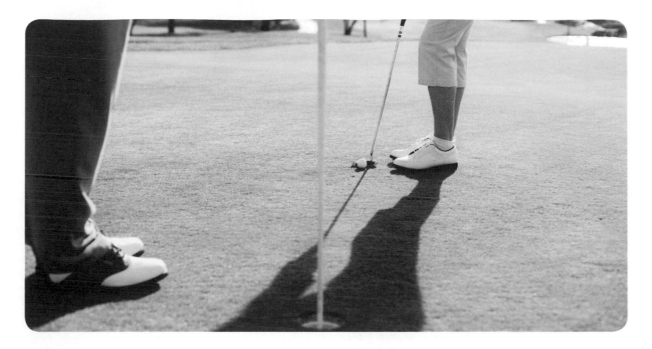

cise can be too much of a good thing and lower your blood sugar to dangerous levels. On the flip side, having too little insulin in your blood while you exercise can make blood sugar build up and potentially cause ketoacidosis. To ensure your safety, check with your doctor about taking steps like the following:

Avoid peak hours. Try to time your workout so that you're not exercising when insulin activity peaks, often within the first hour or two of an injection, depending on which type you use. This may be less of an issue than it has been in the past. With the increased use of insulin pumps and intensive injection therapy, it's possible for people to exercise any time they can fit it in. Talk to your doctor or diabetes educator for specific advice.

Adjust your dose. You may be able to drop your daily insulin requirement by as much as 20 to 30 percent if you cut your dose before a workout. Ask your doctor how much of an adjustment to make based on your current dosage and how hard you exercise.

Inject into the abdomen. Problem: If you inject insulin into the muscles you'll be using, they will absorb it faster and send your blood sugar plummeting. Solution: Unless you're going straight into sit-ups, inject into the softer folds of your midsection. If you're working your abs, wait to exercise until about an hour after your injection to give the insulin a chance to disperse throughout the body.

Have a snack. Eating a small low-fat snack containing about 20 grams of carbohydrate (two rolled fruit snacks, for example) during your workout can help keep blood sugar from falling too low, especially during vigorous exercise or workout sessions lasting an hour or more.

> Try to time your activities so that you're not exercising when insulin is at its peak.

If You Have Type 2 and Use Insulin

The great promise of exercise for people with type 2 diabetes is that—unlike with type 1—it can actually throw the condition into reverse. Boosting your insulin sensitivity could bring your blood sugar back into the normal range, especially if you're controlling your diet as well, and could permanently reduce the amount of insulin you need—or even get you off insulin altogether. Some practical advice:

Proceed with caution. While keeping your eyes on the prize—less insulin or none at all—remember to keep your goals reasonable at first. If you're taking insulin, you stand the same risk of hypoglycemia during exercise that a type 1 person does. Take a look at the above list of recommendations for people with type 1—they also apply to you.

Try not to snack. If you're in danger of hypoglycemia during exercise, you may need a snack to bring your blood sugar back up. But this solution can ultimately work against you because it adds calories you're probably better off avoiding. So instead of relying on snacks to head off hypoglycemia, be diligent about planning to exercise after a meal so blood sugar is high during your workout.

Stick to your meal plan. If you do eat an unplanned snack during your workout, don't make up for it by subtracting calories from your after-exercise meals. It's just as important to keep calories up after a workout as before, since exercise can make blood sugar dip dangerously for as long as a day.

If You Have Type 2 and Use Medication

If you take a drug like metformin to control your blood sugar, you may be able to get by with less—or stop taking it altogether—by adding more physical activity to your life. Once you figure out how exercise affects your blood sugar, you'll want to talk with your doctor about how to adjust your drug regimen accordingly. Keep in mind, though, that exercise and diet aren't automatic substitutes for diabetes drugs—and taking drugs doesn't excuse you from working out. In fact, drugs often work their best only when combined with other measures, such as meal planning and exercise. Some advice:

The Blood-Sugar Exercise Paradox

Why does blood sugar go down sometimes but go up other times after exercise? Muscles use glucose for energy, so as a rule, blood sugar goes down when you're active, as the body moves glucose from the liver and bloodstream into the cells. But that assumes there's enough insulin on hand to help with this transfer. If you take insulin and your dose is too low, glucose can build in the blood during exercise and cause hyperglycemia. That's why it's important to consult your doctor for advice on exercising and to check your blood sugar before and after (and perhaps even during) exercise to understand how physical activity affects you.

Time your workouts. If you're using medication, avoid exercising when the drug is reaching its peak effectiveness, so that your blood sugar doesn't drop dangerously low. If you're working to cut back on or eliminate your drug use, your doctor may start by having you take less (or none) before your workout. In effect, you may be able to exercise in place of taking your medication if the effects on blood sugar prove to be similar.

Be alert to side effects. Some diabetes medications can cause muscle ache or fatigue, while others can make you dizzy or nauseated. Be sure you and your doctor are clear about how intensely you intend to exercise and how your medication's side effects may limit your activities.

Drink plenty of water. It takes about eight 8-ounce glasses of water a day to keep the body hydrated—and you'll need more when you're sweating. Don't wait for thirst to hit before drinking; that's a sign of high blood sugar and could bring your workout to a halt while you check for hyperglycemia. Instead, drink one to two cups 15 minutes before exercising, at least a half cup every 15 minutes during your workout, and another one to two cups afterward.

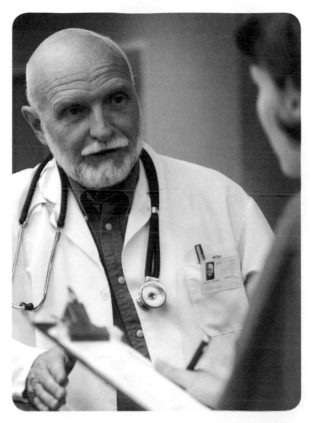

If You Have Impaired Glucose Tolerance

The best evidence for exercise's effectiveness against diabetes comes from research in people with impaired glucose tolerance. In one University of Pennsylvania study, every 2,000 calories burned per week through exercise dropped the risk of diabetes by 24 percent, with people at greatest risk gaining the most benefits. To take advantage:

Get started immediately. Just because full-blown diabetes lies "out there" over the distant horizon doesn't mean you have time to spare. If you don't start making changes now, insulin resistance is only likely to get worse. But if you jump on the exercise bandwagon right away, you can boost your cells' insulin sensitivity within a week, even if you're obese, giving you a good chance of dodging a diagnosis of diabetes.

Track your blood sugar. Don't assume that because you haven't developed diabetes you don't have to worry about blood sugar. You may not need to test as often as a person with a diabetes diagnosis, but you should still keep track of your glucose levels with self-monitoring and regular checkups to make sure your condition remains under control.

> Talk to your doctor about how intensely you intend to exercise and how your medication's side effects may limit your activities.

Keep it up. It's just as important for you to keep workouts regular and consistent as it is for a person with diabetes. Controlling the risk of developing the disease will never be easier than it is now—and you should aim to keep it that way.

Sweat Safely

You'll avoid most hypoglycemia problems with proper planning (by matching exercise to your drug, insulin, and meal regimens), but you should always be prepared for surprise bouts of low blood sugar.

Know when to stop—now. The second you detect symptoms of hypoglycemia, such as confusion, shaking, light-headedness, or difficulty speaking, stop immediately—not after "just one more minute." Be alert to all symptoms, and understand that some of them overlap with natural responses to exercise, such as sweating and rapid heartbeat.

Carry a snack. A quick snack can rapidly bring dropping blood sugar back up in an emergency, but only if you remember to bring one along.

Get a partner. It's not always obvious when hypoglycemia is setting in, so it's wise to work out with somebody else or in a place where other people are available if you need help, especially if you're exercising vigorously.

Pack ID. Even if you're with a friend, you should carry identification with your name, address, and phone number—and those of your doctor. Also have the name of someone to call in an emergency as well as your insulin or drug dosages.

Stay alert afterward. Blood sugar can continue to fall long after you've exercised, so keep your guard up for signs of hypoglycemia up to 24 hours after your workout.

The Active Living Pyramid

This handy, simple guide to exercise is designed to help you understand and internalize how much walking, stretching, strength training, and simple daily movement you really need to achieve optimum health. This exclusive Active Living Pyramid boils down all the scientific research and government recommendations into one easy-to-follow guide.

As with any hierarchy, it's easy to focus entirely on the bottom layers, since that's what you should be doing most. But that doesn't mean the top layers are not essential. You need to stretch and strengthen—and yes, even sit—every day. You just don't need to do them in equal doses. Most important, you need to move, each and every day.

Experts will tell you that moving your body and avoiding prolonged "sitting" time is one of the most important things you can do to live the life you want to live. Study after study show that maintaining adequate levels of physical activity may reduce your risk of depression, dementia, certain cancers, heart disease, and other chronic illnesses.

The trick is integrating movement into your everyday routine. The Active Living Pyramid makes that ultra-simple. Let's start climbing!

Break up your sitting sessions.

If you're like most deskbound keyboard tappers, you need to sit down during the day. Just make sure you get up and stretch on a regular basis. Why? Your body operates much like an idle computer that dims to save power. When you're barely using your muscles, especially the large ones, like those found in your hips and legs, your body starts to shut down at the cellular level. Research shows that when you limit the amount of simple activities like standing and walking, key fat-burning enzymes simply start switching off. Sit for a full day and those fat burners plummet by 50 percent. The solution: Don't sit longer than 30 minutes without standing up, even if it's just to change positions and sit back down. When possible, stretch or walk a few steps around your workspace.

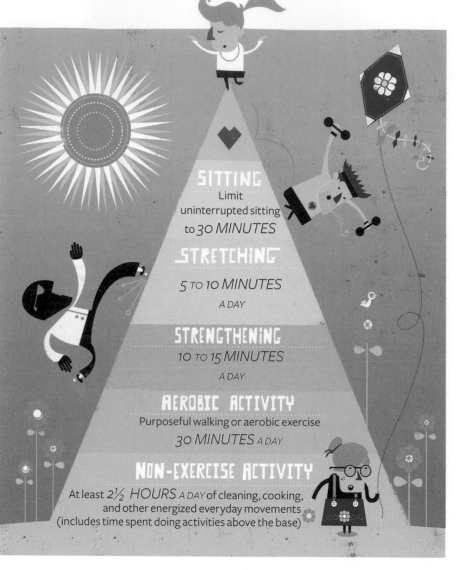

Foundation: Non-Exercise Activity

The science is clear: It's lots of little daily movements—NOT jogging, elliptical training, or body-sculpt boot camp—that your body craves most on the metabolic level. Cooking, cleaning, puttering about, strolling—just standing up—triggers hundreds of thousands of muscle contractions that help your body absorb glucose, regulate cholesterol, and keep your blood flowing clear and clean, avoiding diseases like atherosclerosis and diabetes.

That's why non-exercise activity is the foundation of the Active Living Pyramid. Ideally, you should spend 150 minutes, or about 2½ hours, each day in motion. That may sound like an awful lot, but remember, non-exercise activity is the stuff of everyday life; walking here and there, taking the stairs, cooking, cleaning up, even fidgeting. And because it's spread out throughout the day rather than in one lump sum, you get many little metabolic spikes from morning to night.

Sound difficult? Consider this sample day and see how easy non-exercise activity can be. Notice it doesn't take you much more time to tick off your daily tasks the active way, but you'll move much more—and save money, too.

That's about four hours of daily activity all neatly tucked into a typical day. And the best part? Unlike prolonged sitting, which can actually make you feel more tired, all this movement will keep you buzzing with energy.

	INSTEAD OF	TRY
MORNING	Letting dog out in yard	10-minute stroll around the block
	Drive to Starbucks	Grind beans and make coffee at home
	Turn on TV news	Turn on radio news; sweep or stretch while listening
	Pick up dry cleaning	Hand wash and iron
	Grab a bagel at work	Toast one at home
	Park next to the building	Park in the "latecomers" lot
		TOTAL ACTIVE TIME: 40 minutes
MIDDAY	Buying lunch from office café	Walk to a deli and grab lunch
	Shop online	Head to the sidewalk and shop during lunch hour
	E-mail a coworker	Walk to their office to catch up
	Sit and talk on the phone	Stand and pace while talking
		TOTAL ACTIVE TIME: 60 minutes
EVENING	Picking up take-out food	Shop for ingredients and cook dinner
	Sit at son's soccer practice	Join another parent strolling around the field
	Plop down in front of the TV	Go outdoors and work in the garden or play
	Surf the web	Head to the library, find a good book; surf there
		TOTAL ACTIVE TIME: 90 minutes
NIGHTTIME	Watching TV for 3 hours	Watch for 1 hour, head upstairs and get romantic
		TOTAL ACTIVE TIME: 90 minutes

Level One: Aerobic Activity

If non-exercise activity like mowing the lawn and taking the stairs keeps you living well, purposeful cardio exercise—the next layer in the Active Living Pyramid—keeps you living well longer.

Aerobic exercise—which includes activities like brisk walking, bicycle riding, and swimming—raises your heart rate above its normal, steady thump-thump of daily living and makes it beat faster and harder, which makes it stronger. Making your heart stronger helps you live longer. In a study of more than 73,000 women ages 50 to 79, researchers found that those who walked just 30 minutes a day, five days a week, reduced their risk of having a heart attack by a third, regardless of their age and weight. Even better: Walking worked just as well as jogging or other bucket-sweating exercise for keeping the heart ticking healthfully.

RATING OF PERCEIVED EXERTION (RPE)

1 to 2	Barely moving
3 to 4	Getting the blood flowing; not breathing hard enough to affect speaking
5 to 6	Easy aerobic effort; can still speak in full sentences
7 to 8	Hard effort; can only speak a few words at a time
9 to 10	Very hard; no talking, just breathing

That's why the Active Living Pyramid recommends 30 minutes a day of purposeful activity, in which you make your heart work a little harder. How do you know if you're working hard enough? Many exercise experts recommend using the Rating of Perceived Exertion (RPE). This is a 1-to-10 scale where 1 is just puttering around and 10 is an all-out effort. You typically spend most of your day in the 1-to-4 range. To get the benefits of regular cardio exercise, you should aim to be at least in the 5-to-6 range and, periodically, in the 7 to 8 range. Here's why. A 2015 study presented at the American Heart Association's annual meeting found that short bursts of high intensity exercise were more effective at improving cholesterol, blood sugar, and body weight among people with diabetes than was sustained lower intensity exercise. So pick up the pace and really get your heart pumping for a minute or two out of every five or ten. And try to get your heart rate up periodically over the course of the day, too. At least once in the morning and twice in the afternoon, take a break from work and do 5 minutes of brisk walking or stair climbing. Even jogging or marching in place can help.

And it's never, ever too late to start. A recent study of 1,861 men and women over the age of 70 found that those who did four hours of physical activity a week (which is just over 30 minutes a day) were 12 percent less likely to die between the ages of 70 and 78, 15 percent less likely to die between the ages of 78 and 85, and 17 percent less likely to die between the ages of 85 and 88. The active folks were also better able to perform daily tasks, reported being less lonely, and were more likely to rate their health as good than did those who spent their time in sedentary ways. The best part? The benefits weren't only reaped by long-time exercisers but also by those who first laced up their walking shoes between the ages of 70 and 85.

Level Two: Strengthening

To live life to the fullest requires some heavy lifting—literally. Picking up kids and grandkids, moving furniture, carrying shopping bags, digging in the garden, and so many other tasks in an active life take strength. Unfortunately, muscle tissue is one of the first things to go as we age, to the tune of about half a pound a year starting as early as our 20s.

That may not sound like much, but since muscle is your body's biggest calorie burner, it's like taking your foot off the gas pedal of your metabolism. The result is a creeping weight gain of about a pound a year for the average adult. Worse, if you do nothing to stem the loss, you could lose 40 percent of your muscle tissue by age 65, making you progressively and dangerously weaker during most of your adulthood.

Women, who have less muscle tissue to begin with, are especially at risk. A study of 10,000 American women showed that up to one-third of women ages 40 to

55 struggle with climbing stairs, carrying groceries, and other simple everyday strength-related tasks.

Hands down, the most important benefit of regular strength training is to keep you strong so you can live life to the fullest. A growing body of evidence shows that lifting weights improves your strength, posture, balance, and coordination—as well as keeping your metabolism firing on all cylinders, allowing you to maintain a healthy weight and enjoy youthful stamina and energy.

Increasingly, scientists are also finding that lifting weights can improve your health in other meaningful, and sometimes surprising, ways. One recent study of women ages 42 to 55 found that their total cholesterol, LDL cholesterol, insulin, and artery suppleness measurably improved after just 10 weeks of twice-weekly strength training. Research also shows that strength training can improve insulin resistance and help reverse diabetes.

The Active Living Pyramid recommends 10 to 15 minutes a day, which is the amount of strength training shown in a 2014 study to drive down diabetes risk. That would mean doing about four strengthening exercises each day. Generally, you will do a set of eight to 12 lifts, pause for 20 to 30 seconds, do another set, pause again, and do a final set. Take 30 seconds of rest, then move on to your next exercise.

You want to work out the same muscles only once every three days, so experts recommend targeting different muscle groups with each day's program.

Now, we know that daily strengthening isn't the norm: Regular exercisers often prefer two total-body strength workouts a week, and that's perfectly acceptable. But we still recommend the daily approach, particularly for people who aren't all that passionate about formal exercise routines. Small, daily workouts are not just habit forming but easy: You don't need to change your clothes, you probably won't sweat, and finding the time is much easier. More important for people with diabetes, doing a few moves a day seems to be more effective in keeping your calorie-burning metabolism humming, which is great for better insulin function.

> Hands down, the most important benefit of regular strength training is to keep you strong so you can live life to the fullest.

Level Three: Stretching

Stretching has become the subject of much controversy in the sports medicine world. Long hailed as a way to prevent post-exercise soreness and injury, stretching proved to do neither in a comprehensive scientific review. So should you give up reaching for your toes and reach for the remote instead? No way, say sports docs. Just because it doesn't prevent injury doesn't mean it's useless. Quite the contrary: It's one of the most useful activities you can do for healthy everyday mobility.

As you age, your muscles naturally lose some of their elasticity and suppleness. That leads to shortening and

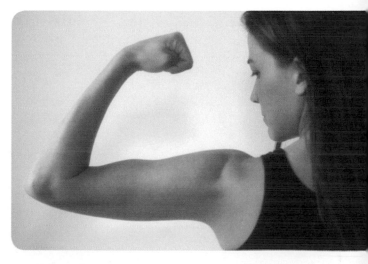

MONDAY THURSDAY	Arms and shoulders
TUESDAY FRIDAY	Chest, back, abs, buttocks
WEDNESDAY SATURDAY	Legs
SUNDAY	Wrists, hands, ankles, feet

tightening that can restrict your range of motion and lead to aches and pains, sending you to the couch rather than the tennis court. To keep motoring through life, you need to "lube your chassis," and that means stretching. When you challenge your muscles to move through a full, extended range of motion, you not only increase the length of the muscle, but also activate the fluids in your joints. Both improve your comfort and mobility.

If you think you're too young to worry about stretching, you're wrong: Muscles can start losing their suppleness in early adulthood if used too little. And if you think you're too old to worry about stretching, you're even more wrong! A recent study of 17 men and women, who were an average age of 88, found that after just eight weeks, those who did twice-weekly stretching improved their range of motion in nearly all their joints and enjoyed a significant improvement in exercise performance. A similar eight-week study of 40 men and women in their 70s found that lower-body stretching, especially in the hip and ankles, improved their walking form and speed.

Stretching works by literally telling muscles to relax. When you sit and try to touch your toes, you'll notice that at first you can't reach very far. But as you hold the stretch, you can go a little deeper and get closer to your feet. That's because you have special receptors in your muscles that are designed to protect them. Reach too far too fast and those receptors, called intrafusal fibers, will signal the muscle to contract, protecting it from injury.

Perform that same stretch slowly, however, and another receptor, called the golgi organ, will take over, signaling the muscle that it's okay to relax. That's why you need to hold a stretch for 30 seconds. That's how long it takes for your muscles to relax and allow themselves to lengthen.

The Active Living Pyramid recommends 5 to 10 minutes of stretching a day. As with strengthening exercises, you can target a different part of your body each time. Or find a simple all-body sequence of stretches and do it daily as part of your waking or bedtime routine.

Your Magic Fitness Number

Knowing a vital number—your heart rate—leads to making the most of exercising. When you tap into your ticker for some inside information during a workout, you'll discover something we call your "magic fitness number," a measure of how fast your heart beats during its optimal rate for exercise. Along with helping to improve fitness and shed weight, this number can be a great help in managing your blood-sugar levels.

The story behind this magic number begins with each and every thump-thump of your heart. Every day, your heart beats about 100,000 times, pushing about 2,000 gallons of blood through 60,000 miles of capillaries, arteries, and vessels. Your heart rate—the number of beats per minute—is a fundamental measure of your heart's fitness. That's why your doctor (or, at least, one of his nurses) always takes your pulse during a visit. The timing of those beats during exercise means the difference between a casual stroll and a fitness-boosting workout. If your heart isn't beating a bit faster during exercise, you're not going to show any improvement in fitness.

For most of us during the course of our day, a typical heart-rate range is 60 to 80 beats per minute. A faster beat can indicate that you just ran up the stairs or did some other physical activity. Fever from a flu or cold can also temporarily elevate your heart rate. A consistently fast resting heartbeat could also be a sign of trouble, such as anemia, thyroid problems, atrial fibrillation, or some other cardiovascular defect.

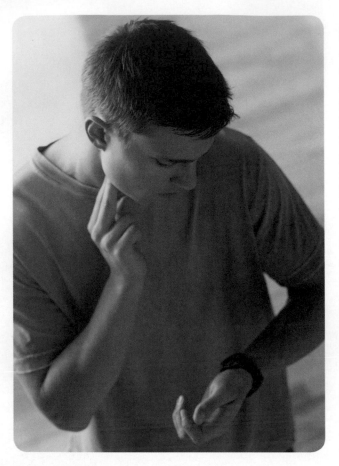

Keeping tabs on your heart rate helps you track how different levels of exercise intensity affect your blood sugar.

Heart rate is a measure of fitness. Those who are less fit will have an elevated heart rate. For example, every minute, the average couch potato's heart beats about 70 to 75 times, a rate of more than a beat a second. On the other hand, an active person's heart is so strong that it can pump the same amount of blood in only 50 beats. So when you exercise at the right amount of intensity, you not only pump up your arm and leg muscles, but you make your heart muscle stronger, too. This kind of conditioning will lead to a more efficient heart—one that will keep on ticking lots longer.

Most fitness experts recommend measuring your heart rate during exercise. The reason: There's a sweet spot, the magic number, where your heart is working just hard enough, but not too hard, to provide a maximum benefit. For most of us, that beneficial area is 60 to 70 percent of our maximum heart rate. For folks who are more fit, it could be as high as 80 percent.

When you work your heart in the 60-percent-of-max zone for at least 30 minutes a day, you're helping build heart fitness, and sticking within this zone has important benefits for people with diabetes, too. You see, the intensity of exercise determines how much blood sugar your muscles use during a workout. By keeping tabs on your heart rate, you can keep track of how different levels of exercise intensity affect your blood sugar and be able to adjust your insulin dosage to avoid crashes when you work out.

How to Find Your Number

To find your magic number, you'll need to know your maximum heart rate. A formula promoted by the American Heart Association (AHA) to determine maximum heart rate is 220 minus your age. So if you are 50 years old, your max heart rate would be 170 (220 minus 50 equals 170).

However, this method often fails to take into account individual differences in fitness and weight. Many trainers and physiologists believe there are personalized methods that can more accurately calculate maximum heart rate. Some of these more precise methods include stress tests where you push yourself to maximum effort while the heart rate is being measured. Other methods involve formulas that incorporate fitness levels, which of course vary person by person.

But whether you have a personal trainer to help find your maximum heart rate or use the AHA formula, you'll still have to do a little more math to determine what 60 to 70 percent of max is. For example, that 50-year-old would need to multiply the 170 max heart rate by 0.60 (for 60 percent) and 0.70 (for 70 percent). In our example, that would mean that to keep the intensity between 60 to 70 percent, the heart rate would need to be between 102 and 119 beats per minute. The heart-boosting benefits don't begin immediately, though. You'll need to stay within your magic number range for at least 10 minutes before your efforts pay off healthwise.

Measure the Beat

How exactly do you track your heart rate? One low-tech way of ensuring that you're exercising in the right heart-rate zone is to take note of your breathing. If you're breathing hard, but can still carry on a conversation, you're likely within that 60 to 70 percent zone. But once your words and phrases are choppy or if you're panting to catch your breath, you're likely over the 70 percent mark. On the too-easy side, if you're able to recite the Pledge of Allegiance without needing to take a breath now and then, you're probably falling below your magic number.

Another low-tech way to check your heart rate is to be an old-school nurse. First, wear a watch with a second hand. Then use the pads of your fingers to find your pulse in your neck or inner wrist. Count the beats for six seconds and then multiply by 10. This will give you a rough idea of your heart rate. For example, if there are 10 beats in those six seconds, your approximate heart rate is 100 beats per minute.

The high-tech, more accurate measurement of your ticker is with a heart-rate monitor. Don't worry, they're not just for hardcore athletes anymore, and they don't cost very much, either. Some models sell for as little as $40. Or you can spend more than $200 to buy a top-of-the-line model that has as much computing power as a GPS, laptop, and watch all rolled into one. If you're just looking for a way keep tabs on your heart rate as you exercise, the less-expensive models will do just fine.

Heart-rate monitors have become very easy to use. With most models, you put a strap or sensing device around your chest against your skin. When your shirt is on, no one can even see it. Then, you'll put the monitor, which looks like a watch, on your wrist. The monitor receives signals from the sensor as it keeps track of your heart. Most monitors are programmable, with features such as an alert that lets you know if you're exceeding or falling below your magic number.

No matter if you're old school or high tech; keeping tabs on your heart rate and sticking to your magic number will give you more efficient workouts. That means the time you spend exercising will actually make a greater difference to your health and blood-sugar management. And your heart will thank you, too.

Walk Away from Diabetes

Taking a long walk is one of life's simplest joys. You can set out with a friend and get caught up on each other's lives. Or you can go it alone and spend your stroll observing, thinking, checking out new music, or listening to the birds chirp. Whatever your preference, going for a walk is more than an escape from daily drudgery—it's a surprisingly effective way to keep blood sugar in check, control your weight, and improve all-around health.

There's no mystery to why walking is so good for people with diabetes. Like any form of exercise, a long stroll forces your muscle cells to burn up reserves of glucose, helping to reduce blood-sugar levels. In fact, regular exercise trains your muscle cells to become more receptive to signals from insulin, the hormone that lowers blood sugar. In one huge study of more than 300,000 men and women, researchers found that devoted walkers cut their risk for type 2 diabetes by 30 percent. If you already have diabetes and take medication, adopting a walking program could help you lower your dose or get off diabetes drugs altogether.

Here's some really good news about taking a stroll: Mile for mile, walking and running burn similar amounts of calories. A well-designed walking program is just as likely to help you lose a belly roll. And you're more likely to stick with a walking routine.

Walking has other vital benefits, of course. It burns calories, reduces stress, stokes your energy levels, lowers blood pressure and levels of bad LDL cholesterol, and raises

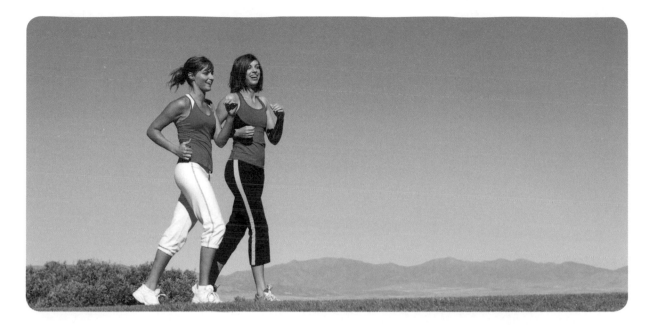

HDL cholesterol—the healthy kind. Start walking five days a week and you'll quickly see these important changes in your blood tests, belt size, and overall well-being. Here's how to make these good things happen.

Get the Right Shoes

A good pair of walking shoes will help you travel farther and faster with more comfort. Your old running shoes may be okay, but be sure they don't have "flared" heels, which are wider than the shoe itself at the base. That provides stability if you're galloping fast but can prevent your foot from rolling normally while walking. Walking shoes should have an "undercut" heel.

Best bet: Go to a respected athletic-footwear store where a skilled salesperson can recommend the ideal shoe for your foot shape and size. Explain what type of terrain you'll be walking on and how many miles you plan to walk a week. Bring along a well-worn pair of sneakers. A savvy salesperson can look at the wear pattern on your shoes to help pick out a style that's right for your foot type. For example, if the inner heel is more worn than the outer heel, your foot probably turns in excessively as you walk. In this case, you'll want some extra arch support and a shoe designed for "motion control."

Try on your shoes and walk around the store. They should hug your heel and not slide up and down as you walk. The shoes should also be flexible but have firm arch support. Most important, the shoes should feel comfortable when you walk. A good walking shoe lasts about 350 miles. If you walk 10 miles a week, that's about eight months.

exercise more today!

Record how long you walk each day.

Use the weekly planner in the Healthy Tools section to record this info. If you choose to wear a pedometer and count your steps every day, write your steps down, too.

Set Strolling Goals

Setting goals for when and how long to walk each day is a surefire way to get the most out of any exercise program. For people who are serious about walking for better health, the right goal is to walk 45 minutes a day, five days of the week. Early morning, during lunch hour, or right after dinner are perfect times; commit to one (or two) of these.

But don't assume you can immediately walk with vigor for 45 minutes. If you have been on the sidelines for some time, you'll need to ease into your program. Create a chart like the one below (or set up a simple spreadsheet on your computer) and record your daily walking time.

Walk This Way

There's walking down a hallway, or in a mall, or to get to your car, and then there's walking energetically for fitness for 45 minutes. You don't need to worry much about your walking technique for the former, but for the latter you want to be sure your stride

WEEK	DAILY WALK TARGET*	S	M	T	W	TH	F	S
1	10							
2	15							
3	20							
4	25							
5	25							
6	30							
7	30							
8	35							
9	35							
10	40							
11	40							
12	45							

* in minutes

and body positioning is right. Following some good habits will boost your payoff and keep your joints, limbs, muscles, and torso healthy.

Warm up and stretch. Before you set off down the road, walk around to warm up your muscles, then stretch for a few minutes. Here's a good basic pre-walk leg stretch: Lean on a pole or other stationary object with both hands. Extend your left leg behind you and bend your right knee. Lean forward until you feel the muscles in your left calf stretch. Now reverse legs. Stretching after your walk is a great idea, too.

Perfect your technique. Using good form when you walk will increase the amount of fat and calories you burn and help prevent muscle and joint pain. Here are some tips for getting the most out of your workout:

▸ Stand tall with your spine elongated and your breastbone lifted. This allows room for your lungs to fully expand. Use the basic rule of good posture: Keep the top of your head as high as you can get it without standing on your toes.

▸ Keep your head straight with your eyes focused forward and your shoulders relaxed. Don't let your shoulders slump or hunch toward your ears.

▸ Roll your feet from heel to toe. If you hear a slapping sound as you walk, you are probably landing on your full foot, not rolling through your step.

▸ As you speed up, take smaller, more frequent steps rather than longer steps. This protects your knees and gives your butt a good workout.

▸ Allow your arms to swing freely. No need to do any unnatural pumping; do what feels right.

▸ Firm your tummy and flatten your back as you walk to prevent low back pain.

Find your pace. You don't have to (and should not) gasp and hurt to reap important health rewards. If you're new to fitness walking, a brisk but comfortable pace will get your heart working hard. If you already walk for exercise, picking up the pace can help you get fit faster. Here's how to set the right pace, whether you're a beginning fitness walker or a veteran of the road.

Beginners: Slow and Easy

Your top priority is regular walking, not setting new speed records. Focus on length-of-time walking more than pace. Once you can comfortably walk continuously for more than 30 minutes, you can shift your attention to speed. Here's how to find out if you've reached your max:

Breathe deeply as you walk to a count of 1-2-3. If you feel breathless and tired during a workout, you may be unintentionally holding your breath. Muscles need oxygen to create energy for movement, so try this as you walk: Inhale by expanding your tummy for a count of three, bringing air to the deepest part of your lungs. Then exhale fully through your nose or mouth, also to the count of three.

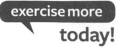

exercise more today!

Strap on a pedometer. These little gadgets tally the number of steps you take in a day. By providing hard data that you can compare one day to the next, pedometers help coax people into walking more. Pedometers are about the size of a book of matches and clip to your belt or waistband, though some tuck into a pocket or are available as a watch or wristband. Simple mechanical versions cost under $20; more elaborate digital versions aren't much more, and often track other data, such as miles covered and calories burned. You can also download a pedometer "app" for an iPhone, Blackberry, or other smartphone.

Take the talk test. Once you're walking for 20 minutes or more each day, aim for a lively pace—the speed you'd reach if you were 10 minutes late for an appointment. Try reciting the Pledge of Allegiance as you walk. If you can get it out phrase by phrase with little pauses for breath in between, you're right on target.

Add in fast bursts. Incorporating brief bursts of faster walking can increase your calorie burn by as much as 60 percent. Move at your usual speed for three to five minutes, then walk even more briskly for one to two minutes. To pick up the pace, take short, quick steps; also bend your arms at 90 degrees and pump them quickly.

> The best walking program is one that's fun and fits into your life.

Start a Walking Routine

The best walking program is one that's fun and fits into your life. Here are some strategies for making walking a regular part of your daily routine.

Roll out of bed and go. You'll want to get dressed and put on some shoes first, of course. And eating a light breakfast first is a good idea, too. But research shows that people who plan to work out in the morning are more likely to follow through than others who plan on exercising later in the day, when meetings, errands, and other distractions can get in the way.

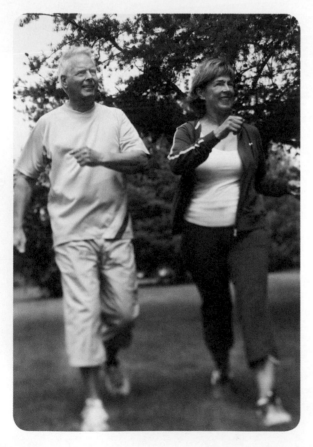

Or walk in the evening. There is something wonderful about after-dinner walks. They get you away from the TV and out in the fresh air where you can say hello to neighbors and watch the sun set. Don't let bad weather stop you, either—that's why jackets, boots, and umbrellas were invented.

Build walks into your lunch routine. As mentioned, eating usually takes just a few moments; use the rest of the time allotted for a stroll. Even if it's just around the perimeter of your office building!

Meet friends for walks, not food. We tend to arrange social events around food or drink. But rather than meeting your girlfriend for coffee or lunch, meet at the park and walk together.

Try a treadmill. If the climate where you live is often just too hot or too cold for comfort, consider investing in a treadmill. Price and space are key considerations, but try to find one with a long walking surface (you'll feel less cramped), good shock absorption (to decrease wear and tear on your legs and feet), and a range of speeds and incline levels.

Nine Walks of Life

Avoid getting bored with the same old walking route or sticking to the same neighborhood. Here are nine ways to make putting one foot in front of another more exciting.

Opt for nice. Walk in the prettiest area in your town (or the next town over), even if it means you need to drive over. That could include downtowns, parks, school campuses, or residential areas. According to studies, you'll be more likely to make it a habit if you like your surroundings.

Take the entire family on your daily walks. You'll be modeling good fitness habits for your children, and it's cheaper than paying a sitter.

Pump up the volume. Research proves it: Listening to music while walking helps you walk longer, probably because you're distracted by the songs and almost forget that you're exercising.

Explore your world. Stroll down streets in your own neighborhood that you've never been on, or check out the hiking trail in a nearby park. Varying your terrain will keep you mentally engaged and work different leg muscles, improving the effectiveness of every outing.

Pick a charity. Sign up for a charity walk. Or donate $1 for every mile you walk for the next two weeks to a non-profit group you believe in. Whoever thought exercise could be tax deductible?

Find a regular walking partner. You're more likely to get out of bed on cold winter mornings or skip the cafeteria in favor of a lunchtime walk if someone is expecting you.

Take a dog with you. Once your dog gets used to your routine, he or she will never let you forget when it's time for your walk. Don't have a dog? Offer to walk an elderly neighbor's dog twice a week.

Walk for entertainment one day a week. Walk through the zoo, an art museum, or an upscale shopping mall. First circle the perimeter of your location at your usual brisk pace. Then wander through again more slowly to take in the sights.

Once a week, complete your errands on foot. If you live far from town, drive to within a mile of your destination, park, and walk the rest of the way there and back.

Go to an indoor track—with cash registers. Many malls open early for walkers. You could also easily walk for 20 minutes in a big warehouse store or at a Walmart or Kmart.

Weather-Proof Your Walking

Walking for health has to be a habit that you practice and practice until it's second nature to get out the door for your daily 45-minute session. In the beginning, especially, it's easy to let nasty weather keep you inside. Do that a few times in a row and—*bingo*—your walking habit is history. Here, some clever tips to help you overcome the most common weather beaters.

Buy a pair of waterproof sneaks. If you live where winters are harsh, your regular walking shoes aren't going to cut it. So put them on the shelf, head for a specialty retailer, and ask for a pair that's "waterproof and breathable." Make sure that describes the tongue of the shoes, too. Some manufacturers cut corners there, and the tongue will lap up moisture. Size the shoes a little bigger to accommodate thicker socks.

Warm your core. When your body senses cold, it decreases blood flow to your arms, legs, hands, and feet to protect vital organs. So keeping your torso warm is the secret to staying comfy. To do this, dress in fours:

exercise more this month!

Buy a good pair of walking shoes.

High blood sugar and circulation problems mean that people with diabetes are at high risk for slow-healing sores that can lead to dangerous infections. That's why good walking shoes aren't a luxury for people with diabetes—they're a necessity.

exercise more
today!

Every little step you take counts.

If you're too busy for your usual 45-minute walk, get out there for 5 or 10 minutes at a time. Every little movement burns calories, and all those minutes will add up.

▸ First, don a snug-fitting base layer made of a fabric (not cotton) that will wick moisture from your skin.

▸ Next, put on a bulkier mid-layer made of a fabric, such as fleece, that will insulate and continue to move moisture out. Vests are ideal for this, plus they free your arms to swing so you don't end up moving like the Michelin man.

▸ Cover everything with a wind-and water-resistant jacket or shell to protect you from the elements. Choose a zippered model rather than a pullover, again for easy venting.

▸ Top off your outfit with a hat. Even though it has recently been shown that we lose only about 10 percent of our body heat through an uncovered head, that's still significant.

Embrace the chill to start. You'll know you're dressed perfectly for winter walking if you're chilled when you first step outside. You should feel like rubbing your hands together or jumping up and down. If you're too warmly dressed, you'll sweat, and evaporative cooling will make you feel cold. If you don't like feeling chilly to start, then add an extra layer you can remove.

Pack some heat. If the cold makes your fingers tingle, put one of those little heat packs that skiers use inside each mitten. But since they're pricey, here's a trick: You can stretch their serviceability from the advertised eight to 12 hours to nearly a week by storing them in a small Tupperware container after each use. Since most brands are activated by oxygen, cutting off the supply preserves it.

Yoga—More than a Stretch

Stand up. Really, stand up. Inhale deeply and reach for the sky as high as you can. Next, slowly blow your breath out, sweeping your arms past your sides and bending toward the floor as you empty your lungs. Draw fresh air into your lungs and slowly roll back up to a standing position, arms by your sides. Feels good, doesn't it?

What you did was just a sample of the art of yoga, stretching and invigorating your body and at the same time clearing your mind to nurture a peaceful, happy attitude.

Developed 5,000 years ago in India, yoga reached American shores with immigrants back in the 1800s. Only in recent decades, though, has our faster-moving, increasingly stressed population embraced this exercise that's more serene than sweat, more meditative than muscle. Today in the United States more than 15 million people include yoga in their regular fitness routines. Its advocates range from rock stars to Supreme Court justices, from NFL running backs to CEOs.

Although some people focus their practice more, um, behind—striving for the coveted firm "yoga butt"—than inward, scientific evidence from the past 15 years shows that this mind-body form of exercise can relieve symptoms of chronic diseases such as cancer, arthritis, heart disease, and yes, diabetes. Even hospitals are getting in on the act. At New York Presbyterian Hospital and Cedars–Sinai Medical Center in Los Angeles, cardiologists routinely steer patients into programs that offer yoga as part of their preventive and rehabilitative care.

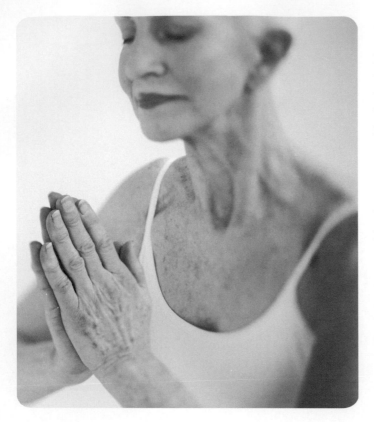

Studies suggest that yoga can help regulate blood-sugar levels and improve insulin receptivity.

Healing Powers

No doctor will tell you that yoga should be used as the primary remedy for a major disease like diabetes, heart disease, or cancer. But without question, what research exists shows that yoga can improve your condition. And like when you eat an organic apple, you can't point to a single negative aspect about yoga. When it comes to yoga, it's all good.

Take the simple pleasures, for example. Yoga is calming for your mind and great fitness for your body. You will carefully stretch and strengthen your muscles, loosen your joints, and align your posture. At the same time, you'll deepen and improve your breathing, slow your heart rate, and improve blood flow throughout your body. All this slows your sense of aging and helps make chronic pain go away—both physical and mental! And it can be done simply, without special gear or training, in the comfort of your own home.

Then there are the medical benefits. A 2011 University of Pittsburgh pilot study showed that when middle-aged sedentary people at high risk for type 2 diabetes took twice-weekly yoga classes for three months, they experienced improvements in weight, blood pressure, insulin, and triglycerides compared to people in a control group who didn't take yoga. Those results are echoed in studies that have shown that yoga can assist in losing weight, lowering blood pressure, and even cleansing arteries. The reasons are often ascribed to the relaxing effect of yoga; the practice calms mind and body and releases feel-good hormones beneficial to your health.

Researchers from India analyzed the results of 17 different studies on the role yoga played in the management of diabetes. They found that yoga helped study participants better manage their fasting blood sugar. A separate research review published in the *Journal of Diabetes Research* looked at 25 randomized controlled trials, finding that yoga significantly improved glycemic control, cholesterol levels, and body weight.

Here's a yoga routine you can easily try at home.

The Sun Salutation Yoga Routine

What will really convince you to take up yoga is its calming joys. There's no better place to start than with the Sun Salutations. A series of 12 graceful, flowing postures, they are considered the core of yoga practice. Each position counteracts the one before, stretching and strengthening the body in a different way so that by the time you're finished, you feel limber and energized from head to toe.

So give it a try. Take five minutes or so, and slowly do the following program. One round of Sun Salutations consists of two sequences, the first leading with the right foot (during stepping poses) and the second leading with the left. See how it goes. See how wonderful you feel afterward. And if you like it, repeat as often as you wish. Yoga lovers sometimes do 12 routines a day, but you can calm stress, increase flexibility, and improve your general well-being by doing them as little as once a week.

If you're new to yoga, some of these poses may be challenging at first; do what you can without taxing yourself. Over time, as your body begins to stretch and strengthen, the moves will come easily. Remember to breathe evenly and fluidly throughout, inhaling and exhaling as you initiate each move. With practice, the 12 steps of the Sun Salutations will flow together as one continuous exercise. Finally, be sure to perform the routine on a comfortably cushioned surface, such as a mat or carpeted floor.

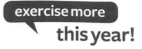

Take a flex test.

When you begin a yoga program, assess your flexibility. Can you touch your toes now? What positions are more difficult? Then, after sticking to yoga for a year, re-check your flexibility to see how much you've improved.

STEP 1 Mountain Pose

1. Stand straight with your feet about hip-width apart and your hands either at your sides or in prayer position in front of your chest.

2. Raise your toes and spread them wide, then place them back on the floor. Your weight should be distributed evenly across the bottom of each foot so you feel grounded, not leaning forward or back.

3. Exhale.

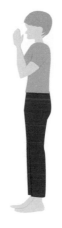

STEP 2 Overhead Reach

1. Inhale as you sweep your arms out to the sides and high overhead until your palms are together.

2. Stretch upward, allowing the fullest expansion of your chest, then arch backward and look up at your hands.

3. Hold the position for a few seconds with your body in pose, holding your breath and keeping your eyes focused and your mind silent.

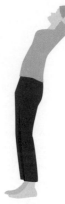

STEP 3 Forward Fold

1. Exhale as you gently bend forward from the waist, keeping your palms together, tucking your head and keeping your back straight and long.

2. When you've bent as far forward as comfortably possible, **grasp** the backs of your legs (anywhere from the ankles to the thighs), **bend** your elbows, and very gently **tuck** your chin to your chest and move your upper body toward your legs.

3. Hold for a few breaths.

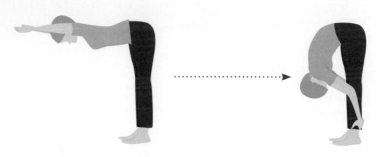

exercise more this month!

Find a yoga teacher.

Most sport centers and health clubs have yoga sessions. If they offer different varieties of yoga, ask an instructor about which one may be best for you and your current fitness level.

STEP 4 High Lunge

1. Step back with your right foot into a lunge, bending your left knee and keeping it directly over your left ankle (you may need to slide your right foot back farther).

2. Lean forward and press your fingertips or palms into the floor in line with your forward foot.

3. Roll your shoulders back and down and press your chest forward while looking straight ahead.

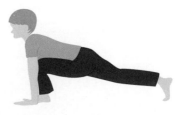

4. Relax your hips and let them sink toward the floor while straightening your back leg as much as comfortably possible.

5. Hold for a few breaths. If it's difficult to reach the floor with your hands in this position, place books on either side of you so you can support your weight with your hands on the books. You may also rest your back leg on the floor if necessary.

STEP 5 Plank

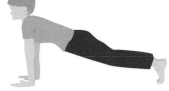

1. Move your left foot back next to your right foot and straighten your body into the plank position.

2. Spread your fingers so that your middle fingers are pointing forward. Your hands should be on the floor beneath your shoulders, as if you're doing a push-up.

3. Tuck in your tailbone so your legs, hips, and torso form a straight line.

4. Press the crown of your head forward, tuck your toes, and press your heels back, stretching down the entire length of the back of your body.

5. Hold for a few breaths. If this is too difficult, perform the move while resting on your knees instead of your toes.

STEP 6 Caterpillar

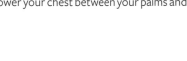

1. Bend both knees to the floor (if they're not already there), then slowly **lower** your chin and chest straight down to the floor.

2. Keep your elbows close to your body as you lower your chest between your palms and lift your tailbone toward the ceiling.

3. Hold for a breath.

STEP 7 Cobra

1. Drop your hips to the floor.

2. Raise your head and chest so your torso is supported on your forearms (if you're very flexible, you can extend your arms).

3. Keep your shoulders down and back, pressing your chest forward and reaching toward the ceiling with the crown of your head.

4. Hold for a few breaths.

STEP 8 Downward-Facing Dog

1. Press your palms into the floor, **straighten** your arms and legs, and **press** your hips up so your body forms an inverted V.

2. Let your head and neck **hang** freely from your shoulders or tuck your chin to your chest.

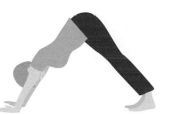

3. Press your heels toward the floor while pressing your hips toward the ceiling for a full stretch. To make this position easier, keep your knees bent. You can also place your hands on a low step.

4. Hold for a few breaths.

STEP 9 High Lunge 2

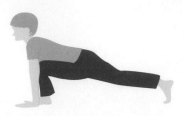

1. Step forward with your left foot. Position yourself so your left knee is directly over your left ankle and your right leg is extended behind you.

2. Support your weight by placing your palms or fingertips on the floor in line with your left foot.

3. Roll your shoulders down and back and **press** your chest forward, looking straight ahead.

4. Relax your hips and let them sink toward the floor while straightening your back leg as much as comfortably possible (if flexibility is a problem, keep your back leg resting on the floor).

5. Hold for a few breaths.

STEP 10 Forward Roll 2

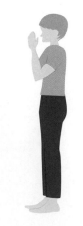

1. Bring your right foot forward to meet your left.

2. Gently **straighten** your legs as much as comfortably possible, letting your hands rise off the floor as necessary.

3. Grasp the backs of your legs (anywhere from your ankles to your thighs), **bend** your elbows, and very gently **tuck** your chin to your chest and **move** your upper body toward your legs.

4. Hold for a few breaths.

STEP 11 Upward Sweep

1. Sweep your arms out to the sides and overhead, stretching them up and back as you expand your chest.

2. Place your palms together and look up toward your hands.

3. Press your feet into the floor and contract your thighs to gently **pull** your kneecaps up (without locking your knees).

4. Hold for a few breaths.

STEP 12 Mountain Return

1. Sweep your arms out to the sides and down, bringing your palms together in front of your chest, and as in Step 1, **stand straight** with your feet hip-width apart.

2. Raise your toes and spread them wide, then place them back on the floor so your weight is evenly distributed.

3. Contract your thighs, pulling your kneecaps up and tucking your tailbone so it points straight toward the floor.

4. Lift the crown of your head toward the ceiling, feeling your spine grow long and straight.

5. Drop your shoulders down and back, pressing your chest forward.

6. Hold for a few breaths; repeat the cycle, starting with your left leg.

Bicycling: Ride for Your Life

That old saying is literally 100 percent true. You really never do forget how to ride a bike. And riding has some fantastic benefits you just can't ignore. These reasons should be enough to make you go out to the garage and sweep the cobwebs off that bike of yours.

BOOSTS YOUR MOOD

Cornell University researchers have found that blue moods make people eat more and more of the high-calorie, high-carbohydrate stuff that packs on pounds. But as little as 10 minutes of cycling can improve your mood, according to a study from Bowling Green State University. Other research shows that just 30 minutes a day of aerobic activity, like cycling, three to five days a week can significantly improve depression symptoms.

And it's never too late (nor are you ever too "unfit") to start! Don't wait another minute.

REDUCES YOUR APPETITE

Riding a bike can make you eat less. The same dopamine that gives you a greater sense of energy also improves your mood, pushing aside the need for other mood boosters like ice cream and potato chips. In addition, British researchers have reported

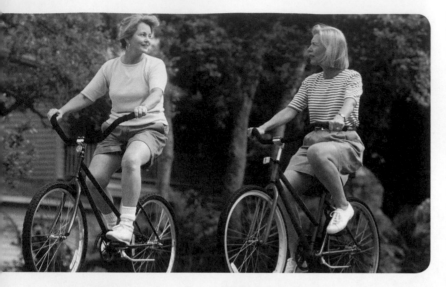

that 60 minutes of vigorous exercise—brisk bicycling, for example—lowers the release of ghrelin (a hormone that stimulates appetite) and increases the release of peptide YY (a hormone that suppresses appetite).

GIVES YOU ENERGY

Tired of feeling tired? Hop on a bike. A study published in the journal *Psychotherapy and Psychosomatics* found that bike riding improved energy levels by 20 percent and decreased fatigue by 65 percent. Though scientists are still studying the energizing effects of exercise, they suspect that dopamine is behind the boost. Cycling triggers your brain to release more of this energy-linked "feel-good" brain chemical. The best part: You don't need to push the pace to enjoy this perk. Those who pedaled at an easy pace reaped the biggest rewards.

But that doesn't mean you won't be a little rusty or that you can't benefit from a few pointers. Especially if the last time you rode a lot, it was on a pink bike with a banana seat and streamers. Try these tips to get rolling the right way.

> Cycling triggers your brain to release dopamine, an energy-linked "feel-good" brain chemical.

Ease Into Riding

We'll be honest. If you're brand-new to biking, or if you haven't rode since you shelved your disco glitter, your butt will be tender at first. Riding shorts will help a lot, as will riding just 20 to 30 minutes to start. That soreness should subside within a week or two.

If it doesn't, look into changing your bike saddle (also known as a bike seat). Your saddle should support your seat bones in the back without placing too much pressure on your sensitive tissues. You'll find women-specific models at your bike shop.

Another note on butt comfort: Riders of all shapes and sizes sometimes suffer some chafing when the tender skin of their butt rubs against the inside of their shorts or against the saddle. Head off unwanted hot spots by applying a gliding cream like Chamois Butt'r to the padding in your shorts.

Get the Right Equipment

For those new to cycling or getting reacquainted with this favorite childhood activity, you'll probably want to put some equipment on your shopping list, especially if you're planning to make a habit out of this oh-so-good for you activity.

Rack it up. If you're lucky, you live in a neighborhood where you can set off from your front door (or garage) and ride away into the sunrise. But alas, many of us can't. We live on busy urban streets; hilly, curvy lanes; or unsafe, narrow roads that just aren't conducive to everyday riding. Don't let this stop you! Bike racks for your car have become cheaper, stronger, easier, and more versatile. We recommend a removable model that holds the bike at the rear of your car. Straps hook to the top of the trunk and to the bumper and are easily tightened for safety and then easily loosened for removal. Throw your bike on, drive to the local park or to a trail, and away you go! Great for taking your bike on car vacations, too. Look for models from established companies like thule.com or yakima.com. A removable, two-bike rack will start at around $100.

Protect your head. No matter how superior your cycling skills are, you absolutely must wear a helmet, even on the shortest bike rides. All kinds of things can cause your brain to hit the pavement—dogs that suddenly race into your path, careless drivers who fling car doors open, or unseen potholes or road debris. These days helmets are a high-tech affair: Smart materials offer incredible protection in case of a fall, and streamlined designs allow lots of air vents that both reduce weight and keep your noggin cool. Focus mostly on fit: Have a professional adjust all the straps so the helmet is I-barely-feel-it comfy, but with minimal wiggle. Pick white or a bright color for visibility, and avoid extreme shapes and thin straps. Since 1999 all helmets must conform to federal safety standards mandated by the U.S. Consumer Product Safety Commission; make sure that your helmet has a CPSC sticker inside.

Get a comfy saddle. The prices are reasonable, and replacing them is easy, so don't be intimidated about changing the seat on your bicycle for one that's softer, wider, or fits your body better. Some seats contain layers of gel across the top, body-friendly contouring, and shock- and vibration-absorbing materials. A comfy saddle can make all the difference between a joyous bike trip and a miserable one.

Dress for success. If you're planning to really go the distance, you might want to dress for it; bike clothes can make the ride more comfortable. Padded shorts are practically a must if you're serious about the sport—they'll help cushion your nether region and keep

Bike Check

If you already have a bike, just keep using it for a few months until you figure out how and where you like to ride before you invest in a new one. If you haven't ridden it in more than a year, take it to your local bike shop for a tune-up before you go any distance on it. Time and disuse can take a toll on a bike's key components (such as brakes and shifters) as well as tires. Your local bike mechanic can tighten up all the nuts and bolts, lube the moving parts, and make sure you're ready to roll safely.

No bike? Consider a hybrid. These are made for casual riding and are equally good for both paved and unpaved roads, since they combine features of mountain and street bikes. Hybrid bikes can feature 15 or more gears so you can easily adjust for downhill, uphill, and uneven surfaces. Tires are wide enough to provide lots of stability, but not so wide that they hold you back if you want to put your head down and go for speed. They start at about $250 and go up from there.

exercise more this week!

Go longer, stronger on weekends.

If you're not into tracking mileage, start out riding 20 to 30 minutes most days, working up to longer rides, especially on the weekends. To get fitter (and lose weight) faster, try adding intervals (short bursts of hard efforts) to your rides twice a week.

you rolling longer. Cycling jerseys, made from special wicking materials, help keep you dry and comfortable. They're also equipped with a zipper in the front for cooling off when the going gets hot, and convenient pockets in the back for stashing your cell phone, some cash, your keys, a snack, or whatever else you might want for the trip.

Slip on gloves. Cycling gloves that cushion your hands are a smart purchase, especially for longer rides. Since your hands support as much as 50 percent of your body weight, you'll be surprised at how your arms and hands can get tired over time. Gloves help ease the pressure and keep your hands feeling comfortable.

Ride for Fitness

While you're unlikely to have forgotten how to ride that bike, you may need to brush up on technique to make sure you get the best possible workout while you're on the road. Take these tips into consideration.

Just keep pedaling. Keep your coasting to a minimum to burn maximum fat. Sure, there'll be some descents and some gradual stops for which coasting is necessary. But make an effort to use your gears to keep power going into your pedals on 90 percent of your ride.

Stay in your comfort zone. A little huffing and puffing on hills or during some purposefully fast pedaling is great for strengthening your heart and burning extra calories, but aim to keep your breathing deep and rhythmic for the majority of your ride so you can go longer without tiring. You should be able to hold a conversation while you're riding. If you can't, you're exerting yourself too much; shift to an easier gear and slow down. The goal is to balance the work of your legs with that of your lungs. They should both be putting out pretty equal efforts.

Shift often. Your bike has gears. Use them. Often. New riders mistakenly believe every pedal stroke should feel hard if they want to burn fat fast. In reality, you'll just fatigue (and quit) fast. You want to keep your pedals spinning at a comfortably brisk

Cycling Calorie Burn

Riding a bike burns lots of calories—even when you're just cruising along soaking in the sunshine. The following chart, drawn from The Compendium of Physical Activities Tracking Guide, shows how many calories a 150-pound rider burns per hour, based on her pace. Heavier riders will burn more.

An hour of riding at...	Burns...
<10 mph, very leisurely	272 calories
10 to 12 mph, easy	408 calories
12 to 14 mph, moderate	544 calories
14 to 16 mph, vigorous	680 calories
16 to 19 mph, very fast	816 calories
>20 mph, racing speed	1,088 calories

BEGINNER RIDING PLAN

Follow this plan and after two months you'll be able to rack up 100 miles in one week! Miles for each day of the week are listed, along with an approximate weekly mileage. For the first four weeks, maintain at least a 10 mph average. After four weeks, try to bump up that average to 12–14 mph.

WEEK	WEEKLY MILEAGE	M	T	W	TH	F	S	S
1	46	5	REST	5	REST	5	8	8
2	48	7	REST	7	REST	7	10	10
3	60	9	REST	9	REST	9	12	12
4	74	11	REST	11	REST	11	15	15
5	74	11	REST	11	REST	11	15	15
6	74	11	REST	11	REST	11	15	15
7	85	13	REST	13	REST	13	18	18
8	100	15	REST	15	REST	15	20	20

cadence—at least one revolution per second. The purpose of bike gears is to help you maintain that pedaling rate, whether you go up, down, or flat. So shift often. Try to feel and anticipate the grade. As you feel the pressure on your pedals increasing, whether it's a small rise or a stiff headwind, shift down to an easier gear. When you feel your legs start spinning too fast because of a slight downhill or tailwind, shift up into a harder gear.

Get your heart pumping. After warming up for 10 or 15 minutes, pedal very hard for one minute. Ease up for one minute. Repeat five to 10 times. Then finish the rest of your ride at a moderate pace. New riders can expect to pedal along at about 10 mph, working up to 14 or 15 mph.

Add intervals. After riding for about a month, it's time to step it up a little with intervals. Here's how:
▸ Warm up for 10 to 15 minutes. Then do the following:
▸ Ride briskly for 2 minutes.
▸ Pick up the pace to very brisk for 1 minute.
▸ Pick it up a bit more and go as hard as you can for 30 seconds.
▸ Ease back to very brisk for 1 minute.
▸ Ease back to brisk for 2 minutes.
▸ Ride along at a moderate pace.

Follow Your Fun

You don't have to be one of those 20-mile-a-day runners or a Tour de France cyclist to be an active person. Focus on sports and hobbies you love. Do them often, and you'll find yourself in better shape—and maybe even a happier person—in no time. And it won't even seem like effort.

People who play tennis every week, take a daily swim in the ocean, or hit the golf links whenever there's an open tee time don't do it for the exercise; they do it because they love it. (That doesn't mean it doesn't sometimes frustrate them to the point of throwing tennis rackets or golf clubs!) You may not love a new sport in the beginning, when your skills aren't quite up to snuff, so give it some time. But do choose a sport or activity you're naturally drawn to—that you simply think is fun or emotionally satisfying—and you'll be much more likely to stick with it and not view it as exercise.

NO NEED TO BE A GYM JUNKIE

Experts conclude that aerobic activity (walking and cycling, for instance) and strength training (lifting weights and doing strength exercises) are almost equally beneficial for controlling blood sugar, so pick whichever most appeals to you. Aerobic activity causes your muscles to burn energy and then draw glucose out of the blood to replace that energy, thus lowering your blood sugar. Strength training gives your body a larger mass of muscle, so there are more cells drawing glucose out of your bloodstream at any one time—another path to lower blood sugar.

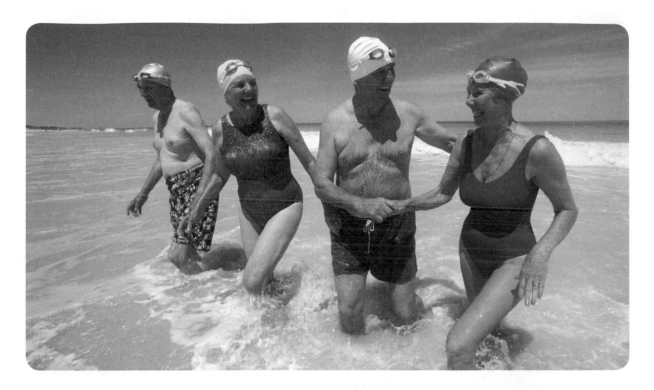

SIGN UP FOR SOMETHING FUN

You might be turned off by the prospect of huffing your way around a running track or grunting your way through a series of weight machines at the gym, so appeal instead to the human desire for fun. Try a swimming-pool aerobics class that plays oldies music, sign up for tango lessons and dress the part, join a hiking club to become one with nature, or volunteer to give walking tours at an arboretum.

INVEST IN LESSONS

You may do a double take when you find out the price of a three-day yoga retreat, but if you're going to splurge on something, your health should be at the top of the list. When you pay an expert to show you how to use weight machines properly, ride a horse, or belly dance, you'll master the skill faster and enjoy your pursuit more. And a lesson is a small price to pay to keep from injuring yourself.

TRY TAI CHI

You don't have to work up a sweat to get a benefit—or three—from exercise. Both yoga and tai chi increase your flexibility and balance. The slow, sure movements and gentle stretching not only benefit your muscles and joints but also your mental health—their stress-relief benefits are proven. Since being stressed can raise your blood pressure and drive your blood sugar down—or more often, up—those 45 minutes in class can do you more good than you realize.

Focus on sports and hobbies you love. Do them often, and you'll find yourself in better shape.

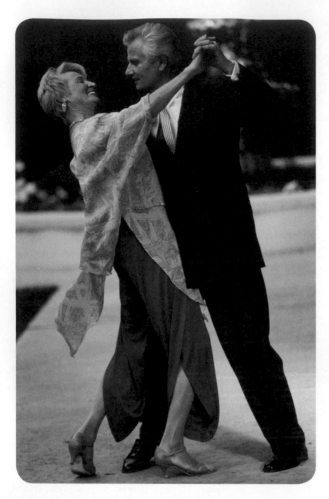

BURN CALORIES WITH ZUMBA

Zumba is one of the fitness world's sizzling hot workout trends—even folks who say they're totally uncoordinated sing its praises. This high-energy aerobic workout came out of Latin America; its founders like to call it a dance fitness party, and fans couldn't agree more. Zumba classes feature Latin and international music; the rhythms are fast and complex, and the dance moves fun and exhilarating. Zumba came into existence in only 2001, but classes can now be found in more than 110 countries, claim the folks at Zumba Fitness. They also say that 10 million people take weekly classes. And of course, DVDs are available for Zumba workouts at home.

Truth is, the Zumba program is a lot of fun, and for music lovers the rhythms are irresistible. But it is also pretty intense exercise; it follows in a long tradition of fast-moving aerobic workouts that have been the mainstay of fitness centers since the days of disco. If you haven't been exercising, start very slowly and carefully. But as they say, if the rhythm sets you free, then enjoy! It's great for your body, and your spirit.

BE SOCIAL

If you've got the gift of gab or are always up for meeting new friends, seek out group activities such as volleyball, shuffleboard, bocce, and bowling. Staying socially connected is a key to keeping your spirits up.

> Aerobic activity causes your muscles to burn energy and then draw glucose out of the blood to replace that energy.

And you know what they say: Laughter is the best medicine. If you have a good time with the people you're exercising with, chances are you'll keep coming back for more.

If you have friends who love to hike or hit the driving range, their enthusiasm is likely to rub off on you. And most sports are more fun when you play them with friends. A study at the University of Iceland found that men whose fathers, brothers, and close friends exercised with them (or who emphasized exercise in their own lives) were more likely to exercise and be fit than those whose friends and family did not participate.

VARY ACTIVITIES

Your passion for racquetball is bound to wane if you keep doing it day in and day out. Give yourself a break from your favorite game and go line dancing or hiking in the great outdoors once in a while for a change of pace. If mountain biking is your thing, trade in your spokes for some strokes at the swimming pool.

SIGN UP FOR AN EVENT

Whether it's a 5K "fun run" or a walk for a good cause, put it on your calendar, then get out there and get ready. Give yourself plenty of time to work up gradually to the amount of walking or running you'll be doing. Having a long-term goal like an event will help motivate you and keep you exercising on days when you might otherwise pack it in.

VOLUNTEER YOUR MUSCLE

That is, offer to do manual labor for an organization that helps less-fortunate people. For instance, Habitat for Humanity (www.habitat.org) will put you to work painting, nailing, and hauling materials as you build homes for the poor. Not only will your body benefit, but your spirit will, too, knowing the good you have done.

The Take It Easy Workout

Would you like a low-impact way to ease into exercise?

Can you spare a half hour? Of course you can. Well, then we can help you rejuvenate your health, spark your energy, and improve your mood. These are just some of the benefits of this 30-minute home-workout routine. No trips to the gym necessary, and the only fitness trainer you need is you. If you haven't exercised in a while, our stretching and strengthening plan is the perfect place to start.

And then there's the diabetes connection. By strengthening and stretching your body, you are training your cells to be more receptive to insulin. Along with a healthy diet, there's nothing better you can do for your diabetes than to get fit.

You've probably read about the benefits of exercise dozens of times. But this time why not really put that knowledge into action? This Take It Easy home routine is simple, fun, habit-forming, and made precisely for people who aren't currently following a fitness program.

We promise: Pair up this routine with a more active daily lifestyle and you will make a huge contribution toward lowering your blood sugar, losing weight, and possibly getting off your medications. You'll love how you look and feel. Let's get started!

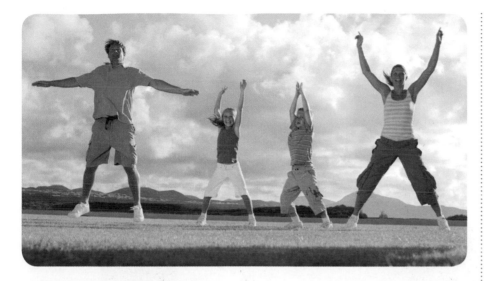

PERFECT FOR PEOPLE WHO...

▸ Have not exercised for two years or more
▸ Are overweight or have limited movement
▸ Are recovering from prolonged injury or exercise
▸ Are new to formal fitness plans

THE PLAN

We provide three 30-minute stretch-and-strengthen routines, each focused on a different part of your body. Do the three routines on consecutive days, then take the fourth day off. That means in a week you will do:

▸ Day 1: Upper-body routine
▸ Day 2: Lower-body routine
▸ Day 3: Core-body routine
▸ Day 4: Rest
▸ Day 5: Upper-body routine
▸ Day 6: Lower-body routine
▸ Day 7: Core-body routine

THE GUIDELINES

1. Do strength exercises first, then stretches.
2. Do the indicated number of sets and reps.
3. Take no more than 2 minutes of rest between sets.
4. To improve endurance, shorten rests to under 30 seconds.
5. Hold stretches for the times noted—never more than 30 seconds.
6. Focus on deep, long breathing throughout the routine.
7. No TV, no eating, and no phone calls during the workout.

What You Need

▸ Light dumbbells (2 to 5 lb)
▸ Towel
▸ Mat, bed, or daybed
▸ Supportive chair
▸ Wall space

DAY 1 & DAY 5 | Upper-Body Strength Exercises

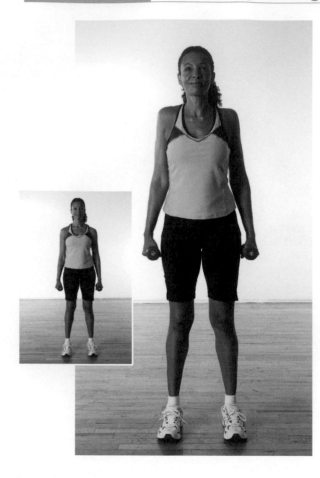

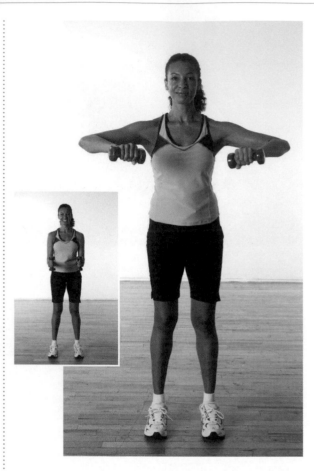

Shrug

TONES UPPER BACK, MIDBACK, SHOULDERS

1. Stand with your feet hip-width apart. **Hold** a dumbbell in each hand and let your arms hang straight down so your hands rest by the side of your thighs, palms facing in.

2. Keeping your arms straight, slowly **raise** your shoulders toward your ears as if you were shrugging. **Roll** your shoulders back as far as comfortably possible. Then return to start.

▸ *DO 2 SETS OF 10 REPS.*

Water Pitcher Raise

TONES SHOULDERS

1. Stand with your feet hip- to shoulder-width apart. Hold a dumbbell in each hand. With your elbows close to your body, **bend** your arms straight out in front of you 90 degrees, keep your palms facing in. It should look as though you're holding two water pitchers.

2. Keeping your hands out in front of you, **raise** your upper arms and elbows out to the side. The weights should **rotate** toward each other as though you were pouring water down in front of you. Pause, then return to start.

▸ *DO 2 SETS OF 10 REPS.*

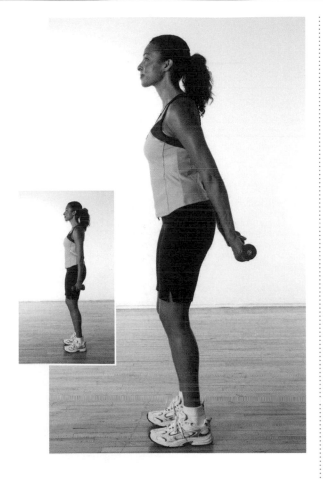

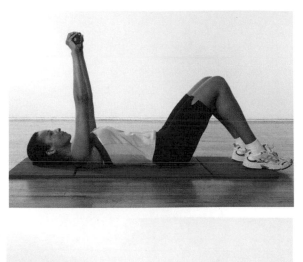

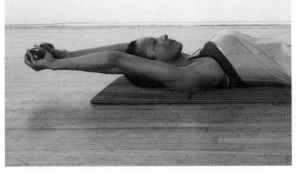

Reverse Raise

TONES TRICEPS

1. Stand with your feet about hip-width apart, knees slightly bent. **Hold** a dumbbell in each hand, allowing your arms to hang naturally by your sides, palms facing in.

2. Keeping your arms straight, slowly **raise** your arms behind you as high as comfortably possible, rotating your palms so they face the ceiling. Pause. Then slowly lower back to start.

▶ *DO 2 SETS OF 10 REPS.*

Pullover

TONES CHEST, BACK

1. Lie back on a supportive bed with your knees bent and feet flat on the ground. **Grasp** a dumbbell by the ends with both hands. Hold it above your chest, so the weight is above your chest.

2. Keeping your elbows straight, **lower** your arms downward and back over your head as far as comfortably possible. (Don't arch your back.) Pause. Then return to start.

▶ *DO 2 SETS OF 10 REPS.*

DAY 1 & DAY 5 | Upper-Body Stretches

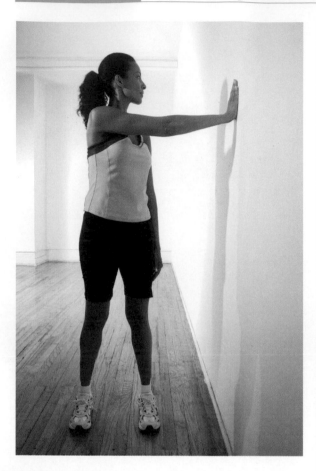

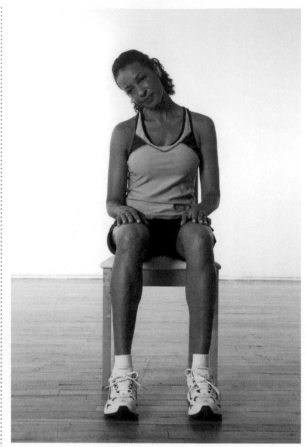

Wall Twist

STRETCHES CHEST, SHOULDERS

Stand to the right of a wall. **Reach out** with your right arm and place your right hand against the wall. Gently **turn** your torso toward the right, away from your arm, as far as comfortably possible.

▶ *HOLD 15-20 SECONDS, THEN SWITCH SIDES.*

Neck Stretch

STRETCHES NECK, UPPER BACK

Sit up straight in a supportive chair. Drop your chin toward your chest. Slowly **drop** your head toward your right shoulder, trying to touch your ear to your right shoulder as you let your shoulders drop.

▶ *HOLD 15-20 SECONDS, RETURN TO CENTER, THEN SWITCH SIDES.*

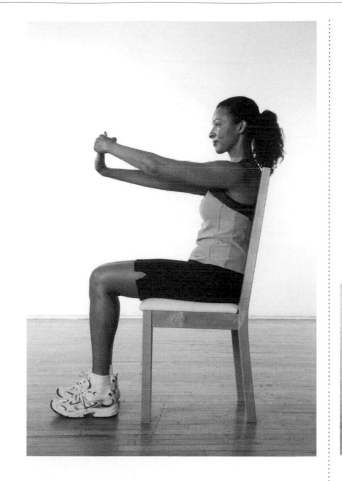

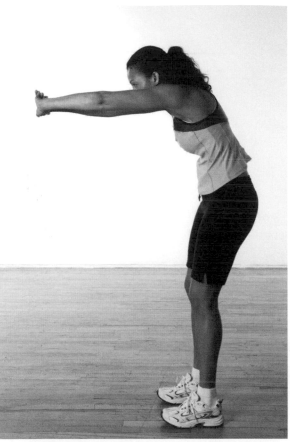

Hand Pull

STRETCHES HAND, WRIST, FOREARMS

Sit straight up in a chair. **Extend** your right arm, wrist flexed, fingers pointed toward the ceiling. Using your left hand, **pull** the fingertips on your right hand back toward your body as far as comfortably possible.

▶ *HOLD 15-20 SECONDS, THEN SWITCH SIDES.*

Back Stretch

STRETCHES UPPER BACK

Stand with your feet hip- to shoulder-width apart. **Extend** both arms straight in front of you and **lace** your fingertips together, turning your hands so your palms face away from you. **Press** your palms away from you, straightening your arms and rounding your back as far as comfortably possible.

▶ *HOLD 20-30 SECONDS.*

DAY 2 & DAY 6 | Lower-Body Strength Exercises

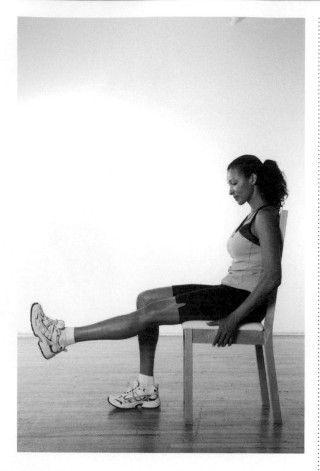

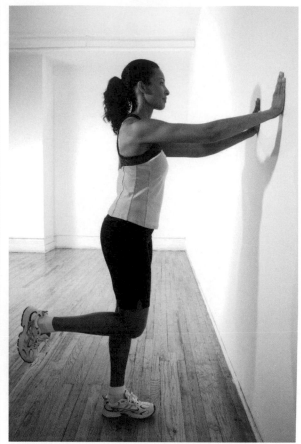

Seated Leg Extension

STRENGTHENS QUADRICEPS

Sit on a chair with your feet flat on the floor. **Hold** on to either side of the chair seat for support. Slowly **lift** your left leg so it's straight out in front of you. Pause for 1 to 2 seconds. Then slowly **lower** your leg. Repeat with the opposite leg. Alternate for a full set to each side.

▶ *Do 2 SETS OF 10 REPS WITH EACH LEG.*

Standing Leg Curl

STRENGTHENS HAMSTRINGS

Stand with your feet about hip-width apart, facing a wall. Place your hands against the wall for support. **Keep** your back straight. Slowly **bend** your right leg at the knee, raising your heel toward your rear until your shin is parallel to the floor. Pause two seconds. Then **lower** back to the starting position. Complete a full set with one leg before switching to your other leg.

▶ *Do 2 SETS OF 10 REPS WITH EACH LEG.*

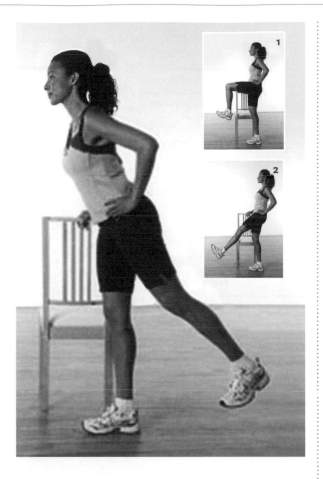

March and Swing

STRENGTHENS LEG, REAR, BACK

1. Stand with your left hand on your hip, and the other on a tabletop or chair back for support. **Lift** your left knee until the thigh is parallel to the floor, with the foot flexed.

2. Straighten your left leg, pressing the heel forward and toward the floor as you **lean** your torso slightly backward.

3. Return to the knee-lifted position, then **straighten** the left leg behind you, leaning your torso forward. That's one rep.

▶ *DO 2 SETS OF 10 REPS WITH EACH LEG.*

Tiptoes

STRENGTHENS CALVES

1. Stand behind a chair with your feet hip-width apart, with one hand planted on the chair for support.

2. Using your calf muscles, slowly **rise up** onto your toes as high as comfortably possible. Pause, then slowly lower your heels back to the floor.

▶ *DO 2 SETS OF 10 REPS.*

DAY 2 & DAY 6 | Lower-Body Stretches

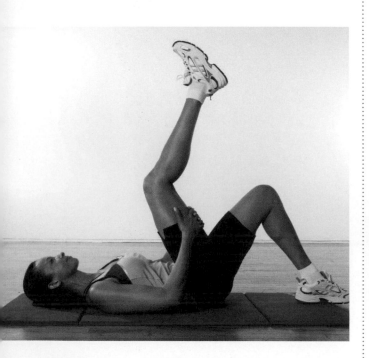

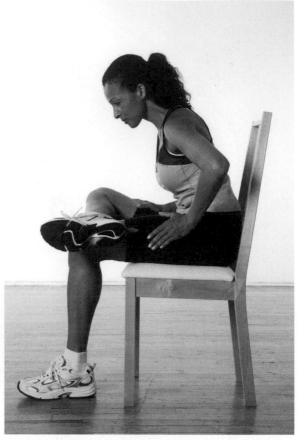

Hamstring Stretch

STRENGTHENS HAMSTRINGS

Lie on your back with your legs bent and both feet flat on the floor. **Lift** your right leg and raise it toward the ceiling. **Clasp** your hands around the back of your right thigh and gently pull it toward your chest (use a towel if you can't reach).

▶ *HOLD 20 SECONDS, THEN SWITCH LEGS.*

Seated Figure 4

STRETCHES GLUTES, LOWER BACK, HIPS

Sit in a chair with your legs bent, feet flat on the floor. **Cross** your right ankle over your left knee, so your calf is parallel to the floor, and your right knee is pointing to the right. Keeping your back straight, **lean** forward from the hips until you feel a stretch deep in your right glute muscle.

▶ *HOLD 15-20 SECONDS, THEN SWITCH LEGS.*

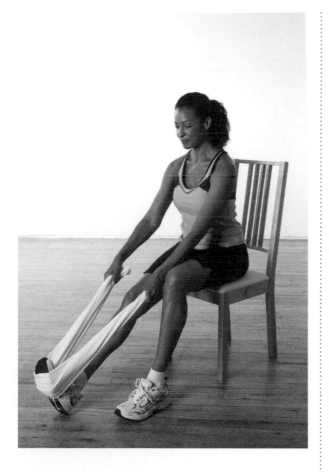

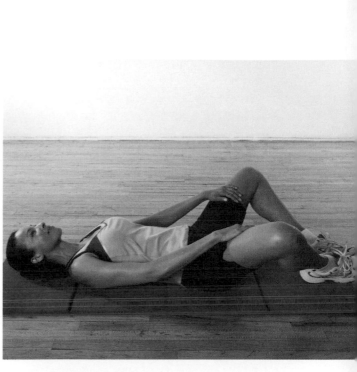

Seated Calf Stretch

STRETCHES CALVES

Sit on the edge of a chair with your left foot flat on the floor, and your right leg extended, foot flexed. **Loop** a towel around the ball of your right foot, and keeping your back straight, gently **pull** your foot toward you as far as comfortably possible.

▶ *HOLD 15-20 SECONDS, THEN SWITCH LEGS.*

Knee Drop

STRETCHES GROIN, INNER THIGHS

Lie back on your bed with knees bent and feet flat. **Place** your hands on the inside of your knees, and gently let your knees fall out and down toward the bed. Then gently **press** down to deepen the stretch as far as comfortably possible.

▶ *HOLD 15 SECONDS, RELAX, THEN REPEAT.*

DAY 3 & DAY 7 Core Strength Exercises

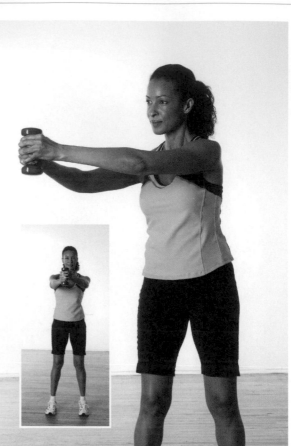

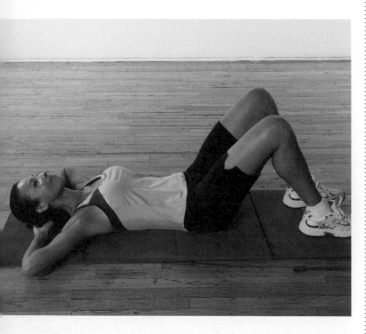

Pelvic Tilt

1. Lie flat on your back with your knees bent and hands behind your head, elbows extended out to the sides.

2. Lift your pelvis up and toward your rib cage, **tightening** your lower abdominal muscles and gently **"pushing"** back into the floor. **Hold** for 2 seconds. Relax and let your pelvis rotate back to its normal position. Repeat the exercise in a slow, controlled manner.

▶ *Do 2 sets of 10 reps.*

Standing Twist

1. Stand straight up with your legs hip- to shoulder-width apart. **Hold** a dumbbell with two hands and **extend** your arms straight out in front of you, keeping your elbows soft.

2. Keeping your arms extended, **contract** your abdominal muscles, and **turn** your torso to the right as far as comfortably possible. Pause. Return to start. Repeat to the opposite side. Continue alternating for a full set of reps to each side.

▶ *Do 2 sets of 10 reps.*

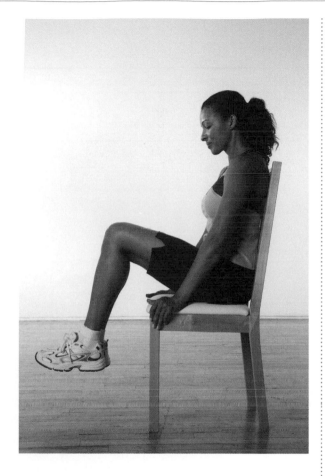

Seated Toe Lift

Sit straight up all the way back in a chair. **Place** your hands on the sides of the chair seat in front of your hips, or on the arms of the chair. **Contract** your abdominal muscles, and slowly lift your feet off the floor as far as comfortably possible. Pause. Then lower your feet back to the floor.

▶ *Do 2 sets of 10 reps.*

Navel Pull

Sit in a chair with your hands on your stomach. **Contract** your abdominal muscles, and pull your navel in toward your spine. Keeping your abs tight, slowly **inhale** for 4 to 5 seconds, and exhale for 8 to 10 seconds. Relax and repeat.

▶ *Do 2 sets of 6 reps.*

DAY 3 & DAY 7 | Core Stretches

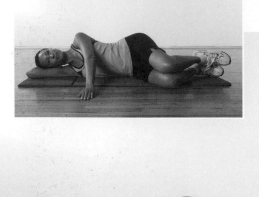

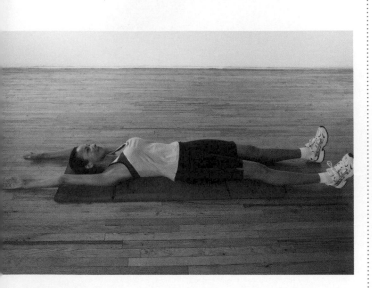

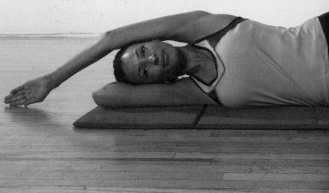

Morning Stretch

Lying on a bed, **reach** your arms overhead and **extend** your legs so your body forms a straight line from your heels to your head. **Imagine** strings are pulling your arms and feet in opposite directions, and try to reach your limbs out as far as you can. Keep your feet flexed.

▶ *HOLD FOR 10 SECONDS, RELAX, THEN REPEAT 3 TIMES.*

Lying Rotation

Lie on the bed on your right side with your right arm bent and right hand under your head. **Bend** both legs (you can put a pillow between your knees for added comfort). **Extend** your left arm straight in front of you. Then slowly **rotate** it up toward your head and all the way around (your torso will naturally roll back, and your palm will flip so it's facing up; but keep your lower body stable) past your head, behind your back, and over your hips until it's back to the starting position.

▶ *SWITCH SIDES AND REPEAT. DO THE SEQUENCE 5 TIMES.*

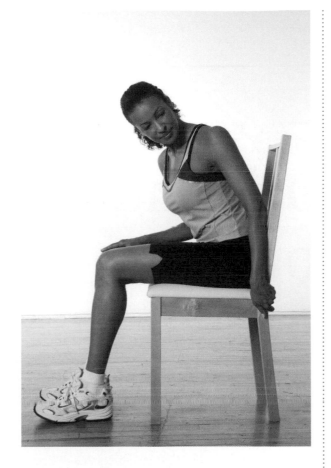

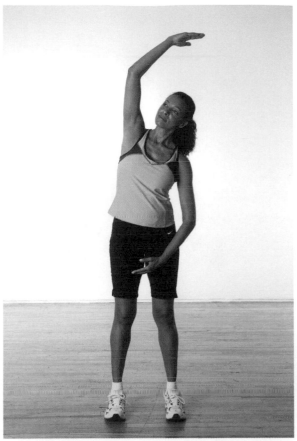

Side Stretch

Sit in a chair (preferably one with no arms), and **grasp** the back of the seat by your left buttock with your left hand, palm facing your body. **Hold** on as you gently **lean** forward and drop your right ear toward your right shoulder.

▶ *HOLD 15 SECONDS, THEN REPEAT ON THE OTHER SIDE.*

Reach and Bend

Stand up straight with your feet about shoulder-width apart. Gently **lean** to the left as you **reach** your right arm up toward the ceiling, curving it slightly overhead, palm facing down.

▶ *HOLD 15 SECONDS, THEN REPEAT TO THE OTHER SIDE.*

The 10-Minute Fit Workout

Want in on a secret? The reason most people gain weight year after year is not because they're eating more but because their metabolism is slowing down. Just glance around at your next high school reunion to see what the results look like. But that doesn't have to be you. You can turbocharge your weight loss and reverse your diabetes at the same time by building up muscles that gobble up fuel—calories and blood sugar. One Canadian study found that combining strength training with aerobic exercise reduced A1C levels more than aerobic exercise alone.

Improving blood sugar through exercise could delay your need for medication, help you lower your dose, or delay the need for a higher dose. When you're really pressed for time, you can spend 10 minutes every morning working just a few muscle groups. It takes far less time and if you do it right, it may work even better.

The trick is to perform the moves circuit-style—that is, one exercise following the next with minimal rest in between. In a study of 10 exercisers, researchers found that those who did their workouts circuit-style burned nearly twice as many calories as the standard-style lifters, who rested between sets. What's more, circuit-style lifting keeps your heart rate in an aerobic fat-burning zone.

Ready to start? Do one three-move circuit each morning, performing 10 to 16 reps of each move unless otherwise indicated. Perform each circuit three times (do all three moves before starting over with the first). One day a week, you'll do a yoga circuit, which adds some stretching to your strengthening for well-rounded fitness.

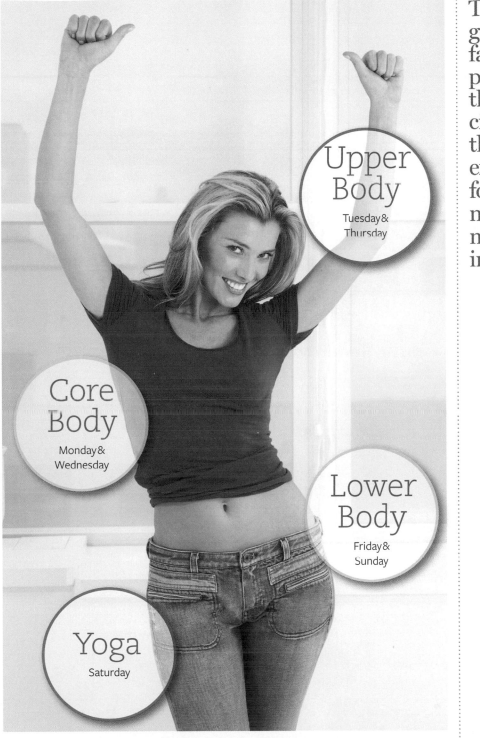

The trick to getting fit faster is to perform the moves circuit-style—that is, one exercise following the next with minimal rest in between.

DAY 1 & DAY 3 | Core Body

PERFORM THIS CIRCUIT 3 TIMES.

Extensions

TONES BACK AND GLUES

1. Lie facedown with your arms at your sides, hands on outer thighs.

2. Keeping your head and neck in a straight line, **lift** your torso off the floor as far as comfortably possible. Pause and return to the starting position.

3. Next, keep your torso on the floor and **contract** your glutes (your buttocks muscles) and **lift** your legs off the floor as high as comfortably possible. Pause and return to start.

4. Finally, **lift** your torso and legs simultaneously. Pause and return to start.

▶ *PERFORM 6 TO 8 REPS.*

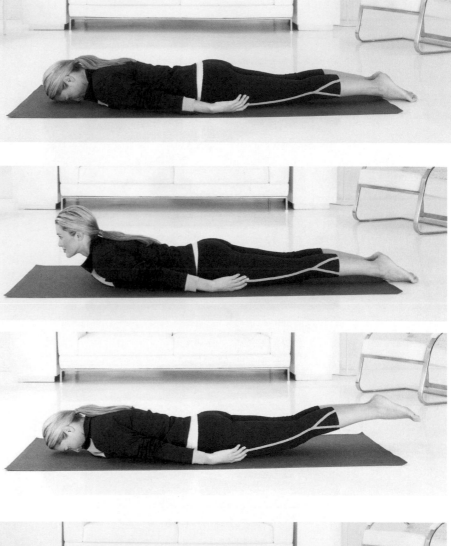

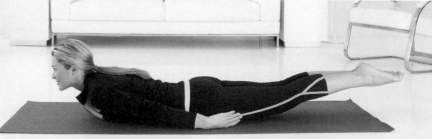

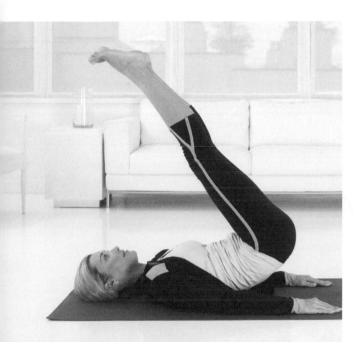

Rear Lifts

TONES ABDOMINAL MUSCLES

1. Lie on your back with your arms at your sides, palms down. Keeping your legs extended and your feet flexed, **lift** your legs off the floor so they form a 90-degree angle with your body. (If you have tight hamstrings or a history of back pain, bend your knees about 45 degrees.)

2. Keeping your upper body stable, **contract** your abs and **lift** your butt off the ground. Hold. Lower to the starting position.

3. To tone your oblique muscles at the same time, **twist** your hips to the right as you **lift** your butt off the ground. On your next rep, **twist** to the left side. **Rotate** between right and left twists as you go through your set.

▶ *PERFORM 10 TO 16 REPS.*

Rolling Like a Ball

TONES CORE

1. Sit on the floor and hug your knees to your chest. Balancing on your tailbone, **lift** your feet, pointing your toes.

2. Pull your abdominal muscles in and **roll** back onto your upper glutes and lower back.

3. Contract your abs and pull yourself back to the starting position. If the move is too difficult, **loosen** your arms, so your knees are pulled less tightly to your body. Keep it to a small range of motion if necessary.

▶ *PERFORM 10 TO 16 REPS.*

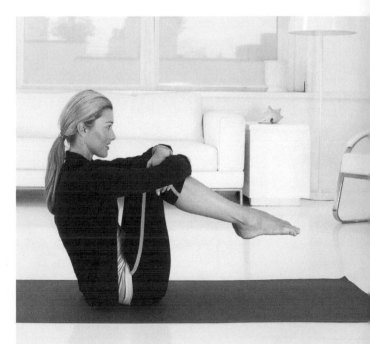

DAY 2 & DAY 4 | Upper Body

PERFORM THIS CIRCUIT 3 TIMES.

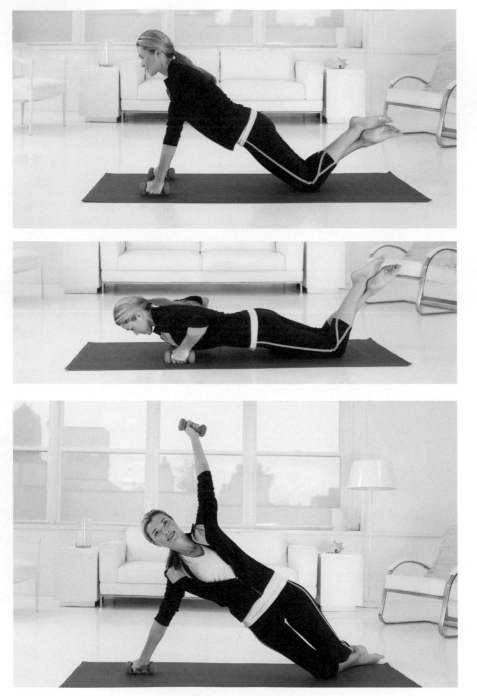

Push and Plank

TONES CHEST, CORE, UPPER BACK, SHOULDERS, AND ARMS

1. Grab a light dumbbell in each hand and **assume** a modified push-up position with your arms extended, hands directly under your shoulders (the weights should be parallel to your body), your knees bent, and your ankles crossed.

2. Bend your elbows and lower your chest until your upper arms are parallel to the floor.

3. Press back to start, immediately rotating your body to the left and raising the right arm straight up toward the ceiling.

4. Return to start, and continue alternating arms. To make the move harder, perform it from your toes with legs extended.

▶ *PERFORM 10 TO 16 REPS EACH ARM.*

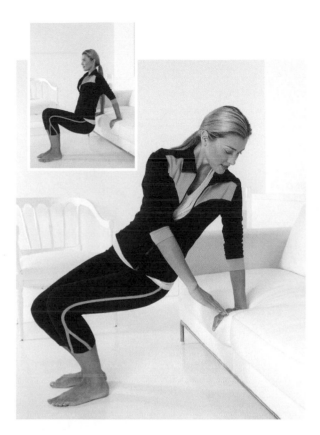

Triceps Dip Lift

TONES ARMS, SHOULDERS, CORE, AND BACK

1. Sit on the edge of a sturdy chair or hard sofa. **Grasp** the seat with your hands positioned wider than shoulder-width apart. **Inch** your butt off the sofa, keeping your legs bent and your feet flat on the floor. Bend your arms about 45 degrees.

2. Straighten your arms, tighten your abdominals and glutes, and lift your torso upward. Immediately **raise** your right arm straight up (balancing your weight on your left arm), bring it across your body, and reach over and touch the sofa by your left hand.

3. Return to the starting position, bending elbows again, and repeat to the opposite side. Continue alternating arms.

▶ *PERFORM 10 TO 16 REPS.*

Boat Curl and Press

TONES CORE, ARMS, AND SHOULDERS

1. Sit on a bench, holding a light dumbbell in each hand, arms hanging at your sides, palms facing forward. (The floor will do if there's no bench available, in which case, place the weights on either side of your hips.) **Lean back** slightly, pulling your knees to chest height with your lower legs parallel to the floor; you'll be balancing on your tailbone.

2. Curl the weights to your shoulders, then immediately **rotate** your wrists so your palms face forward and **press** the weights straight overhead.

3. Return to the starting position.

▶ *PERFORM 10 TO 16 REPS.*

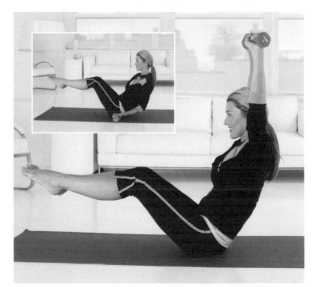

DAY 5 & DAY 7 | Lower Body

PERFORM THIS CIRCUIT 3 TIMES.

Touchdown Lunge

TONES LEGS AND BUTT

1. Stand with your feet hip-width apart, hands on your hips. **Bend** your knees 45 degrees so that you're partially squatting.

2. Take a giant **step back** with your left leg, bending both knees until your back knee grazes the floor. Simultaneously **reach** down and **touch** the floor next to your right foot with your right fingertips (your left hand shouldn't touch the floor).

3. Push back to the starting position. Repeat then switch sides. To make it easier, instead of stepping back to the starting position, stay in the lunge position and simply straighten and bend legs to perform "stationary" touchdown lunges.

▶ *REPEAT 10 TO 16 TIMES EACH SIDE.*

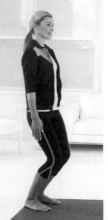
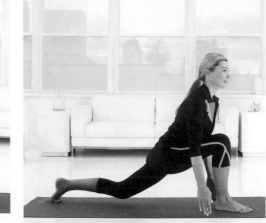

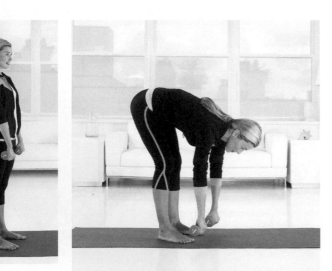

Deadlift

TONES LEGS AND BUTT

1. Stand with your feet hip-width apart, knees slightly bent, holding dumbbells in front of your thighs, palms facing in.

2. Keeping your lower back straight throughout the move, slowly **bend** at the hips, lowering the dumbbells toward the floor as far as comfortably possible. Keep the weights close to your body as you lower.

3. Return to the starting position. If you have lower-back problems, skip the dumbbells (and avoid this exercise altogether if it hurts).

▶ *DO 10 TO 16 REPS.*

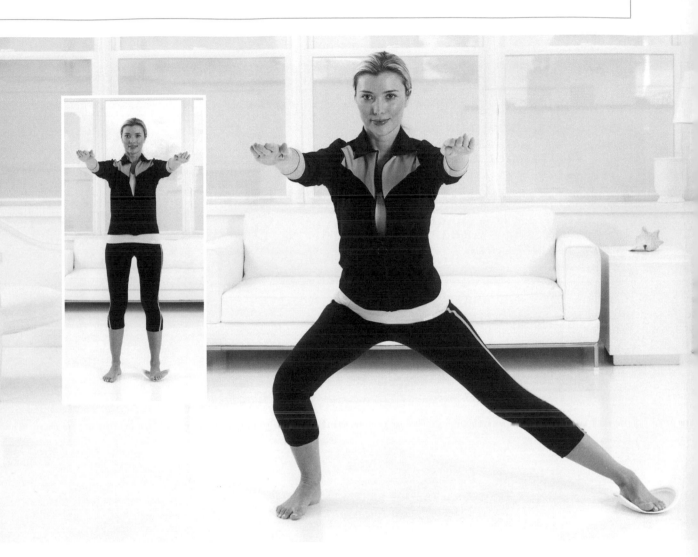

Sliding Side Lunge

TONES LEGS AND BUTT

1. Stand on a bare floor with your feet hip-width apart. **Place** a paper plate underneath your left foot. **Shift** your weight to your right leg and **extend** your arms straight out in front of you for balance.

2. Bend your right knee and **squat** back 45 to 90 degrees while sliding the foot on the paper plate out to the left as far as comfortably possible. Keep your right knee behind your toes as you lower.

3. Slowly **pull** the left leg back to the starting position while straightening the right leg.

▶ *REPEAT 10 TO 16 TIMES, THEN SWITCH SIDES.*

DAY 6 Yoga

PERFORM THIS CIRCUIT 3 TIMES.

Sweeping Forward Bend

WORKS BACK, ARMS, AND LEGS

1. Stand tall with your feet together, arms down at your sides, palms facing forward. **Sweep** your arms out to your sides and overhead, stretching tall.

2. Bend forward from the hips (bend your knees if you need to) and push your tailbone back, while you **sweep** your hands back out to the sides and down to the ground, placing your fingertips under your feet. **Allow** your head to hang, and breathe deeply and evenly while contracting your quads to help relax and lengthen the hamstrings.

3. Hold. Then bring your hands to your hips, press your tailbone down, and hinge back to a standing position with a long, straight torso.

▸ *HOLD 30 TO 60 SECONDS.*

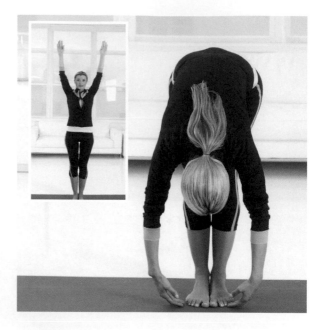

Cobra

WORKS ABS, ARMS, CHEST, AND BACK

1. Lie facedown with your feet together, toes pointed, and your hands on the floor, palms down just in front of your shoulders.

2. Lift your chin and gently extend your arms, contracting your glutes and lifting your upper body off the floor as far as comfortably possible.

3. If you feel any strain in your back, **alter** the pose so that you keep your elbows bent and your forearms on the floor.

▸ *HOLD 30 TO 60 SECONDS.*

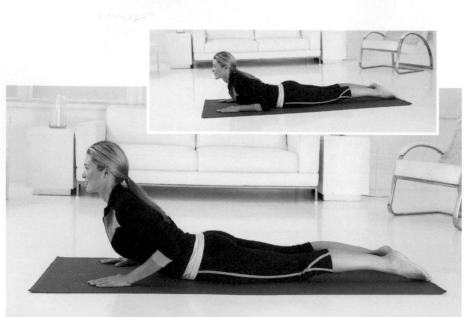

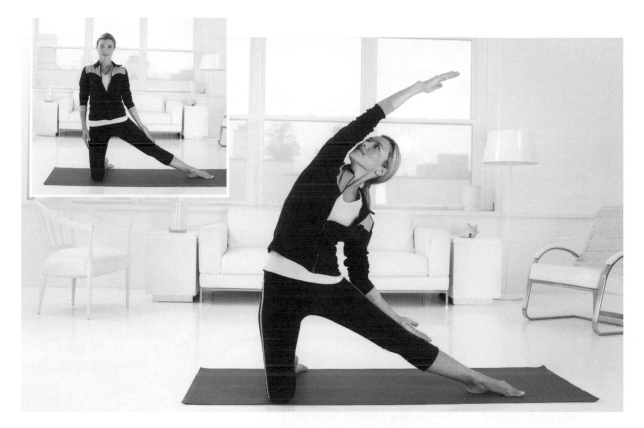

Gate

WORKS LEGS, ARMS, AND CORE

1. Kneel on the floor with your knees hip-width apart. **Stretch** your left leg out to the left side and turn the foot so the sole is flat on the floor, toes pointed to the left. **Keep** your right knee directly below your hip. **Align** your left heel with your right knee. Turn pelvis to the left so the right hip comes forward. Turn upper torso to the right. Point kneecap to ceiling.

2. Move arms out parallel to the floor with your palms facing down. **Bend** left over the left leg and place your right hand on your shin, ankle, or floor along the outside of your left leg. **Contract** the left side of the torso and stretch the right. Place your right hand on the outer right hip and push your pelvis toward the floor. **Slip** the hand up to the lower right ribs then left toward the shoulder.

3. Sweep your right arm over the back of your right ear. Without pushing your right hip, **roll** it slightly forward and **turn** the upper torso away from the floor.

4. Inhale as you return to the starting position.

▸ *HOLD 30 TO 60 SECONDS.*

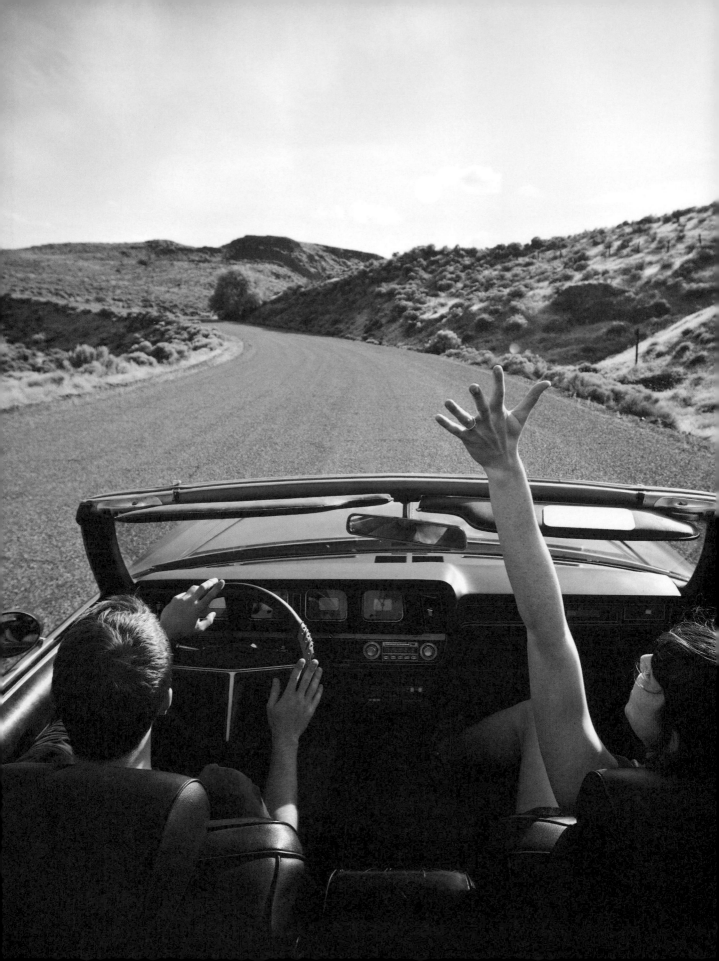

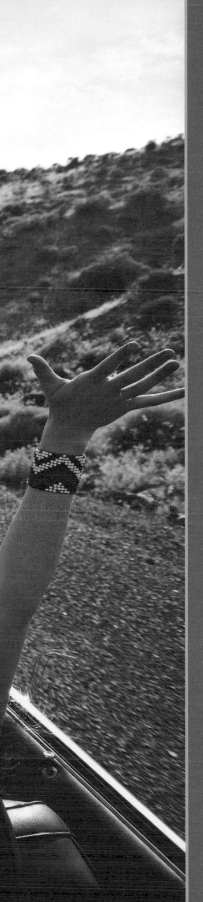

PART 4

Live Well

Refreshing sleep. Deep, daily serenity. Renewed motivation. Extra support if you're feeling burned out. Real help if you're depressed. This chapter will help you take care of your body and your mind in ways that make it easier for you to manage your diabetes and your overall health. Yes, taking care of your disease is a choice you make right now, this week, this month and forever. We're here to help you make that choice again and again. Need an extra dose of information and motivation? Start here!

▼▼▼▼▼▼▼▼▼▼▼▼▼

Reverse Diabetes Forever by **Staying Motivated**

Keeping up a strong motivation is proven to help people with diabetes.

We all love before-and-after stories. That's why there are a bazillion reality TV shows. But between the humble beginnings and the dramatic, uplifting endings, there's a lot of hard work that goes on. And to achieve it takes lots and lots of motivation.

Of all the elements you need to master, motivation may be the most difficult, because imprinting healthy new behaviors is challenging. Here's where persistence will pay off, as will getting the support you need from reading this chapter (over and over again, if necessary!). Keeping up a strong motivation is proven to help people with diabetes not only keep blood sugar within a healthy range but also prevent diabetes complications.

This motivation can take many forms, such as compliments from friends who noticed you wearing more flattering clothes to seeing how a new diet lowers blood-sugar levels. Some of the more surprising motivators that help successfully reverse diabetes include getting enough quality sleep and busting stress. It turns out that nurturing your mind and spirit also are self-care essentials that help keep you motivated and reduce the stress hormones that raise blood sugar and pack on belly fat.

Along with dieting and exercise, recent medical advances now present several options for those who want to lose weight. Such procedures can put you on the right track for weight loss and help keep you motivated to stay there. In addition, how we cope with potentially stressful situations such as being sick and traveling can help avoid motivation pitfalls. So here you'll learn how to stay motivated to manage diabetes so that your "after" you stays happy ... ever after.

Live Well > Right Now

Sneak away this moment for 10 minutes of quiet, peaceful time. Commit to doing this a few times a day. It's essential for normalizing blood sugar, maintaining or achieving a healthy weight, and staying on track as you make healthy lifestyle changes. Learning the art of relaxation is worth the investment in time.

Live Well > Today

Or tonight, actually. You may not think of sleep as a key weapon against diabetes. In fact, you may even think you're doing yourself a favor when you cut back to just five or six hours a night, in the hopes of getting more done during the day. But the exact opposite is true: Now we know that seven to eight hours of sound sleep a night is proven to help people with diabetes control their blood sugar. Research shows it is a powerful strategy for shedding unwanted pounds and keeping them off. Being well rested also will help you accomplish other motivation and weight loss goals with ease.

Live Well > This Week

Count up your TV viewing time during the week. It should be at or less than 14 hours, or an average of two hours a day. Limiting TV viewing ensures that you have plenty of time for sleep, exercise, and relaxation. Need extra incentive to turn off the tube? Harvard University researchers estimate that TV viewing burns even fewer calories than reading a magazine, sewing, or playing a board game!

Live Well > This Month

Sometime in the next 30 days, make a date to stock up on sick-day foods. Even if you don't have an appetite, it's important to eat regularly to keep your blood sugar steady. Start with foods that are already part of your healthy diet, such as oatmeal, chicken soup, applesauce, or toast. Stash a supply of broth-based soups, along with saltine-type crackers.

Live Well > This Year

Being consistent from day to day, especially when it comes to diet and exercise, is key to managing diabetes. But over the course of a year, we have special occasions, travel and (unfortunately) sick days. From time to time as your routine changes, you'll face challenges that can affect your blood sugar and other aspects of your health. Having the ability to manage such unusual circumstances is an invaluable skill. Tips in this section give you those tools.

Live Well > Forever+

Maintaining a positive, can-do attitude can also significantly cut your risk for diabetes complications. In a study of 165 people with type 2 diabetes, those who were motivated to take charge of their diabetes were 55 percent less likely to have a heart attack, 53 percent less likely to have a stroke, and 50 percent less likely to have severe kidney damage over 7½ years. Their blood-sugar levels were lower, and their blood pressure and cholesterol levels were healthier than people who were less motivated to care for themselves.

Recharge with Restful Sleep

If you frequently toss and turn at night, you'll spend your days feeling like a zombie. That's bad enough, but here's an even better reason to find a fix for your sleep problem: It could cause or worsen diabetes. Studies have long hinted that people who struggle with sleep are top candidates for developing diabetes. But until recently, no one was sure just how much getting too little shut-eye can mess up your metabolism and raise your risk for developing the disease. And some doctors still poohpooh the idea that sleep deprivation plays an important part in triggering diabetes.

It's getting harder and harder to ignore the connection, however. In 2010 researchers in England looked at stacks of studies and found "unambiguous and consistent" evidence that having insomnia puts you at risk for diabetes. They determined that people who sleep less than five or six hours a night are significantly more likely than sound sleepers to develop diabetes. And don't think that just because you drift off quickly every night you're in the clear. The study found that people who can fall asleep, but frequently wake up in the middle of the night and end up eyeballing the ceiling for hours, were an alarming 84 percent more likely to develop type 2 diabetes. These findings proved true for men and women, as well as people of all races. A 2014 study of more than 8,500 Canadians found that people with sleep apnea—a condition that causes you to briefly wake and gasp for air during the night—were 30 percent more likely to develop diabetes over six years than people without the condition.

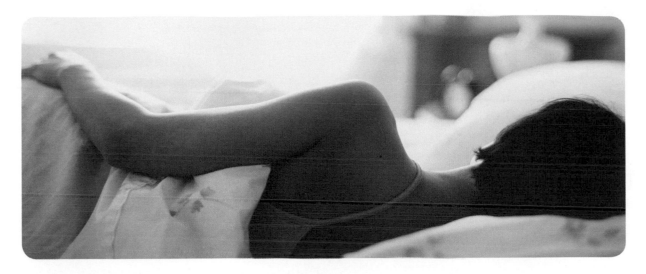

It's not entirely clear why insomnia and sleep apnea may trigger diabetes, though it's known that getting too little shut-eye causes certain hormone changes that interfere with good control of blood sugar. In fact, sleep problems are deeply connected with insulin resistance, high blood sugar, and hormone changes that lead to weight gain. A lack of sleep is also guaranteed to raise your stress levels during the day. It's tough staying calm and centered when a tired mind meets an emotional challenge—whether it's an angry boss, a rude driver on the road, or a broken dishwasher at home.

Better sleep leads to better health. Get this one right, and the rest—from reducing stress to taking control of top blood-sugar challenges—will be far easier.

Create a Sleep-Friendly Environment

Many of us don't get enough sleep, simply because we choose to stay up late (there are always bills to pay and late-night TV for laughs). Or if we do hit the hay on time, we toss and turn, replaying the day's worries, fighting the lingering effects of that late-afternoon cup of coffee, or trying to ignore the noise of a sleeping spouse or the discomfort of a sagging mattress. If that's you, a deep, refreshing night's sleep is just a few fixes away. These strategies will help you prepare your mind, body, and bedroom for a full dose of slumber.

Wake up at the same time every morning. This is one of the surest ways to train your body to fall asleep at the same time every night. Experts say that keeping a regular sleep schedule is critical to keeping insomnia at bay. A 2015 study published in the *Journal of Clinical Endocrinology* recently found that a regular sleep schedule keeps the metabolism running smoothly. So hit the sack and wake up at the same time on weekends as you do during the workweek.

live well this week!

Check your blood sugar more often.

See if you're hitting the target goals you've set with your doctor. High and low blood sugar can affect sleep quality. And take one more step: Set your alarm for 3 a.m. for another check. If your levels are normal, that's great; if they're low, it might explain why you're waking up in the night. (If sugar levels are below 75 mg/dL, have a small snack. Discuss any ongoing pattern of low blood sugar at night with your doctor.)

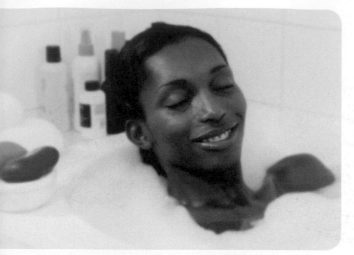

Build a nighttime routine that relaxes your body and tells your mind that sleep is up next.

Beware Sunday night insomnia. Staying up late on Friday and Saturday nights and sleeping in on Saturday and Sunday mornings is frequently the gift we give ourselves on weekends after a hard week at work. Yet that little gift—small as it is—is enough to mess with your biological clock. Even if you get to bed early on Sunday night, you will not be ready to sleep, and you will not end up being the happy camper you were expecting come Monday morning.

Get some exercise every day. Physical activity improves sleep as effectively as powerful sleeping pills called benzo-diazepines in some studies. On average it reduces the time it takes to get to sleep by 12 minutes, and it increases total sleep time by 42 minutes.

Wait till you're pooped. Ever find that you get really sleepy at 10 P.M., that the sleepiness passes, and that by the time the late news comes on, you're wide-awake? Some experts believe sleepiness comes in cycles. Push past a period of sleepiness and you likely won't be able to fall asleep very easily for a while. If you've noticed these kinds of rhythms in your own body, use them to your advantage. When sleepiness comes, get yourself to bed, pronto.

Don't sleep on a full tummy. If you know that you have a busy day planned for tomorrow, have your big meal at lunchtime and a lighter meal as early as possible in the evening. If you find you are still hungry before bedtime, avoid sugar; try a small handful of nuts.

Relax before you turn in. According to a National Sleep Foundation poll, during the hour before bed, around 60 percent of us do household chores, 37 percent take care of children, 36 percent do activities with other family members, 36 percent are on the Internet, and 21 percent do work related to their jobs. A better plan: Read a book, listen to music, take a warm bath, or do some light stretching. The goal is to build a routine that relaxes your body and tells your mind that sleep is up next.

Curfew the computer. Researchers at Stanford University have found that the light from your monitor right before bed is enough to reset your whole wake/sleep cycle—and postpone the onset of sleepiness by three hours. PS: That goes for all your electronic toys: readers, tablets, games—and the TV.

Be cool, real cool. Lowering the temperature in your home or bedroom will signal to your body that it's time to sleep, experts say. It's generally agreed that 65°F is the optimal temperature for great sleep.

Blacken the room. You sleep better in the dark. If your eyelids flutter open as you move from one stage of sleep to another, even streetlights or a full moon can wake you. Why? Blame it on melatonin, the hormone that makes you sleepy. Darkness encourages high levels, but light shuts it down—even dim light or brief light exposure.

No more night-lights. That goes for clocks, too, as well as any blinking lights from electronic devices. Turn your clock's face or digital readout away so you can't see it. We wake slightly throughout the night. Your brain can misinterpret even such dim lights and wonder if it should wake you up. Do all you can to keep things dark—researchers say it tells your brain to stay asleep. If you have to get up to visit the bathroom at night, keep the path from bed to toilet clear so you can navigate it with a minimum of light (use enough to stay safe, of course!). A night-light in the bathroom is a good idea.

Relax your body. If your mind is relaxed but your body is tense, do some low-intensity stretches and exercises to relax your muscles, especially those in your upper body, neck, and shoulders. Try the relaxation routine and progressive muscle relaxation exercises you'll find later in this chapter.

Keep a worry book. Put a small journal and a pen on your bedside table. If you wake up in the wee, small hours and begin worrying, jot down your thoughts. Then close the book, put it on your nightstand, turn out the light, and go back to sleep.

Don't just lie there. Snoozing from 11:30 P.M. until 2:00 A.M., tossing and turning until 4, then sleeping until 6 gives you eight hours in bed but only 4½ hours of sleep—and letting yourself toss and turn at night to the point of frustration creates anxiety about sleep that can make insomnia worse. If you wake at 3:00 A.M., get up and go read a book or magazine in the living room. Don't go back to bed until you feel sleepy enough to fall asleep. It's tempting to stay in a warm, cozy bed even if you're not asleep, but remind yourself that it's important to get out of bed when you're awake. If you don't, a part of your mind will begin to associate the bed with being awake rather than being asleep, making falling asleep more difficult.

Train your pets to sleep elsewhere. Up to 25 percent of insomniacs may have their pets to blame for their lack of snooze time, say Mayo Clinic researchers who interviewed

---

live well today!

Take a walk for deeper sleep.

Studies at the University of Arizona show that walking six blocks at a normal pace during the day significantly improves sleep at night for women. Just make sure you finish your walk at least two hours before bed. Any later and the energizing effect of the activity can keep you up.

Is Your Bed Dead?

When a consulting firm surveyed 400 adults for the Better Sleep Council, they found that 8 in 10 thought a bad mattress could cause sleep problems. Ironically, nearly half also confessed that their current mattress was "bad" or even "very bad."

You need a new mattress if:

▶ Yours is 10 years old or older.

▶ The topography of your mattress resembles a mountain range, with all its peaks, valleys, and slopes.

▶ You wake up feeling sore or stiff, despite not being physically active the day before.

How to buy a mattress you'll like:

▶ Try it in the store. Lie on it. Roll over. Get into your typical sleeping position and stay there for at least five minutes. Go by what's comfortable. *Consumer Reports* found that firmer mattresses don't resist permanent sagging any better than softer mattresses; and that the more padding there is, the greater the possibility the mattress will sag.

▶ Buy one that's larger than you think you will need, especially if you sleep with someone else. If you're used to a queen and feel cramped when you sleep, invest in a king.

▶ Once you get it home, turn it over and upside down at least every three months.

Sleeping Pills or Therapy?

The first line of sleep aid should be therapy. When researchers at Johns Hopkins University compared 21 studies using drugs or cognitive behavioral therapy for insomnia, the therapy emerged as the clear winner. It reduced the amount of time it took people to fall asleep by 43 percent; drugs reduced it 30 percent. Therapy shortened the length of wake-ups at night 56 percent; drugs, 46 percent. Therapy improved overall sleep quality 28 percent; drugs, 20 percent. The therapy bonus: no side effects. And other studies show it keeps on working for months or years.

However, if therapy doesn't do it, the newer versions of sleeping pills may be the answer. Talk to your doctor and ask for a prescription to try sleeping pills for a few nights. The new and widely advertised insomnia drugs—including zolpidem (Ambien), zaleplon (Sonata), and eszopiclone (Lunesta)—appear to be as effective as older, habit-forming sleeping pills, with fewer side effects, probably because the body metabolizes them faster.

Taking them for a few nights can help quell your anxiety about being unable to fall asleep and get you out of the habit of dreading the bed. But don't rely on them as a long-term solution. A report from the National Institutes of Health warns that few prescription drugs for insomnia have been tested in long-term studies of a year or more—yet many people take them for years on end. And recently the FDA required warnings on 13 prescription sleep aids about risks that people may attempt to drive, cook, and eat while asleep.

---

live well
right now!

**Go up a wall
to lower stress.**

Legs-up-the-wall is a favorite stress-reducer of yoga practitioners. Place a pillow next to a wall and position yourself so your hips and low back are on the pillow, your head and shoulders are on the floor, and your legs are resting against the wall. Your body will be in the shape of an L. Close your eyes and breathe deeply for about a minute. If having your legs straight up a wall is uncomfortable, you can do the move by draping your legs up on a sofa or chair.

300 patients at the clinic's Sleep Disorders Center. Pets wake us up by walking around at night, jumping on the bed, and demanding to be let outside for middle-of-the-night bathroom breaks. Consider investing in a white-noise machine to cover up their sounds, shut your door and insist they sleep elsewhere, or talk with your vet about introducing your animal to sleeping in a pet crate. Healthy pets can also be trained gradually to wait till morning for a bladder break; your vet can help you do this the right way.

Sleep in to counteract periodic sleep deprivation. Yes, a regular sleep schedule is important, but we all occasionally can't help disrupting it every once in a while. Maybe you were up all night with a sick kid. Or perhaps you lost sleep during a red-eye. Whatever the reason, make up for the sleep debt by getting extra shut-eye two days in a row. A 2016 study found that two consecutive nights of extra sleep helped to reverse the negative effects of this type of periodic sleep loss.

Cut out caffeine. In a study of thousands of Australians, those who got 240 milligrams of caffeine a day—about the amount in two 8-ounce cups of coffee or 2½ shots of espresso—had a 40 percent higher risk for insomnia than those who skipped it. Caffeine blocks the action of a sleep-inducing brain chemical called adenosine. It takes three to seven hours for your body to metabolize just half the caffeine in a cup of tea or coffee. If you can't live without it, relegate your caffeine to the morning.

Fight Insomnia the Smart Way

Tossing and turning again? You're not alone. At least one-third of all adults have a hard time falling asleep—or staying asleep—at least one night per week. When does "I can't get to sleep" qualify as insomnia? Experts say you've crossed the line and may need treatment if on three or more nights each week you need more than 30 minutes to fall asleep and/or you awaken in the middle of the night and have trouble getting back to sleep.

If that's you, be sure to start with all of the sleep tactics on the following pages. Experts recommend them for people with insomnia, too, because they'll help your mind and body establish a healthier sleep schedule. If you still feel you're losing out on zzzzs, move on to these strategies.

Rewire your circuits. The most successful treatment for insomnia is called cognitive behavioral therapy (CBT). In more than 20 studies involving 470 patients with insomnia from a variety of causes, CBT worked just as well as sleeping pills at increasing sleep and improving sleep quality—and it was better than sleeping pills at helping study participants fall asleep faster.

CBT involves meeting with a trained therapist to discover information about what keeps you from sleeping (the "cognitive" part) and learn how to alter your behavior (the "behavioral" part) so that you can improve your sleep. It may take as few as four or five 30-minute sessions to effect change; some people will need three months of sessions to conquer insomnia.

Unfortunately, certified cognitive behavioral therapists are scarce. To find one, visit www.academyofct.org and click on "Find a Therapist." Fill in your zip code or city and state on the pop-up, and a list of therapists in your area will appear. If none do, or if you don't have time for even the small number of sessions CBT requires, you can visit www.cbtforinsomnia.com. For a fee ($34.95 at press time) you can take an online tutorial based on a Harvard University CBT insomnia program to retrain your brain for a better night's sleep.

Limit your time in bed. It sounds crazy, but one of the most effective strategies to combat insomnia is to restrict the number of hours you spend in bed.

The reason is that most people who have been struggling with insomnia will do seemingly practical things like go to bed a couple of hours early to try to sleep. It rarely works, researchers have found, so most of those people end up spending seven hours in bed but only sleep for five.

Be drowsy before hitting the hay. Don't go to bed until you truly feel like you can fall asleep. And remember what we said previously: Don't stay in bed when you're awake or the association you make (bed = awake) can program you for insomnia. Get up, go into another room, and do something boring and quiet for awhile. When you're really sleepy, go back to bed.

It sounds crazy, but one of the best ways to fight insomnia is to spend less time in bed.

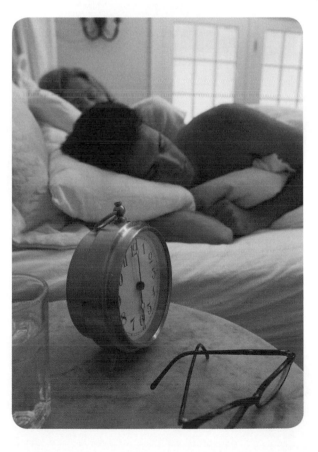

Sleep Apnea and Diabetes

If you wake up in the morning feeling tired, irritable, sad, forgetful, and headachy, there's a good chance that you have sleep apnea, a sleep-related breathing disorder that affects millions of people—including many with diabetes.

When you have sleep apnea, your breathing actually stops or becomes very shallow as you sleep. Hundreds of times every night, your breathing may pause for 10 or more seconds, depriving your body of oxygen, increasing your heart rate, and preventing you from entering the important stages of deep sleep that restore mind and body. You may awaken slightly as you struggle to take a breath. By morning you may not recall any of your nighttime awakenings. But they have a profound affect on your blood sugar, your heart, and your brain.

Most sleep apnea is a type called obstructive sleep apnea, or OSA. It occurs when the soft tissue in the back of the throat relaxes and blocks the passage of air until your airway opens—often with a loud choking or gasping sound—and you begin to breathe again. Getting your sleep apnea diagnosed and treated will help you get a good night's sleep and feel refreshed. It can also help you control your blood sugar and reduce your odds for diabetes-related kidney damage, one recent study shows.

SYMPTOMS OF SLEEP APNEA

If you have one or more of the following symptoms, you may have sleep apnea. Consult your doctor for a diagnosis.

You snore loudly. About half of all people who snore loudly have OSA. It's a sign that your airway is partially blocked. Ask your sleep partner if you snore loudly at night, and whether he or she has noticed if you seem to stop breathing during sleep, then catch your breath again with a loud snort.

Sleep Soundly with a Snorer

Sure you love your spouse or partner, but studies find one of the greatest disrupters of sleep is that loved one dreaming away next to you. He might snore; she might kick or cry out or whatever. One study found that 86 percent of women surveyed said their husbands snored, and half had their sleep interrupted by it. Men have it a bit easier; 57 percent said their wives snored, while just 15 percent found their sleep bothered by it.

The best solution? Have one of you sleep in the guest room. If you absolutely will not kick your partner out (or head to the guest room yourself), then consider these anti-snoring tips:

▸ Get him (or her) to stop smoking. Cigarette smoking contributes to snoring.

▸ Feed him (or her) a light meal for dinner and nix any alcohol, which can add to the snoring.

▸ Buy some earplugs and use them!

▸ Present your partner with a gift-wrapped box of Breathe Right strips, which work by pulling the nostrils open wider. A Swedish study found they significantly reduced snoring.

▸ Make an appointment for your sleeping partner at a sleep center. If nothing you do improves his or her snoring, your bedmate might be a candidate for a sleep test called polysomnography to see if sleep apnea is the cause.

You have a large neck. The size of your neck can be a telltale sign because it's a reflection of being overweight—and carrying extra pounds is a major risk factor for sleep apnea. Women with OSA often have a neck size of more than 16 inches; men, 17 inches.

You wake frequently for bathroom breaks. If you're not drinking loads of water before bed and you're not taking high-dose water pills, you shouldn't wake more than once or twice a night to use the bathroom. People with OSA often visit the bathroom three or more times each night.

You feel sleepy in the morning after eight or more hours of sleep. Or you become dangerously drowsy during the day. People with OSA can become so sleepy that they fall asleep while driving.

HOW TO FIX SLEEP APNEA

If you nodded your head to any of the above, then chances are, you have sleep apnea. Don't ignore the situation—tackle it head on. Here's how.

See a sleep specialist. A sleep doctor will check your mouth, nose, and throat and make a recording of what happens with your breathing while you sleep. This may require an overnight stay at a sleep center

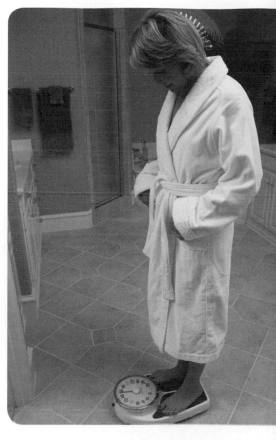

Lose weight. Dropping pounds can reduce sleep apnea. When University of Wisconsin Medical School researchers tracked 690 Wisconsin residents for four years, they found those who lost 10 percent of their body weight saw apnea improve 26 percent. Almost any amount of weight loss helps. Extremely overweight people who underwent surgical weight loss procedures to drop 25 to 50 percent of their body weight saw a 70 to 98 percent drop in sleep apnea in one study. And among people who lost just seven to nine percent of their weight (about 14 to 18 pounds for someone weighing 200 pounds), sleep apnea scores fell by about 50 percent. Weight loss usually is not a replacement for CPAP or surgery, if you need them, but it can help make those treatments even more effective.

Ask about continuous positive airway pressure (CPAP). This "gold standard" treatment uses a small, quiet air compressor to gently push air through a mask over the sleeper's nose. The extra pressure keeps airways open, so you breathe normally all night. When researchers analyzed 36 CPAP studies involving 1,718 people with sleep apnea, they found that those who used this system improved daytime alertness by nearly 50 percent, cut the number of sleep interruptions by eight per hour, and boosted the amount of oxygen in the blood significantly.

In one Chicago study, people with diabetes and apnea saw blood-sugar levels drop three months after starting CPAP therapy. Other research shows it can also lower blood pressure and even improve the size, shape, and pumping action of the heart—good news because people with sleep apnea often have enlarged hearts. Talk to your doctor about this therapy and whether it might be right for you.

Studies show that dropping pounds can reduce sleep apnea.

Plan Time to Relax

You know how your body responds to stress—your head starts to throb, you sweat, or your neck muscles tense up. But what you may not realize is while you're feeling stressed on the outside, something much more insidious is going on inside. Your body reacts to stressful situations by pumping a torrent of chemicals into your bloodstream designed to power you up to avoid the stressor. That worked great back in the day when your stressor was a club-wielding enemy or a predatory animal.

Today's stresses are less life-threatening but more pervasive, so your stress response can get stuck in overdrive. That means that you're continually pumping out hormones and other chemicals designed to release glucose into your blood, among other things, so you have enough energy to sprint away from danger. End result is a body-wide assault that results in the kind of subtle inflammation that doctors now say contributes to diabetes and a host of other chronic conditions—think arthritis, even some cancers.

That's why it's essential to learn how to regularly evoke your body's relaxation response—an innate, natural ability we have to enter into a physical state of total relaxation. Doing so can blunt the physical effects of stress—and it just plain makes you feel good. With a little practice, you can teach yourself to elicit this relaxation response wherever and whenever you like—even when you're stuck in traffic! Here's how to get there.

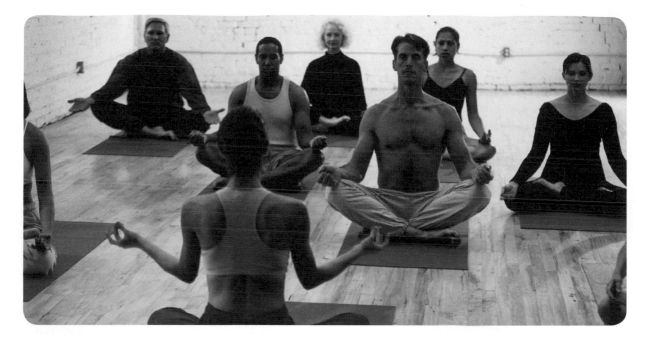

How to Chill: Eight Cool Ways to Relax

No matter which one of these tension-taming techniques you choose, commit to practicing it regularly—every day if possible. The more you do, the better and faster it will work, and the easier it will be for you to turn on your body's relaxation response when you need it. These are great ways to melt tension at the end of the day and can help you avoid spiraling into high anxiety when something stressful does happen in your life.

1. TRY PROGRESSIVE RELAXATION.

One study after another has demonstrated that progressive muscle relaxation blocks the chemical effects of stress, anxiety, and 24/7 living on your brain. To do it, lie down or sit in a comfortable chair that supports your head. Close your eyes and start by mentally scanning your body for places that feel tense. Now, starting at your toes and working your way very slowly up to your scalp, do this: Focus on an area, and tightly clench each muscle in it for five seconds. Take about 20 seconds to gradually release the tension, consciously relaxing your muscles as much as possible, then move on to the next area. Move up from your toes, to your feet, to your ankles. Focus all your attention on each area, willing its muscles to relax. Continue slowly moving up your body until you finally focus on the tension in your forehead and your scalp. When you've finished with the entire sequence, silently repeat a soothing thought, such as "I am totally relaxed."

2. USE IMAGERY TO ERASE TENSION.

You can't just physically escape to a beautiful, peaceful place whenever stress rears its ugly head. But you can imagine such a place—including all the sights, sounds, smells,

> Close your eyes and mentally scan your body for places that feel tense.

and even the temperature, and that imagining allows you to experience its relaxing benefits. The scenario you choose is up to you. Here's one example.

Picture yourself on a mountaintop surrounded by lush tropical vegetation but open to the sky, so you're bathed in sunlight. Note the deep blue color of the sky, feel the sun's rays soothing your body, smell the fragrance of the flowers all around, and hear the patter of drops falling off leaves after a recent rain. Look far below and see the shore of a tranquil beach on a placid lake. Take yourself to the shore of the lake and imagine walking along the soft sand. You're completely alone, but you find a boat tied to a dock. After untying the mooring rope, lie down on soft blankets inside the boat and watch the clouds as you drift on the calm water. The boat rocks gently, and waves gurgle under the hull as you drink in the warmth and feel the soft movement of a breeze. You feel a deep sense of relaxation as you drift between the water and the clouds.

3. BREATHE IN SERENITY, BREATHE OUT TENSION.

A simple meditation that focuses on your breath can melt stress in as little as three to five minutes. Sit quietly with your feet flat on the floor and your back supported (don't slump). Close your eyes. Inhale slowly, feeling the air move through your mouth or nose and your abdomen filling up. Pause for a second or two, then exhale slowly. When your mind wanders (and it will!), gently direct your attention back to your breathing. This is a shortened version of mindfulness-based stress reduction, a meditation technique proven (when practiced for longer periods of time every day) to improve long-term blood sugar levels in one Duke University study.

4. USE MOVEMENT TO RELAX.

> One of the most effective ways to defuse stress is to run away from it—or at least walk briskly.

One of the most effective ways to defuse stress is to run away from it—or at least walk briskly. In one study that asked 38 men and 35 women to keep diaries of their activity, mood, and stress, volunteers reported that they felt less anxious on days when they were physically active than on days when they didn't exercise. Even when stressful events occurred, people in the study said they felt less troubled on their physically active days.

5. TURN YOUR WORKOUTS INTO STRESS REDUCERS.

Virtually any kind of physical activity seems to relieve stress, although some researchers think that activities that involve repetitive movements—walking, running, cycling, or swimming, for instance—may offer the best defense. Many people consider swimming to be one of the most relaxing exercises, a soothing way to literally

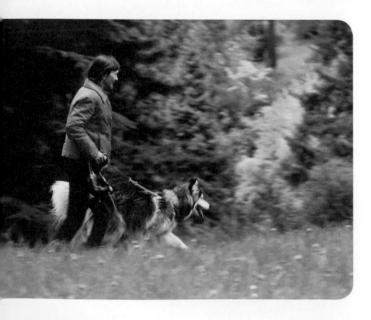

go with the flow. Repeating a physical movement over and over again somehow seems to ease mind and body.

6. TAKE IT TO THE NEXT LEVEL.

Think about some ways to make your workout even more relaxing. If you're a walker, be aware of the way your arms swing from front to back and the rhythm of your gait. Repeat a soothing word or phrase each time you exhale. If you work out on an exercise cycle or stair machine at a fitness club, ignore what's on the big TV screen in the room. Scientists have found that watching television makes people more jittery, not less. If you can't turn off the TV, look elsewhere and focus on your breathing, or plug yourself into some soothing music.

7. DISCOVER YOGA.

Looking for a simple way to relax, refresh your energy, become more limber, and strengthen muscles at the same time? Yoga may be just the ticket. Exercise scientists have long known that yoga offers a great way to stretch, increase strength, and improve balance. And believe it or not, yoga holds promise for reducing the risk factors for type 2 diabetes, say University of Pittsburgh researchers. In their 2011 study, they learned that people who attended yoga classes for three months lost weight, lowered their blood pressure and triglycerides, and even improved their insulin levels, which prompted them to declare that yoga holds promise for people with diabetes.

How to get started? Try a yoga class at a local fitness center or yoga studio to see if it's right for you. Don't give up—there are plenty of yoga styles out there; you're sure to find one that's to your liking. If you're just beginning, consider "restorative yoga," which is super-relaxing and gentle.

8. ESTABLISH A DAILY STRETCHING ROUTINE.

Stretching isn't just relaxing; it's also great for your whole body. Get in the habit of spending just 5 or 10 minutes stretching in the evenings, and you may find yourself sleeping better before you know it—and craving your stretches the next day. Try the stretches starting on the next page.

Learn to Let Tension Go

There's the life-changing stress: moving, losing a job, getting divorced. Doctors call this chronic stress, because it continues on for a long time. Then there's the daily stresses that go hand-in-hand with living—the annoyances, hassles, rude comments, and deadlines that can keep your anxiety level boiling all day if you let it.

Fortunately, you don't have to let everyday living drive you nuts. By mastering a couple of instant tension-tamers, you can head off stress before it gets a grip on your mind and body. All of the following strategies can work. Find two or three that seem

---

live well right now!

Practice acceptance. You've probably heard of the Serenity Prayer: "God grant me the serenity to accept the things I cannot change, the courage to change the things I can, and the wisdom to know the difference." This prayer about acceptance is a great reminder that some parts of our lives are not ours to control, but others are. For instance, you can't change the fact that you have diabetes, but you can find the courage to alter your lifestyle in ways that will help you control your diabetes better. When you're feeling worried, sad, or irritable, stop and say this little prayer. Afterward, ask yourself what you need to accept and what you can change.

live well
this month!

Chart your stress.

Studies find that stress affects blood sugar differently from one person to the next. How do your sugar levels change when you're all charged up? To find out, each time you check your glucose level, rate how stressed you feel at that moment on a scale of one to 10, with one being a sunny day at the beach and 10 being just about the worst day of your life. Write the number down next to your reading. After four weeks, look at the numbers together (plotting them on a graph can help) to see how much your blood sugar swings in response to various levels of stress. If yours shoots up in response to stress, take the tips in this chapter seriously and make an extra effort to follow them.

to fit you best, then test-drive them for a few days to see if they melt away the nuisance tensions in your life.

Smile on. Studies show that the physical act of smiling—even if you don't really mean it—causes chemical changes in your body associated with happiness.

Think joy. Write down five or 10 things that make you happy or thankful—friends, a beloved pet, a roof over your head, a sunny day—and reflect on each of them for a minute.

Schedule some "ah" time. Massages not only relieve muscle tension, they trigger the release of serotonin, a brain chemical associated with a feeling of well-being, and reduced levels of the stress hormone cortisol. Bonus: Lowering your stress hormones may even lower your blood sugar. Many day spas and nail salons now have chair massages that cost as little as $10 for 10 or 15 minutes. If you can't get a massage from a professional, ask your partner to rub your shoulders, or rub your own feet.

Employ aromatherapy. Scents have an amazing impact on your mood. Sprinkle a few drops of an essential oil such as lavender, bergamot, or lemon on a tissue or handkerchief and inhale the scent. Or slice up some lemons, simmer in a pot, and breathe in the steam. Lavender is known to relieve anxiety; citrus scents lift your mood.

Try some tunes. Whether it's soothing classical music, soulful blues, cool jazz, or rousing rock and roll, music can change your mood faster than you can say "feeling groovy" or "here comes the– sun."

Don't sweat little nuisances. When something goes wrong, ask yourself whether it's really a big deal. Will you remember it years from now? What's the worst thing that can happen as a result? Is it likely to happen?

Picture your beloved. Sometimes diverting your thoughts momentarily to those who love you, who matter more, who bring you pleasure, helps you instantly put things in perspective during very stressful moments.

Play with your pet. Playing with a dog for just a few minutes raises levels of the brain chemicals serotonin and oxytocin—both mood elevators. You don't even need to own a dog to experience these feel-good effects. Your neighbor's dog would probably love the attention. Or stop by your local animal shelter. Who knows? You may even end up taking a pooch or kitty home.

Post a stop sign in your brain. When you catch yourself in the midst of stressful thinking, shout "Stop!" to yourself and picture a stop sign. Replace the distressing thought with another thought that's more positive and rational. For example, if the stressful thought is, "I can't do this; I'm worthless," instead say to yourself, "There are many valuable things I can do."

Stay Motivated No Matter What

While it's true that you will have to live with diabetes for the rest of your life (unless medical science surprises us all with a cure), we'd like to remind you that you can reverse both of the main factors behind it—insulin resistance and lack of insulin secretion. But remember this: The better you take care of yourself, the less likely you are to experience the complications that account for most of the suffering that goes with diabetes.

Take Care of Number One

Reversing diabetes requires daily attention, which can often seem overwhelming. Before you pull the motivation genie out of the bottle, realize that you first must focus on your own needs—something, frankly, few of us are trained to do. As responsible adults, we know all about sacrifices, right? Our families, our children, our friends, our coworkers, our clients, our community—these things usually come first.

It's a noble sentiment, widely shared. But it's also complete hooey. You're surrounded by people who manage to make time for their own good health. If they can do it, so can you. Here's how.

Convince yourself that it's important. Remember how you felt physically and emotionally the last time you lost a few days to a cold or flu? Good! Let it remind you that the best way to fulfill your obligations to others is by taking good care of yourself. Your children, your coworkers, and pretty much everyone you touch in a day want you to be healthy, rested, and happy. Not only because they care for you, but because they rely on you.

Look for heroes. Presidents do it. So do many chief executives, entrepreneurs, scientists, artists, educators, moms, and other everyday heroes. What they all do is find time in their day to exercise, and then a little more time to relax. If such accomplished people can do it, so can you. Find a few of them, read their stories, or talk to them directly about it. Ask specifically about what they feel are the benefits of living healthfully. Their answers will likely be inspiring.

Stop using time as an excuse. Taking care of your health need never come at a sacrifice of other priorities. Often, it's about choices that require no extra time at all. This is particularly true when it comes to nutrition: Choosing a salad rather than a cheeseburger for lunch makes a huge difference to your health, at no impact to your schedule.

Inspect your schedule. Be honest: How much time did you spend today watching TV, browsing the Internet, texting or phoning friends, or playing digital games? The national average for such activities has skyrocketed in recent years, well past three hours daily. If you can cut back by one hour per day, you will have built in enough time to take a long walk, have a revitalizing stress-relief break, and get more sleep, without sacrificing any other commitment.

Don't think health, think joy. Healthy living is about great food, being outdoors, laughing, relaxing, even having sex. If the goal of good health doesn't motivate you, then let your goal be more fun. The two often go hand in hand.

Talk to your diabetes educator. Unlike doctors, who have limited time to spend with you, certified diabetes educators (CDEs) have more time to answer questions and are there to help you solve frustrations. If you're feeling overwhelmed with your medication regimen or you don't understand why you're not seeing better results, don't keep it to yourself; diabetes is a big issue to tackle, and there's no reason to go it alone.

Join an online diabetes community. Sometimes there's nothing better than talking with someone who knows what you're going through. Through online forums (or "discussion boards") you can find people who share the very same challenges you're facing—and listen to how they solved them. You could create your own blog and post how you are doing each day, or take part in an existing one. Either way, you'll have a place where you can go whenever you feel you need to soak up some support or to get out of your own head by helping others with diabetes. The message boards of the American Diabetes Association at www.diabetes.org are a good place to start.

Look for a stress management class at a nearby hospital. Chronic stress might be especially harmful to people with diabetes because it can raise blood sugar and shelve your motivation to eat healthy and exercise. Plus, depression, which is a common response to stress, raises the risk of heart disease. When Duke University researchers provided more than 100 people with diabetes-education classes—some with and some without stress-relief training—those who got the stress-relief training improved their blood sugar significantly compared to those who didn't.

---

live well today!

Exercise whether you feel like it or not.

The biggest benefit to regular exercise is a significant improvement in mood. In a study of more than 150 men and women aged 50 and over with major depression, regular aerobic exercise over the course of four months (30 minutes of moderately intense walking or jogging three times a week) was shown to be just as effective as antidepressant medications. A single exercise session can also boost your mood and help give you the energy to do it again.

Angry? Scared? Pretend that you are a caring friend, and write yourself a letter. You will have days when you just don't want to have diabetes. That's completely normal. It's when you closet your worries, fears, and frustrations without addressing them that they eventually get bigger. It's great to be able to call a friend when you're feeling lousy, but if no one is around, be your own best friend. Grab a piece of paper or sit down at your computer and send yourself an e-mail message. What would you say to someone who was feeling the way you are? Be kind, gentle, and supportive.

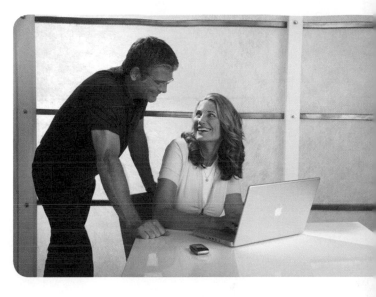

Visualize success. Thinking about your dreams and aspirations for the future can help stoke the fire that keeps your motivation strong. Sit down, close your eyes, and imagine what you want to be doing in the future. Do you want to be alive and healthy in 20 years to enjoy your grandchildren? In 10 years for a healthy, active retirement? In five years, so that you can start a family or enjoy the one you have?

Can't figure out what's eating you? HALT! It's an oldie but goodie: Anytime something's eating at you—you're irritable, feeling sad, or can't shake a feeling of doom—stop and ask yourself if you are Hungry, Angry, Lonely, or Tired (HALT). If it's been too long since your last meal, you might be feeling irritable because your blood sugar is low. If it's anger you're feeling, you need to pinpoint what's upsetting you, so you can work through it. Lonely? Call a friend. Finally, have you been getting enough sleep? Being overly fatigued can throw off your mood.

Are You Burned Out?

Many people newly diagnosed with diabetes start out motivated to make all the necessary changes to take care of themselves. But as time goes by, it's common to start feeling drained or overwhelmed, something experts refer to as "diabetes burnout." To help determine if you might be experiencing burnout, ask yourself if the six statements below are true or false.

1. My diabetes is taking up too much of my mental and physical energy every day.
2. I feel too exhausted, fatigued, or "burned out" by the constant effort it takes to manage my diabetes.
3. I feel like I am often failing with my diabetes regimen.
4. I feel like diabetes controls my life.
5. I'm not motivated to keep up with my diabetes treatment plan.
6. I feel completely overwhelmed by my diabetes.

> Through online forums you can find people who share the very same challenges you face—and learn how they solved them.

live well
this week!

Schedule some laugh-it-up dates.

Get together with a rowdy group of friends once a week or make a date to go see a comedian with your spouse. Just taking yourself out to a comedy club or renting a funny movie can perk you up when you are feeling down. Bonus: Laughing boosts your heart health, according to a study from the University of Maryland Medical Center in Baltimore. Researchers there found that of 300 adults, those who had heart disease were 40 percent less likely to laugh than those without heart troubles.

If you answered true to more than two of the above, you might be experiencing burnout. Your first step is to talk to your doctor, a certified diabetes educator, or a counselor. Maybe your medications or shots can be adjusted so that you don't have to take so many throughout your day. Or maybe counseling will help you learn new strategies for easing stress and improving your mood. Follow these tips.

Remind yourself that when it comes to blood sugar, better control equals a better life. One study, published in the *Journal of the American Medical Association*, compared quality of life in people with diabetes who had good blood-sugar control with peers who didn't. Those with good control had milder symptoms, felt better, and were more likely to feel mentally sharp than the other group. As a result, they tended to be more productive and less restricted in every aspect of life. Don't you want to be one of those people?

Take charge of your future. Remember that diabetes is very manageable and that most aspects of diabetes management are under your direct control. Don't accept complications or worsening blood sugar as inevitabilities—even if friends or relatives with diabetes have suffered serious diabetes-related complications. It doesn't have to happen to you.

Know what's at stake. An estimated three out of five people with diabetes have one or more complications associated with the disease, ranging from heart disease to vision loss to nerve pain to kidney damage. The key to avoiding complications is keeping your blood-sugar levels in check—which *Reverse Diabetes Forever* aims to do. Stick with it and you'll see results—we promise!

Back out of one activity. If you're having a rough day and feeling overwhelmed, cut yourself some slack. If you have a mental to-do list, prioritize the items and move the bottom one to a day or two later. If your mother calls, tell her honestly that you don't have time to talk and will call her back tomorrow when you can spend more time with her on the phone.

Bounce Back from Adversity

The art of becoming more resilient can enable you to weather the ups and downs of life with diabetes. The best news: You can learn and practice the ability to draw on your inner strength and to bounce back from whatever life throws in your path. Developing a positive attitude, maintaining a sense of humor, and knowing when to reach out for help are crucial. You'll learn how to master all three.

Anyone can be happy on a gorgeous spring day when all you have to do is stroll through a garden and hear the birds singing. But it's another thing altogether to be joyful, content, and upbeat on a slushy winter day when your car's broken down, your blood sugar is too high, there's little time for exercise or choosing healthy foods, or you haven't quite reached the goals you've set for yourself.

That's when you need resilience, the ability to deal with life's curveballs and challenges. It's a trait anyone can cultivate—and one that helps people with diabetes to thrive. In one recent University of Texas at Austin study of people with type 2 diabetes, those who took weekly resilience-training classes for just one month saw improvements in their cholesterol levels, blood pressure, and fasting blood-sugar levels—and they felt less stressed.

Researchers have identified four common traits of resilient people, traits that this chapter will help you develop.

▶ Seeing a challenge as an opportunity, not a threat.

▶ Having a strong value system to guide their decisions and actions.

▶ Being genuinely committed to the people in their lives and activities in which they're involved.

▶ Feeling a sense of control and believing they have the power to make things better.

Even if you're on the low end of the resiliency scale now, you can take the following steps today to build your inner resiliency.

Don Your Rose-Colored Glasses

It's hard to relax and feel good about yourself when your inner critic is constantly feeding you negative messages. Here's how, as the old song goes, you can accentuate the positive and eliminate the negative—and, in the bargain, start reclaiming the joy in your life.

Stop dwelling on "poor me." Almost everyone has at least one major problem to deal with in life, be it a health problem, a financial challenge, or marital trouble. If you catch yourself having a pity party because of your diabetes, remind yourself that no one's life is perfect. Then take a few minutes to remind yourself of the future you've visualized, and tell yourself that it's up to you to make it happen by eating healthy, staying active, and monitoring your blood sugar (and acting on the results).

Spend 10 minutes in the morning contemplating the day ahead. Sit with your cup of coffee, tea, or juice, and set positive and conscious intentions for how you want your day to go and what you'll need to do to make sure it happens. Do you have your medications organized and your monitor ready to go? When will you fit in your daily walk?

Do You Need an Attitude Adjustment?

Having a can-do attitude starts with being willing to make some changes in your life to improve your health. But being diagnosed with a chronic disease like diabetes can send a person through a series of emotions similar to the stages of grief. It's not a linear process; you may find yourself skipping stages or regressing to stages you already went through. The most productive stage, of course, is acceptance.

Denial: "This can't be happening to me!" If you are feeling disbelief or numbness about your diabetes, you might be in denial. A certain level of denial in the beginning can be positive because it protects you from over-worrying about all the possible outcomes of having a progressive disease.

Anger: "Why is this happening to me?" It's true that you didn't cause your own diabetes; your genes played a big part. So it's not unnatural to be angry at having the condition. But anger is most useful when you channel it in a positive way—like becoming determined to do absolutely everything in your power to beat the disease.

Bargaining: If you're a person of faith you may catch yourself making deals with God, such as, "I'll be extra careful about eating healthy and exercising if you'll keep me off insulin." That's bargaining.

Depression: "I don't care anymore." This is the worst stage to get stuck in because when you're depressed you're much less likely to take good care of your health. If your depression lasts more than two weeks or becomes severe, call your doctor for help.

Acceptance: "I'm ready for whatever comes."

If you haven't packed a healthy lunch, what's your game plan for buying one? If you have a hectic day ahead, think about specific strategies you'll use to help you stay calm, such as deep breathing. Remember that keeping your stress levels in check will help you manage your blood sugar better. You can write down your thoughts and answers, just think about them, or pray to a higher power to help you succeed.

Get in the habit of giving thanks. Before you get out of bed in the morning, prior to eating a meal, and when you're preparing to go to bed, take a moment to appreciate the things you might typically take for granted, such as having shelter, regular meals, clean water, clothes, and friends. And don't forget to be grateful for access to health insurance, top-rate medications, and the ability to improve your well-being with diet and exercise. Counting your blessings will make you more aware of how lucky you really are.

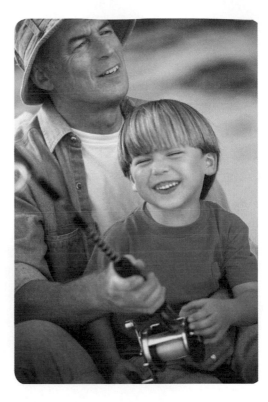

Say "no" to your inner skeptic. When a "downer" thought threatens to drag you into the deep, fight back. If you find yourself thinking that you'll never lose weight or get your blood sugar under control, tell yourself "no!" in your firmest, most commanding voice, whether you do it in your head or out loud. Sometimes this is all it takes to stop nagging, negative thoughts from snowballing into a defeatist attitude.

Now think again. Once you've successfully stalled a negative thought, it's time to put something more positive in its place. If you were thinking along the lines of, "I'll never change," or "I'll always be sick," try to be more objective, specific, and fair with yourself. Are there other ways for you to look at the situation? For example, "I'm feeling lousy right now. Maybe my blood sugar is low. I'll check it and see if I should have a snack."

Avoid toxic people. You've met them...they're the ones at the water cooler sharing the most downbeat of the office scuttlebutt. Or they're the parents constantly finding fault with your child's school, or they're the relatives or friends whose topics constantly focus on the depths of their unhappiness. Instead of these "Debbie Downers," seek out friends with optimistic attitudes and intact senses of humor. They'll help you brighten up, even on your worst days.

Focus on all the reasons that you'll succeed, not the reasons that you'll fail. You're eating better, you've started exercising more, your doctor recently put you on a new drug or changed the dosage, you're checking your blood sugar on schedule, and in general, you're a competent person who's succeeded at other things in life. In short, the deck is stacked in favor of you succeeding at managing your diabetes. Focus on these "success" cards in the deck, not on any perceived "doomed-to-fail" cards, like your weakness for bagels or past problems with your weight.

As the old song goes, you can accentuate the positive and eliminate the negative to reclaim the joy in your life.

A sense of humor is part of the resiliency toolbox. And when it comes to your blood sugar, laughter is good medicine, too.

Keep a deity, a peace lily, or a worry stone on your desk. Choose a tangible object that symbolizes positive energy, tranquility, or victory to you, and keep it where you can see it during your day. Most times, it really doesn't take much to "check yourself back into" an attitude you can capitalize on and move forward with. Maybe your object is simply a shell from a beautiful beach or a trinket that's a sign of your faith. If you hit a rough patch in your day, hold, touch, or look at your object and think about what it means to you.

Post a picture of an inspirational person on your refrigerator or bathroom mirror. People who were successes despite huge obstacles are great reminders that "you can do it!" no matter what you face. Your hero might be Rosa Parks, Gandhi, or your own grandfather. You'll get an instant morale boost when you stop to comb your hair or make a meal and you see his or her face.

Don't say anything to yourself that you wouldn't say to someone else. Many of us are so used to being hard on ourselves that we don't even notice that we're doing it. What

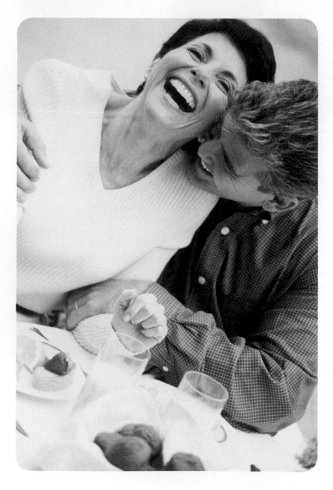

do you say to yourself when your blood sugar spikes or you forget to take a pill? Is it helpful or belittling? A good way to check is to ask, "Would I say this out loud to a friend?" If the answer is no, it's a good sign that you're not being fair to yourself or helpful to your cause. Instead, think of what you would say to a friend to be helpful and encouraging, and use that dialogue with yourself.

Pamper yourself at least once a month. Indulging in regular manicures, pedicures, massages, or facials will boost your self-esteem. Taking the time to give yourself some TLC reinforces the idea that you're worth it.

Manage your expectations. Don't expect that every aspect of managing your health, or your life, will always go perfectly; it won't. For instance, if you expect everything to be smooth when you travel by airplane these days, you're setting yourself up for disappointment. Instead, anticipate delays and lost luggage; bring extra reading material or playing cards, and don't put anything you can't live without—especially your diabetes medications—in your checked luggage.

Pinch yourself every time you hear yourself using words like "never" and "always." As in, "I always seem to eat foods I shouldn't" or "I'm never going to get my blood sugar under control or lose weight." Such thinking leads to a black-and-white, all-or-nothing defeatist mentality that's sure to make you stumble in your efforts to reverse diabetes. If you mess up one day, forgive yourself. Remind yourself that everyone's human and that at least you're trying. Then vow to do better tomorrow!

Set daily goals. You need a sense of accomplishment every day to strengthen your own belief in yourself. These goals could be small—eating one extra vegetable serving, going to bed 15 minutes earlier—but don't worry, they'll add up. And remember that success often breeds more success.

Smile First, Then Laugh

A sense of humor is part of the resiliency toolbox. And when it comes to your blood sugar, laughter is good medicine, too. That's the conclusion drawn by scientists at the University of Tsukuba in Japan who kept tabs on the blood-sugar levels of 19 men and women with high blood sugar after they attended two radically different events: a boring lecture and a hilarious comedy show. The study was published in the journal *Diabetes Care*.

Before both events, volunteers each ate a 500-calorie meal. Afterward, their blood sugar was tested. Sugar levels were significantly lower after the comedy. Why is mirth magic for your sugar levels? Laughter makes us move (ever try to sit perfectly still while you laugh? Impossible!)—and muscle cells absorb more blood sugar when they're active, the researchers speculate. Comic relief may also influence hormones that play a role in blood sugar absorption.

Of course, having a sense of humor also makes it far easier to sail through the ups and downs of daily life. It vaporizes fear, relaxes your mind and body, helps you keep things in perspective, and gives you an outlet for negative emotions. It might even help you lose weight.

Have fun! When is the last time you had fun? If a recent memory doesn't pop into your mind, it's time to ink some fun onto your calendar. It doesn't have to be elaborate, just something you look forward to. Once a week, set up a golf date, rent a funny movie, go to a comedy club, or take your kids or grandkids to the park. You'll feel less bogged down by daily life if you regularly reward yourself with good times.

Find absurdity in annoyance. You can blunt all but the day's worst trouble spots with a healthy dose of humor. Boss ignoring you in a meeting? Focus on his silly comb-over. Stuck in a too-long line when you're late? Silently pretend you're with the fashion police, then rate everyone's outfit.

Watch a comedy instead of a tearjerker. University of Mississippi researchers have found that study volunteers munched 30 percent more buttered popcorn while watching the classic romance *Love Story* compared to when they guffawed their way through the comedy *Sweet Home Alabama*. So put comedies at the top of your list when you're heading to the video store or choosing a movie on TV or online. These

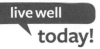

live well today!

Feeling burned out or downright depressed? Take a short walk. Numerous studies show that regular exercise improves depression. In one, getting 30 minutes of moderately intense activity three times a week for four months was as effective as antidepressant medication. (If you have depression and take medication, a walk is a great add-on therapy.) A single walk can boost your mood and give you motivation to do it again tomorrow.

live well
forever+

Maintain a positive, can-do attitude.

By looking on the bright side, you can significantly cut your risk for diabetes complications. In a study of 165 people with type 2 diabetes, those who were motivated to take charge of their diabetes were 55 percent less likely to have a heart attack, 53 percent less likely to have a stroke, and 50 percent less likely to have severe kidney damage over 7½ years. Their blood-sugar levels were lower, and their blood pressure and cholesterol levels were healthier than people who were less motivated to care for themselves.

10 top the American Film Institute's list of the 100 Funniest Films: *Some Like It Hot, Tootsie, Dr. Strangelove, Annie Hall, Duck Soup, Blazing Saddles, M*A*S*H, It Happened One Night, The Graduate,* and *Airplane!*

Call your funniest friend. Everybody has someone who makes them laugh. Keep your funniest pal's phone number on speed dial so you can chat regularly—both of you will get a boost.

Choose funny books. Act like a kid at the library or bookstore and head for the humor section instead of the serious literature. Stock up on a few by your favorite humor writers, such as Dave Barry or David Sedaris. Or try a few authors you've never read before. Not only will you get a few laughs, you'll also get an education in seeing the hilarious side of things that would normally frustrate or upset you.

Laugh at your foibles. Finding humor in your own life doesn't mean laughing at who you are. It means finding the funny side of what you're doing, what you're thinking, or what's happening to you. Did you get lost on your walk when exploring a new neighborhood? Silly you! But hey, it made you walk a few extra blocks—so you benefited in the end.

When a person upsets you, respond with humor, not hostility. For instance, if someone is always late, say, "Well, I'm glad you're not running an airline." Life is too short to turn every personal affront into a battle. If someone in particular constantly offends you, take it seriously and take appropriate action. But for occasional troubles, or if nothing you do can change the person or situation, take the humor response.

Cultivate the humor habit. Have a ha-ha bulletin board, where you post funny sayings or signs. Every night at dinner, ask family members to share one funny moment of their day. Develop a silly routine to break a dark mood. It could be something as silly as speaking in a crazy accent, doing a little dance, or repeating a funny punch line from a movie or TV show that always cracks you up. And add an item to your daily to-do list: Find something humorous. Don't mark it off until you do it.

Recognize Depression

Let's get right to the heart of the matter. There are three things you absolutely must know and, more important, believe, about depression.

1. IT IS A REAL DISEASE.

Depression is *not* a prolonged period of moodiness, or a downbeat reaction to the world around you, or a perpetually negative disposition. It's a formal disease. Meaning there is a physical component (out-of-balance brain chemicals), a set of common symptoms, a way to diagnose it, and a way to cure it.

2. DIABETES AND DEPRESSION ARE LINKED.

Having one significantly increases your likelihood of developing the other, according to a study in the *Archives of Internal Medicine*. The link goes in both directions. People diagnosed with depression have a greater risk of getting type 2 diabetes, and if you have diabetes, your chances of having clinical depression are more than double those of people of the same age and general condition who don't have diabetes.

3. IF YOU HAVE DIABETES, YOU ARE DEFINITELY AT RISK.

In one recent overseas study, fully one-third of patients attending diabetes clinics met the criteria for having depression. Yet few were diagnosed or getting care for the condition. While there hasn't been a parallel study done in the United States, some estimates put the rate of depression among people with diabetes at over 20 percent.

Why does this matter? Because depression is far more serious than just a few days or weeks of feeling down. Not only does it make your life so much less than it can be, depression also raises your risk of other chronic conditions, including heart disease, pain, and obesity. And depression has a ripple effect, making life harder for those you love and those around you.

Most cases of depression go undiagnosed, yet it is one of the most treatable mental health conditions. The keys to it all? Patience and persistence. Just as it takes time to arrive at the right mix of medications and lifestyle adjustments to best manage your diabetes, it will take time for you and your doctor to find the right combination of treatments for your depression. Expect to feel like your old, depression-free self again, and be sure to tell your doctor if you don't. It's worth the effort—and the collaboration. Trying to work out depression on your own can be dangerous, and it's not necessary. Your doctor can help.

While everyone will have occasional days when they feel so wiped out that they won't have the energy to make a healthy salad for lunch or get out and walk, you should know when your symptoms mean something more serious. If you've been experiencing five or more of the following signs and symptoms for two weeks or longer, you could be clinically depressed and should see a doctor or qualified mental health professional for evaluation and help.

▸ You feel persistently sad or anxious.
▸ Your sleep patterns have changed (wanting to sleep all the time or not being able to fall or stay asleep).
▸ You're experiencing a loss of appetite and weight loss or an increase in appetite and weight gain.
▸ You have lost your pleasure and interest in previously enjoyable activities.
▸ You are frequently restless or irritable.
▸ You have difficulty concentrating, remembering, or making decisions.
▸ You feel constantly fatigued or drained of energy.
▸ You constantly feel guilty, hopeless, or worthless.
▸ You are thinking about suicide or death.

While building resiliency may help you lower your risk for depression, it's important to watch out for signs of depression, understand when it's time to seek help, and know what you can do on your own. Self-care strategies can be helpful, but don't substitute them for regular visits with your doctor.

Busting the Blues

Fortunately, many approaches can lift your mood. The trick is to find the ones that work for you. You'd be a rare person if you tried just one of these strategies and it worked—for most people, a sustained combination approach will be the most suc-

live well
right now!

You deserve to feel better.

The trouble is, most people with depression aren't getting the help they need. Thanks to wrong-headed beliefs that this mental health problem is a sign of weakness (or something you can "tough out" on your own) and to doctors who don't routinely check or treat depression, millions of us just continue to slog along. If that sounds like you or someone you know, stop now. Call your doctor, ask for an evaluation, and sign up for treatment. No one should go through life feeling sad and hopeless. There's just too much at stake.

Depression and Medication

For many people, medication can help jump-start a happier outlook. And with scores of different antidepressants available worldwide, chances are one will work for you if you need it. Two of the main drug classes—tricyclics like amitriptyline (Elavil) and imipramine (Tofranil) and selective serotonin-reuptake inhibitors (SSRIs) like fluoxetine (Prozac) and paroxetine (Paxil)—work equally well. But SSRIs tend to have fewer side effects such as weight gain and dry mouth, and studies find that patients are more likely to stick with them. New data suggests that two SSRIs together often work significantly better than one alone.

One of the newest antidepressants is venlafaxine (Effexor). Unlike an SSRI, which works only to increase the amount of the mood-related chemical serotonin in the brain, Effexor increases the amounts of serotonin and norepinephrine. When researchers pooled data from eight well-designed studies that compared Effexor to SSRIs or a placebo, they found that scores on three depression scales declined more in people taking Effexor than in those taking SSRIs or placebos.

You may have to try several drugs or drug combinations to find one that relieves your depression without unacceptable side effects. That said, some doctors are hesitant to switch patients from one antidepressant to another without first increasing the dosage or giving it enough time to work. Generally, if you don't show any improvement within two to four weeks of taking the highest recommended dose (which could be six weeks or more after you start taking the drug), it's time to switch. Note that most side effects abate within one to two weeks of starting the medication.

cessful. And as with any chronic illness, don't expect overnight miracles. It will take a few weeks, perhaps even months of diligence before you begin feeling well again. Don't think that if one or two approaches don't work that you're doomed to suffer with depression. If after several weeks of diligence, whatever you're trying isn't working, talk to your doctor and try something else. Most likely, he or she will tap into a combination of these eight approaches.

Mindfulness classes. Mindfulness-Based Stress Reduction (MBSR) is a structured, eight-week long program that combines aspects of meditation and yoga. It began back in 1979 and was developed by Jon Kabat-Zinn, PhD at the University of Massachusetts Medical Center in Boston. In a 2007 study conducted at the Jefferson Medical College of Thomas Jefferson University in Philadelphia, researchers studied a small group of people with type 2 diabetes and discovered that taking an MSBR course decreased their feelings of depression, anxiety, and distress. What's more, the course actually improved their A1C levels and their blood pressure. Scores of studies have attested to the practice's promise for reducing depression and its ability to improve well-being. Leading medical centers around the world now offer the program. To learn more and find a program near you, visit http://w3.umassmed.edu/MBSR/public/searchmember.aspx.

Therapy. A well-trained, experienced therapist listens incredibly well, and is full of insights, compassion, and wisdom that truly can help you change your outlook on life, and how you react to its challenges. Look for a therapist who practices cognitive behavioral therapy or interpersonal therapy, in which you learn to cope better with stress, improve your interactions with others, and deal with the effects of depression. Studies find these two forms work best. If after three months, your mental state remains unchanged, you may need to see a psychiatrist who can offer talk therapy and prescribe appropriate antidepressants.

Workouts. The same endorphins that contribute to "runner's high" can provide natural relief for depression, and help prevent a relapse, if you can just manage to get yourself off the couch. In one study that pitted brisk walking or jogging against sertraline (Zoloft) or a combination of the drug plus the exercise, after 16 weeks all three groups had about the same improvement, but at six months, the people who kept up the exercise had the lowest rates of recurring sadness. Just 50 minutes of exercise a week reduced the risk of relapse by 50 percent. It doesn't seem to matter what form of exercise you do: Aerobics, strength training, and flexibility exercises like yoga all seem to provide similar benefits.

St. John's wort. This wild yellow flowering plant (*Hypericum perforatum*) has been used as a mood-enhancing medicine for centuries, especially in Europe. And under the spotlight of modern science, it is holding up fairly well. St. John's wort has been shown in studies to be as much as 71 percent more effective than placebos for treating mild to moderate depression. Trials comparing St. John's wort to antidepressants found they both worked about the same, although patients were less likely to drop out of the trials if they took the herb, because it had fewer side effects. Note that the herb has not been proven effective for what doctors call major depression.

SAM-e. SAM-e is short for S-adenosyl methionine, a naturally occurring molecule found in the cells of plants, animals, and humans. With age, our bodies produce less of this chemical, and some experts believe that taking it as a supplement to treat certain diseases makes sense. As it turns out, research suggests that it provides some benefit in the treatment of depression—which makes sense, because SAM-e is necessary

Kick the Habit

If you're a smoker with diabetes, getting cigarettes out of your life should be your top priority. Diabetes is already putting your heart and blood vessels at risk; they don't need any more trouble from tobacco. Need even more incentive? Some 90 percent of people with diabetes who need to have a foot amputated are smokers. Your best quitting strategies:

Counseling programs and cognitive behavioral therapy. These train you to solve practical problems related to quitting (for instance, if you always light up when you pour your morning coffee, maybe you need to switch to tea or have your coffee in a nonsmoking environment); include social support, such as pairing you with a nonsmoking "buddy" you can call when you feel the need to smoke; and help you set up social support outside of therapy. Ask your doctor for a referral.

Nicotine replacement. These include gums, patches, lozenges, inhalers, and nasal spray. It doesn't matter if you get your nicotine fix with a prescription product or an over-the-counter product; both are equally effective.

Bupropion. This antidepressant doubles the success of the nicotine patch compared to using the patch alone. And it seems to reduce the weight gain so common after quitting.

Exercise. Exercising three times a week may work even better than a behavioral therapy program (of course, doing both is ideal). One study found that nearly 20 percent of the exercisers were still smoke free after a year compared to 11 percent of the therapy group.

for the production of the mood-boosting brain chemicals serotonin and dopamine. What's more, it also helps boost production of glutathione, a potent antioxidant.

A major review of studies on this supplement found that SAM-e improved symptoms of depression 27 to 38 percent better than placebos. The review also found that SAM-e was as effective as tricyclic antidepressants. And a study released in 2010 by researchers at Harvard Medical School and Massachusetts General Hospital in Boston suggested that SAM-e might help depressed patients who don't respond to prescription antidepressants.

Qigong. One activity worth trying, particularly if you're 60 or older, is qigong (pronounced chee-guhn), an ancient Chinese martial art that combines steady, slow movements with breathing patterns. In a Hong Kong study, people diagnosed with depression who participated in qigong surpassed the control group in every measure after eight weeks.

Omega-3 supplements. The same fish oil, or omega-3 fatty acid supplements, that can help your heart may also have the power to ease depression. In fact, in a 2011 pilot study, researchers from Harvard Medical School discovered that when women suffering from major depressive disorder and menopausal hot flashes took two grams of an omega-3 supplement, their depression scores on a standard test plummeted—from 24.2 before treatment to 10.7 eight weeks later. In fact, 70 percent of the women responded to the treatment, and depression went into remission for 45 percent. As a bonus, their hot flashes also improved significantly.

And in one review of 10 studies, researchers found that high doses of fish oil improved depression significantly better than placebos, though the researchers noted that more large-scale, well-controlled trials are needed due to problems with the existing studies. You may need to take as much as four grams daily, so check with your doctor before starting.

Electroconvulsive therapy (ECT). Though it sounds like the treatment of last resort, modern ECT is far removed from what was depicted in movies like *One Flew Over the Cuckoo's Nest*. Today, ECT treatments use lower bursts of electricity and are given along with sedatives, and seem to cause changes in brain chemistry. Often, severe cases of depression and other mental illnesses respond immediately—especially for people who've been resistant to other therapies.

live well
this month!

Connect with a cognitive behavioral therapist.

Worrying too much and ruminating too long on your troubles often underlies depression, and cognitive behavioral therapy (CBT), a form of psychotherapy aimed at changing thoughts and behaviors that may be contributing to depression, can help change such habits. After a few weeks of such continued worrying, it's likely time to call on professional help. Find a certified practitioner at www.nacbt.org, the website of the National Association of Cognitive-Behavioral Therapists.

Prepare for the Unexpected

Disruptions to your routine can make managing your blood sugar tougher. When you travel, difficult schedules, security concerns, jet lag, and crowds can cause even dedicated diabetes managers to be temporarily thrown off course. Illness can alter your eating and exercise habits and make it more difficult to take medications at the right times—and both can increase the risk of raising your blood sugar or causing hypoglycemia. Planning ahead will make it easier to take good care of yourself should either one arise. Here's what you need to know and to do.

Your Prescription When You're Sick

Being sick is no fun for anyone, but it takes a special toll if you have diabetes because it can throw off your blood sugar and put you at risk for short-term complications. The best way to deal with sick days is to plan for them before you're laid up. Speak with your primary-care physician, endocrinologist, and dietitian to work out the details of a strategy you can put into action the next time a cold, the flu, or something else strikes.

Illness is a form of stress that—like emotional stress—rouses the body's defenses. One effect is that the liver steps up glucose production to provide more energy. At the same time, stress hormones are released that make cells more insulin resistant.

The net result is that blood sugar can rise dramatically when you're ill. To keep your blood sugar in check and help yourself feel better faster, follow these steps.

Step up your monitoring. It's more important than ever to keep careful track of your blood-sugar levels, so you'll probably need to test yourself more often than you usually do—at least every three to four hours. If your blood sugar goes higher than 240 mg/dL, do a urine ketone test as well. If ketone results are positive, or if your blood sugar consistently hovers above 240, call your doctor.

Talk to your doctor. Call the doctor's office if you're unable to eat, have diarrhea, have been vomiting for more than six hours, have a fever that's not improving, or have flushed skin for more than two days. Know the signs of ketoacidosis (which include stomach pain, vomiting, chest pain, difficulty breathing, feelings of weakness, sleepiness, fruity-smelling breath, and blurry vision) and of dehydration (extreme thirst, dry mouth, cracked lips, sunken eyes, mental confusion, dry skin). Call your doctor right away if you experience symptoms of either of these conditions.

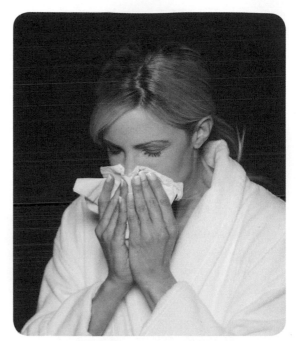

Get plenty of fluids. This familiar advice is doubly critical when you have diabetes because water is drawn into excess glucose and excreted in the urine, which can cause dehydration. Aim to drink a cup of fluid (which includes soup broth) every half hour or so. If lack of appetite is making it difficult for you to consume enough food to meet your energy needs, sip sugared drinks like non-diet soda, fruit juices, or sports beverages instead of plain water to make sure you're getting at least some calories into your body.

Stay the drug course. Unless your doctor instructs you otherwise, it's important to keep taking your medications or giving yourself insulin even if you're not up to eating. In fact, your doctor may want you to take more insulin when you're feeling under the weather, with the exact amounts depending on your blood-sugar readings and how sick you are. Even if you have type 2 diabetes and don't normally take insulin, your doctor may want you to keep a vial of short-acting insulin on hand in case he thinks it's necessary when illness strikes.

Watch the OTC remedies. Some common over-the-counter medicines, such as decongestants with pseudoephedrine, can raise blood sugar. Check with your doctor before taking any drug, herbal remedy, or dietary supplement when you're ill.

Rest in bed. It isn't safe to exercise when you're sick, diabetes experts say. Instead, do your immune system and blood sugar a favor by dimming the lights and hopping into bed. It's a good idea to arrange in advance to have your spouse or a close friend or neighbor take over household responsibilities when you're sick, so that you can rest

Planning ahead for a vacation or an illness will help you take good care of yourself when you're temporarily thrown off course.

Stock up on diabetes essentials.

Sometime in the next 30 days, make it a point to stock up on sick-day foods. Even when you don't have an appetite, it's important to eat regularly to keep your blood sugar steady. Start with foods that are already part of a healthy diet, such as oatmeal, chicken soup, applesauce, or toast. Stash a supply of broth-based soups, along with your favorite whole-wheat crackers.

and recover. See if the kids can spend the evening with a neighbor (offer to reciprocate as soon as you can) and ask if your spouse could make dinner and do laundry.

Your Prescription on the Road

Planning a family vacation or a business trip? Make sure that while you're getting away from it all, your blood sugar isn't. Your mantra: Plan ahead. Let your doctor know your itinerary. Depending on how long you'll be gone, she may want to give you a thorough examination before you depart. And to ensure smooth sailing, heed the following advice.

Anticipate airport security. With the increased security at airports, expect your supplies to get a thorough once-over. The U.S. Transportation Security Administration (TSA), as of press time, allows you to board a plane with insulin, syringes, and insulin-delivery systems. It's okay to carry lancets on board as well, as long as they're capped and you also carry a glucose meter with a manufacturer's name printed on it. The American Diabetes Association recommends that you notify the screener at security checkpoints that you have diabetes and are carrying your supplies with you. For the most up-to-date information about security and diabetes, see the Fact Sheet: Air Travel and Diabetes online at http://www.diabetes.org.

At press time, the TSA doesn't require prescription labels or a doctor's letter, but it's a good idea to have prescription drugs labeled and to be sure that nonprescription items essential for your diabetes care are also clearly labeled in original containers. It will make security screening faster. Be sure to call ahead for current policies before you leave or check the TSA website, www.tsa.gov.

Keep glucose goods close at hand. If you are traveling by plane, pack your medications, insulin, syringes, test strips, lancets, ketone strips, and other supplies in your carry-on bag so there's no chance of losing them. Consider bringing extra supplies in your checked luggage. Some experts recommend packing twice as much as you think you'll need—it's easier to carry extra than to get more on the road. Also ask your doctor if he wants to prescribe a glucagon kit, which contains an emergency dose of a hormone that someone with you can inject if you have a hypoglycemic emergency and are unable to swallow or you lose consciousness. Again, make sure all medications bear the original pharmacy prescription labels.

Bring extra prescriptions and a medication list, too. In case you do need to restock while you're away, have your doctor give you prescriptions for refills. It's also a good idea to have him provide a printout of all your medications in case you need to see a doctor while on the road.

Wear a medical-alert bracelet. If you don't already have one, get a medical ID bracelet or necklace that alerts people that you have diabetes and provides a number to call in an emergency.

Pack a snack. Wherever you go, take a tote-able snack like an apple, an energy bar, a banana, raisins, or cheese and crackers in case your blood sugar starts to dip when you don't have immediate access to other food. If you sample your snacks en route, replenish your supplies as soon as you can.

Maintain regular mealtimes. When traveling, try to stick to your regular mealtime schedule to keep your blood sugar stable. If that's not possible, carry glucose tablets along with you and be alert to symptoms of low blood sugar, such as nervousness, sweating, and crankiness. If you feel a hypoglycemic episode coming on when you're driving, pull over and take several glucose tablets. Wait at least 10 to 15 minutes for the feeling to pass before continuing on.

Monitor insulin needs carefully. Traveling across different time zones can throw your normal insulin and meal schedule completely out of kilter, but you can compensate for the disruption if you're careful. When adding hours to your day by traveling west, you may need to take more insulin. When losing hours by traveling east, you may need less. Check with your doctor for specific recommendations. As for timing your injections and meals, keep your watch set to your home time as you travel to your destination, then switch your watch—and your schedule—to the local time the morning after you arrive.

Walk, don't nosh. Catching a plane involves a whole lot of hurry up and wait. While you're waiting to board your plane, use that spare half-hour to stroll around the terminal rather than heading to the newsstand for an overpriced candy bar. If you combine the calories you'll burn moving your feet and the calories you save not chomping the chocolate, you'll end up saving over 400 calories.

Organize for overseas. If you're traveling outside the country, be aware that insulin you find abroad may be sold in weaker strengths than the insulin available in the

Foot Care for the Diabetes Traveler

Put together a small foot-care kit.

When you're traveling, you want to see and do everything you can in a short time. But zipping from vista to landmark not only can wear out your feet, it can make you susceptible to "hot spots" and blisters. Although they seem innocent enough, blisters can lead to infections that can quickly become serious for someone with diabetes. To keep your feet feeling fine, fill a ziplock bag with a few sheets of moleskin, several large and small adhesive bandages, and round-tipped scissors. As soon as you feel a hot spot developing, cut off a piece of moleskin large enough to cover the spot and stick it on. If you discover a full-fledged blister, cover it with a bandage.

Pack two pairs of comfortable shoes.

This way you can air out one pair while you tool around town in the other. Also bring a pair of brown or black closed-toe flats for dinners and other more formal occasions. All the shoes you bring should be broken in before your trip, so leave your new ones at home. If you're heading to the beach, bring aqua shoes. These stretchy-soled booties will protect your feet from hot sand, rough sidewalks around the pool, and sharp pebbles underfoot.

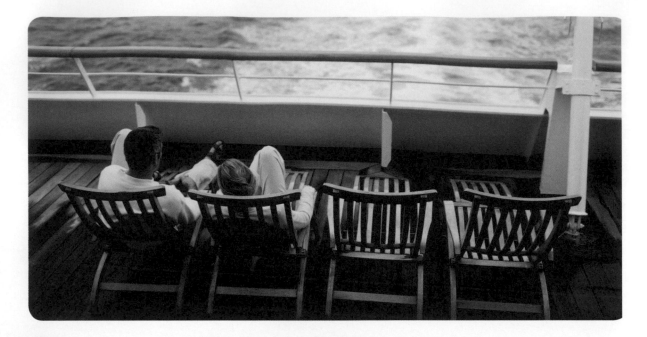

There's no reason diabetes should hold you back from traveling, as long as you take some reasonable precautions.

United States, which has standardized its insulin in a dose known as U-100. Each insulin strength (such as U-40 and U-80) requires specially matched syringes. Filling a different type of syringe with your U.S. insulin will make your dose inaccurate. Best bet: Stick to your own supplies. If you must buy insulin that's a different strength, also buy syringes to match.

Bring sunscreen. Certain diabetes and blood pressure drugs make the skin more sensitive to the sun, so it's especially important that you protect yourself. A bad sunburn can even raise your blood sugar and may take longer to heal than it would for someone else. Choose a sunscreen that has an SPF of at least 15 and look for a "broad-spectrum" brand that protects against both UVA and UVB light. These often contain ingredients such as Mexoryl, Helioplex, zinc oxide, or avobenzone (aka Parsol 1789).

Exercise on the go. It's tough to stay physically active when traveling—but not impossible. Try to keep your body in gear by planning ahead and snatching opportunities as they arise. If your hotel doesn't have an exercise room or pool, bring along a jump rope or elastic resistance band so you can exercise in your room. Definitely pack your walking shoes, and ask at the front desk about where you can take a safe and scenic stroll.

Pack comfortable "nice" clothes. If you're not attending a formal event, try to pack outfits that do double duty as walking gear and meeting or travel clothing. That way, you'll be able to seize small amounts of walking time with ease. Do the same for your feet, by bringing shoes you can wear to meetings and events and also walk in.

Alternative Remedies

You're following a meal plan, watching your weight, getting exercise, and possibly taking drugs or insulin for your diabetes. Are there any other tools that can help you to manage your blood sugar? Maybe. Some herbs and supplements show promise for bringing down blood sugar and protecting the eyes, nerves, kidneys, and heart. Therapies, such as biofeedback, massage, and acupuncture, can help reduce stress and relieve pain, including nerve pain. Should you try them? Before you decide to try them, here's what you need to know.

American doctors sometimes refer to nontraditional treatments as "CAM," which stands for complementary and alternative medicine. CAM emphasizes the fact that alternative therapies may sometimes be useful as an addition to, rather than a substitute for, traditional medical care. These days, a growing number of practitioners use the word "integrative" to refer to the fact that they borrow, in a mix-and-match style, the most studied and effective therapies from alternative and conventional medicine.

Be sure to ask your doctor about any supplement or alternative treatment you want to try, or at least inform your medical team of anything you're using. Many alternative treatments, especially herbs, can interfere with other medications and may affect how your doctor treats your diabetes.

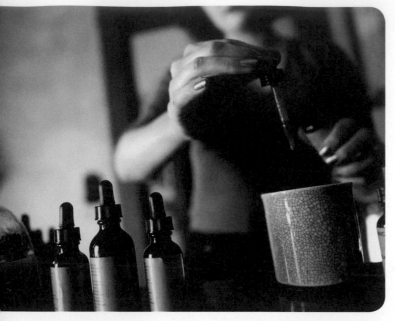

The Natural Medicine Cabinet

Some of the most popular alternative therapies for combating diabetes or its complications are herbal, vitamin, mineral and other dietary supplements.

Whether to use herbal remedies is a personal decision you'll need to make with the help of your doctor. Don't assume that "herbal" means "safe" or "effective" because, in most cases, herbal products don't undergo the same level of research that pharmaceutical drugs do. Because herbs cannot be patented, companies are less likely to invest in researching them. That's not to say herbs haven't been studied, though. Many have been, in Europe and in some American studies funded mainly by university medical centers.

The Federal Drug Administration (FDA) permits the sale of herbs under the Dietary Supplement Health and Education Act (DSHEA), which calls on manufacturers of all supplements (herbs, vitamins, and other dietary supplements) to ensure that their products are safe. Manufacturers also must make sure that product label information is truthful and not misleading. Responsible manufacturers do their best to ensure quality. To identify quality products, check the label for:

▶ The botanical name if the product is plant-based, and what part of the plant was used
▶ The recommended dose in milligrams (or in drops, if the product is a liquid tincture or extract)
▶ A batch or lot number and expiration date
▶ The manufacturer's name and address

> Whether or not to use herbal remedies is a personal decision you'll need to make with the help of your doctor.

Glucose Control through Herbal Therapy

The major goal of herbal therapies for diabetes is the same as for drugs and insulin: to bring down high blood sugar. Here's where it's important to remember that these therapies are complementary: Even if they work, you should never take them as a substitute for your insulin or regular medication, though they might be useful in lowering the doses you require.

It's extremely important that you monitor your blood sugar closely if you take these remedies, for two reasons. First, you won't know how effective they are unless you measure their impact on your glucose. Second, if they're able to bring blood sugar down, you need to be on the alert for an increased possibility of hypoglycemia. Third, if an herb does work for you, let your doctor know; she may be able to lower your medications. Unless otherwise noted, follow label directions on each product for appropriate dosage. Each of these herbs needs to be taken regularly for several weeks before you'll see a difference in your blood sugar.

Among the herbs that show the most promise for lowering blood sugar are:

Gymnema (*Gymnema sylvestre*). A staple in traditional Indian medicine (Ayurveda) for treating diabetes and obesity, this herb seems to lessen your ability to taste sweet substances—and may decrease your appetite for up to 90 minutes. In one 1990 study, insulin requirements were cut in half for 27 people with type 1 diabetes who took a 400-milligram extract of gymnema for 6 to 30 months, while the insulin needs of the control group didn't change. Researchers suspect gymnema might work by boosting the activity of enzymes that help cells use glucose or by stimulating insulin-producing beta cells in the pancreas. Safety studies haven't been done (so be cautious if you're pregnant or nursing or have liver or kidney disease), but the herb has no history of serious side effects.

Cinnamon (*Cinnamomum verum*). This spice rack favorite has a use beyond seasoning cookies and pies. Turns out, it can lower blood sugar, especially for people with metabolic syndrome or prediabetes. A landmark, gold-standard clinical study conducted in 2003 by USDA researchers showed that people with type 2 diabetes who consumed about ¼ teaspoon of cinnamon a day experienced drops in blood sugar ranging from 18 to 29 percent. What's more, folks in the cinnamon group also lowered their triglycerides by 23 to 30 lb, their total cholesterol by 13 to 20 percent, and their LDL (bad) cholesterol by 10 to 24 percent. A more recent review of several studies confirmed these results. However, cinnamon doesn't seem to help people on metformin or people with type 1 diabetes. Sprinkle it on toast or in cereal; do not exceed ¼ teaspoon a day.

Fenugreek (*Trigonella foenum-graecum*). A pea-family relative, fenugreek is used to flavor Indian dishes, including curries. In a 2014 study of 88 people with type 2 diabetes, participants who consumed 10 daily grams of fenugreek seeds lowered their fasting and average blood sugar levels over 8 weeks, compared to participants who didn't consume the seeds. Don't take fenugreek supplements if you're pregnant or have liver or kidney disease, and don't ingest it within two hours of taking an oral diabetes medication, because it may interfere with the body's absorption of the drug. Also be cautious if you're taking blood thinners; fenugreek may interact with these.

Bitter melon (*Mormodica charantia*). Not an herb but a vegetable, bitter melon has long been a folk remedy for diabetes in the East, and a number of studies in people suggest it may indeed have some benefits. In one study of 18 people with type 2 diabetes, 73 percent of those who drank about a half cup of bitter-melon juice (don't do this at home—it tastes terrible) saw significant drops in blood-sugar levels. In another study, five people who took 15 grams of bitter melon capsules brought their blood sugar down by 25 percent in three weeks. Substances in bitter melon may block

live well
this week!

Shop smart for herbal products.

If you're out on your weekly shopping run and you're looking for herbal supplements, don't buy herbal products that contain a laundry list of ingredients. Often, multi-herb combos contain too little of each herb to be effective.

sugar absorption in the intestine. Bitter melon may cause gastrointestinal distress and headaches; don't take it during pregnancy.

Ginseng (*Panax ginseng*, or Asian ginseng; *Panax quinquefolius*, or American ginseng). This ancient medicinal herb is said to have whole-body effects that make it broadly useful for building resistance to disease, recovering from illness, combating the physical effects of stress, and even promoting longer life. For this reason, herbalists classify ginseng as an "adaptogen," meaning it helps your body adapt to stressful conditions. Though the research into ginseng's effects on diabetes is far from conclusive, it's unusually strong and has appeared in respected peer-reviewed journals. In one University of Illinois study, published in a 2002 issue of the journal *Diabetes*, overweight mice with type 2 diabetes who were injected with an extract of Asian ginseng normalized their blood sugar, dropped 10 percent of their body weight, and lowered their cholesterol by about a third. A University of Toronto study published in the *Annals of Internal Medicine* in 2000 found that 10 people who took three grams of American ginseng 40 minutes before eating reduced their post-meal glucose levels by about 20 percent compared with a control group. Finally, an earlier study reported in *Diabetes Care* found that taking ginseng lowered A1C numbers in people with type 2. More recent research confirms these findings. Potential side effects may include headache, increased blood pressure, and insomnia. Ginseng can interfere with certain heart drugs and the blood thinner warfarin. Avoid bargain brands, which are unlikely to contain the purest ginseng.

The Nutritional Pharmacy

Certain vitamins and minerals may help control blood sugar and reduce the risk of complications. They're best when they come from foods—but should you get more of them from supplements? Here are three you might consider.

Biotin. The body needs only about 300 micrograms (a unit measuring one-millionth of a gram) of this B vitamin every day from foods like egg yolks, corn, and cauliflower for normal metabolism (including the breakdown of carbohydrates, fat, and protein from food). But preliminary studies suggest that much larger amounts of 8 to 16 milligrams per day may lower blood sugar. In one study, type 2 diabetes patients who took 9 milligrams of biotin a day for one month lowered their fasting blood-glucose levels by an average of 45 percent. Biotin seems to work by boosting insulin sensitivity and helping the body use glucose. It may also help protect against nerve damage. Biotin is probably safe because the body excretes what it doesn't need.

Chromium. Some studies find that taking this trace mineral in amounts upwards of 500 micrograms bring down blood sugar (though other studies find no benefit). It's possible that chromium helps cells use insulin. The amounts used in studies are higher than the government's estimated "safe and adequate" limit of 200 micrograms. You can probably go above this amount, although no one knows exactly how much is too much.

Magnesium. This mineral lends a hand to many chemical processes in the body, and it may help cells use insulin. Deficiencies (common in people with diabetes) may lead to eye damage. The official daily value is 400 milligrams, but some research finds that taking as much as two grams a day helps people with type 2 diabetes use insulin more effectively. Drawback: Doses that high often produce diarrhea. Avoid high doses if you have kidney disease or are pregnant.

Super Supplements

You're eating right, you're exercising—is there more you can do to protect your health? You bet! These four supplements can help protect your heart, guard against brittle bones and high blood pressure, and plug the occasional nutritional deficit.

Multivitamin. A multi can't make up for a poor diet, but it may help fill in nutritional gaps—especially for nutrients that become more difficult to absorb as we age. For people with diabetes, multivitamins can provide critical nutrients, such as magnesium, in which many diabetics are deficient, and B vitamins, which help protect the heart and nerves. If you're a man or a postmenopausal woman, choose a multivitamin without iron. Make sure it contains 400 mg of folic acid, as well as no more than 100 percent to 150 percent of the recommended daily value for other vitamins and minerals. Note: Take with meals for best absorption.

Calcium. In addition to protecting bones, calcium can help keep blood pressure in check and protect against heart disease. In a 2014 study, people with type 2 diabetes whose diets were low in calcium had elevated levels of inflammation. But so did those whose diets were high in calcium. So stick with the sweet spot of 400 to 600 mg of calcium a day, from food and/or supplements. Calcium citrate is easier than other forms for people over 65 to digest.

Fish oil capsules. People with diabetes have an elevated risk of heart disease. Fish oil guards against off-rhythm heartbeats, slows blood clotting, and keeps arteries supple. Take 1,000 mg of EPA plus DHA once or twice a day. Talk to your doctor before taking it, especially if you're on a blood-thinning drug such as Coumadin.

Vitamin D. Deficiency of the sunshine vitamin is widespread in people with diabetes, and suboptimal levels boost your risk for heart disease. A 2013 study found that people with higher blood levels of this vitamin had better insulin function than did people with lower levels. Take a 1000 to 2000 IU supplement every day, especially during the winter months when your skin may not be able to manufacture enough D from sunlight.

Beyond Dieting

Some books and magazines talk about weight loss as if it's a simple few-week excursion to a "bikini body." If only that were true. The reality is that two-thirds of people with diabetes are obese—a medical term that means overweight to the point of being considered a disease. For a typical American, that means 30 to 100 pounds overweight. And one in five is morbidly obese, meaning so overweight that they are putting their life at risk. For these individuals, getting to a healthy weight is a long, challenging path.

However, it's a path they can't help but walk. Living inside a severely overweight body not only makes blood-sugar control difficult, it raises the risk for life-threatening health problems including heart attacks, strokes, high blood pressure, and some forms of cancer.

Just watch any episode of *The Biggest Loser* and you'll understand in a flash that losing serious body fat takes more than foregoing a pat of butter here, a scoop of low-fat ice cream there, and fitting in a little exercise. While every little bit helps, for most people with substantial weight issues, it takes professional intervention to succeed.

We've pulled together the latest research on weight-loss methods for obesity. Here's what you need to know about how these programs, pills, and procedures really stack up.

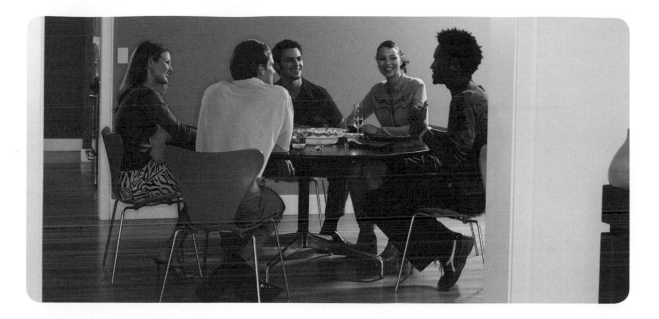

Portion-Controlled Meals

These offer plenty of support. Accountability—from weekly weigh-ins (private, of course) to reviews of your diet-and-exercise journal. These days, programs far and wide use this winning formula to help even extremely overweight people with diabetes lose pounds and not regain them.

If you haven't tried one yet, a well-organized, healthy weight-loss program ought to be your first stop on the road to a slimmer you. Plenty of research proves that they can work, even if you're severely obese. The catch? You'll need to change how you live, starting with low-calorie eating and almost daily exercise. But the beauty of twenty-first century weight loss programs is that they don't stop there. The best also use tools like meal-replacement bars and shakes, diabetes medication changes to encourage weight loss, even the judicious addition of weight-loss medications. And through weekly classes, you get support and new skills that can help you keep the weight off.

Case in point: the 12-week Why WAIT program at the Joslin Diabetes Center in Boston. It helped people with an average BMI of 38 drop 24 pounds in 12 weeks. They trimmed three and one-half inches from their waistlines, reduced their A1C (a measure of long-term blood sugar) by nearly one percentage point (impressive), and saw improvements in blood pressure and cholesterol, too. And a year later, most had kept off 18 pounds—enough to keep blood sugar under better control.

▶**Options:**

There are many hospital-based weight-loss classes and programs, private weight-loss clinics, even commercial weight-loss programs such as Weight Watchers and Jenny Craig. Look for one that meets National Institutes of Health (NIH) guidelines for

> A well-organized, healthy weight-loss program might be your first stop on the road to a slimmer you.

Know your BMI.

If you don't already know what your Body Mass Index is, time to find out, because it's an important number. Medical professionals use BMI as the measurement that defines obesity. The BMI calculates your weight compared to your height. A tall, skinny teenager might have a BMI of 12 to 15. A BMI below 25 is considered healthy. Overweight is a BMI of 25 to 30. Obesity is defined as having a BMI of 30 or above.

What does that mean in pounds? If you're five foot seven, you're obese if you weigh 195 pounds or more. If you're five foot eleven, you're obese if you weigh 210 pounds or more.

Morbid obesity is a BMI of 40 or higher: for example, weighing 218 pounds if you're five foot two, or weighing 311 pounds if you're six foot two.

Calculate your BMI at www.cdc.gov/ healthyweight/assessing/ bmi.

healthy weight loss (1/2 to about two pounds per week), and that has at least some of these proven components: an exercise program that can be geared to your capabilities; regular meetings for support, information, and building new skills; weekly weigh-ins; expertise in diabetes; and the option to try healthy meal-replacements.

Finally, beware of diet programs that sound too good to be true. Fast, dramatic weight losses from extremely low-calorie diets may lead to weight regain later on. And some programs may use drugs or supplements that are dangerous if you have high blood pressure or heart disease.

▶ **Cost:**

Fees can range from $125 for a 10-week-long hospital weight-loss class to several hundred dollars per month for a private arrangement.

▶ **Consider it if...**

You haven't been able to lose weight on your own; then a structured program is a great step. Talk with your doctor about your chosen program before you start to be certain it's right for you, and to brainstorm ways to adapt it to meet your needs.

▶ **Benefits:**

Expect to take off five to ten percent of your body weight in the first half year. If you stick with your healthy new habits, you can keep most of it off, too, or keep on losing.

▶ **Affect on blood sugar:**

Plenty of research shows that this well-rounded approach yields big blood-glucose benefits. In one nationwide weight-loss study of 5,100 morbidly obese people with diabetes (their average BMI was 36), a diet-and-exercise program helped people lose and keep off 8.6 percent of their body weight in one year—that's 24 pounds if you weigh 275—and saw blood sugar improve significantly.

▶ **Side effects:**

Not in the traditional medical sense. But be prepared for the effects a serious weight-loss program will have on your life. You likely will struggle with the food limitations, exercise programs, and brutal honesty these programs mandate. You also might love your new-found energy, confidence, and shape, and make some new friends along the way.

Prescription Drugs

Weight-loss drugs approved by the FDA work by blocking absorption of calorie-laden fat or by blunting your appetite. Sounds good, but in one nationwide study of over 5,000 overweight and obese people with type 2 diabetes, those who took a weight-loss drug for six months saw their bathroom scales barely budge. Some lost an extra one percent of their body weight (about two pounds if you weigh 200), while others lost *less* weight than people who depended on low-calorie eating and exercise alone.

One study isn't the final verdict, of course. According to the American Diabetes Association, weight-loss drugs could give you the support you need to make a serious diet-and-exercise program work a little better. And a little matters: Trimming just 5 percent of your body weight can make you less insulin-resistant, improve blood-sugar control, and even lower your blood pressure.

▸ **Options:**

Currently, two types of drugs are approved by the FDA for weight loss. Orlistat—(Xenical) and the over-the-counter, lower-strength version (Alli)—is taken with meals and blocks absorption of 30 percent of fat from food, so you take in fewer calories. The FDA has approved orlistat for up to one year of daily use, though participants in a four-year study took orlistat daily without added side effects.

The other approved choices are appetite suppressants: phentermine, diethylpropion, and phendimetrazine. They're stimulants that blunt your appetite. FDA-approved for up to 12 weeks of daily use, these drugs shouldn't be used by people with heart disease, high blood pressure, an overactive thyroid, or glaucoma.

The antidepressants fluoxetine and bupropion are often used for weight loss, even though they have not been specifically approved by the FDA for that purpose.

▸ **Cost:**

A 30-day supply of orlistat can cost $285; phentermine can cost $37 to $67; antidepressants can cost $4 to $35. Insurance may cover the cost in some cases.

▸ **Consider it if...**

You have diabetes and a BMI of 27 or higher, according to the NIH. Often, doctors will suggest adding medication if you haven't lost much weight after several months of dieting and regular exercise.

▸ **Benefits:**

Using a weight-loss drug along with diet and exercise could help you lose five to 10 percent of your body weight—10 to 20 pounds if you weigh 200. Results may be less for people with diabetes: Orlistat could help people with blood-sugar problems lose and keep off about five to six pounds, say researchers citing studies involving 2,036 people with diabetes. But in two studies, people with diabetes who took orlistat and followed a reduced-calorie diet and exercise routine didn't lose any more weight than people who took a placebo (fake) pill or no pill at all.

Meanwhile, average weight loss with phentermine is about eight pounds. An antidepressant could help you lose six to 11 pounds, studies show. The catch: You may gain the weight back when you stop using the medication.

▸ **Affect on blood sugar:**

Somewhat. In one study, people with diabetes lost the same amount of weight with or without orlistat, but got better blood-sugar improvements with orlistat. Users reduced their A1C (a measure of long-term blood-sugar control) from 8.1 percent to a healthier 6.5 percent, while those taking a fake pill saw smaller blood-sugar improvements. Meanwhile, people with diabetes who used fluoxetine and lost weight saw their A1C drop by an impressive 1 percent.

▶ **Side effects:**

Orlistat can trigger oily diarrhea, spotting, a sudden urge to have a bowel movement, or an oily discharge when you pass gas—especially if you eat more fat than is recommended. It may also cause stomach pain, nausea, dizziness, and in rare cases, severe liver injury. Phentermine and other appetite suppressants can cause nervousness and sleeplessness (phentermine can also raise blood pressure and heart rate). Fluoxetine may cause nervousness, sweating, nausea, sleep problems and diarrhea, and bupropion may cause dry mouth.

Weight-Loss Surgery

Imagine spending an hour or two on an operating-room table, then heading home (perhaps after a few days of recovery) to a diet-and-exercise program that—*at last!*—helps you shrug off 40, 50, 60 or more pounds. You'll slide into a smaller size. Feel your energy (and spirits) soar. Best of all? Better blood-sugar numbers.

It *can* happen. Bariatric surgery—defined as surgery done on obese people for the purpose of weight loss—is generally successful, and new approaches and refinements are occurring regularly.

But there's more to the weight loss surgery and diabetes story that you should know. The claims—and hopes—are huge, perhaps too huge. Yes, these surgeries can lead to a transformational improvement in your health. But it isn't the surgery itself that provides the benefit, but how it changes your eating and digestive patterns. Undergo one of these procedures, and you can never eat the same way again. Meals become much smaller, because you are physically unable to eat much. And so making smart, nutritious decisions is key—and that is entirely in your hands.

Before you sign up, here's the latest on the promise and controversies surrounding this increasingly popular weight-loss option for people with type 2 diabetes.

▶ **Options:**

Two types of bariatric surgery are most widely used in the United States. *Gastric bypass* reduces your stomach to the size of a golf ball and re-routes the connection from your stomach to your small intestine, bypassing parts to reduce calorie absorption. This has been the standard approach for several years. But recently, the FDA approved a new surgery approach—called *Laparoscopic adjustable gastric banding*—for people with a BMI as low as 30 and one or more health problems (such as diabetes). In this approach, doctors cinch your stomach with an adjustable, salt water-filled silicone belt that creates a tiny stomach pouch, allowing you to feel full with very small, lower-calorie meals.

Other choices include the *bilio-pancreatic diversion with duodenal switch*, which narrows your stomach and bypasses 60 percent of your small intestine. And *vertical sleeve gastrectomy* or "stapling," which reduces the size of your stomach by 85 percent.

What about liposuction? While it is a popular cosmetic surgery—it involves "vacuuming" away fat that has gathered under the skin—liposuction can remove only a small amount of fat from a particular spot on your body. More important, it does nothing to change your eating habits, so the weight usually comes right back. Plus, liposuction does nothing to reduce the fat around your organs, which is the more medically troubling fat. For these and other reasons, liposuction isn't used for obesity.

▸ **Cost:**

Gastric banding may cost $16,000 to $25,000, and gastric bypass can range from $18,000 to $35,000. Insurance, including Medicare and Medicaid, may cover some or even all of the cost if your doctor deems the procedure medically necessary and if you meet NIH requirements.

▸ **Consider it if...**

The FDA says weight-loss surgery may be a good option if you have diabetes and a BMI of 30 or higher. But stay tuned. Researchers are now investigating whether people with BMIs as low as 27 could see dramatic blood-sugar improvements with gastric bypass. This new, experimental approach is called "metabolic surgery" because it alters digestive hormones that help regulate blood sugar, rather than relying on weight loss alone to get the beneficial effects.

▸ **Benefits:**

About 60 to 77 percent of your excess weight in the first year—if you stick with a strict low-calorie eating plan and exercise regularly, say Australian researchers who reviewed 43 weight-loss surgery studies. Weight loss may be slower with gastric banding and faster with gastric bypass, but results evened out after five to eight years in one large study.

▸ **Affect on blood sugar:**

But be wary of reports that bariatric surgery makes diabetes "vanish" or that you'll never need diabetes drugs again. Blood-sugar levels do plummet soon after surgery for at least 80 percent of people with diabetes, thanks to strict low-calorie eating, a new zeal for exercise, steady weight loss, and with gastric bypass, a dramatic shift in digestion-related hormones.

But be sure to keep checking your levels and consulting your family doctor or endocrinologist—often, people need to resume medication at some point. In one large study, 42 percent who had gastric banding and 30 percent who had gastric bypass resumed blood-sugar drugs within two years after surgery.

Hoping you can go drug-free? You're more likely to keep diabetes in remission after surgery if you lose at least 60 to 70 percent of your excess weight (and keep it off), if you used oral diabetes drugs (instead of insulin) before your procedure, and if your diabetes was recently diagnosed, studies show.

▸ **Side effects:**

Overall, the complication rate in one large New York University study was 9 percent for laparoscopic gastric banding and about 24 percent for gastric bypass. This included short-term problems like fever, dehydration, nausea and vomiting, and more serious problems such as infection, bleeding, and glitches that required further surgery.

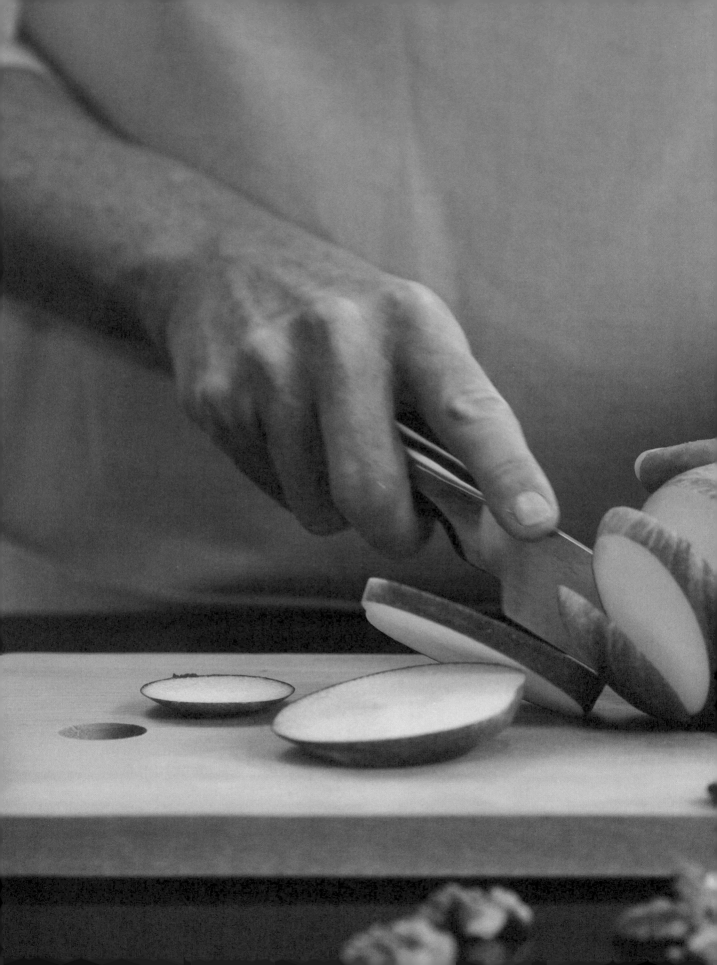

PART 5

Cook
Better

You wouldn't start a vacation without an idea of where you're going or what to take— and you shouldn't eat that way either. Without planning meals, you could be tempted to eat foods that will send your blood sugar on a roller-coaster ride. When you plan ahead and make cooking at home a centerpiece of family life, everyone in the household benefits. Choose recipes from this section to plan meals that will help better manage your diabetes— and that everyone in the family will enjoy.

▼▼▼▼▼▼▼▼▼▼▼▼

Reverse Diabetes Forever with **Delicious Recipes**

In your own kitchen, *you* control the amounts of calories, fat, and carbs in meals.

Managing diabetes begins in your kitchen. After all, diabetes is a disease that is closely linked with the foods you eat day to day, even hour to hour. A 2015 Harvard study of more than 100,000 men and women found that people who prepared their own meals at home—cooking 11 to 14 meals a week—dropped their risk of developing type 2 diabetes by 13 percent, compared with people who ate out more often. Home-cooked meals allow you to steer clear of high-carb, high-sugar foods that spike your blood sugar and make your condition worse.

Start by taking the time to prepare healthier meals at home. In your own kitchen, *you* control the amounts of calories, fat, and carbs in meals. You can ditch old standby recipes and eating habits. By replacing your ho-hum meals with some of the wonderful new recipes in this section, you can eat healthier and discover some great new tastes to boot!

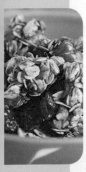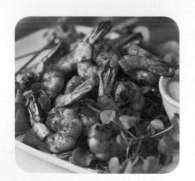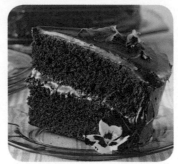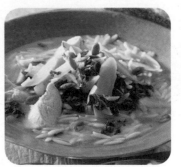

Live Well > Right Now

This moment, go to your cupboards and clean out every single food or snack that's sugary, fatty, or made of simple carbs. We're talking candy, cupcakes, pretzels, and even crackers that aren't whole wheat. Throw them out, or put them in a large bag and take them to the break room at work. You'll be taking a big step toward controlling your blood sugar. Once your shelves are cleaned of the bad stuff, pick a few of these recipes that sound good, and get ready to cook.

Live Well > Today

Breakfast is the easiest meal of the day with the recipes on the following pages. Easy and quick to prepare, they include many high-fiber choices, which can help control your blood sugar all day. Start the first meal of the day off right with a serving of fruit (Fruity Nutty Granola, p. 244). If you're pressed for time, keep fruit handy to toss on top of your cereal or oatmeal.

Live Well > This Week

For most of us, meal planning is done on a weekly basis. As you make your plans, consider creating themed days. For example, Sunday can become Salad Day (check out Green Vegetable Salad with Ginger and Garlic, p. 261). Thursdays could be Greek Day (try some Babaganoush, p. 251). And Fridays are traditionally fish days (see Stuffed Fish with Corn Salsa, p. 272).

Live Well > This Month

At least once a month, experiment with a new food. By expanding your culinary horizons, you'll find fruit, vegetables, and even meats that can help you control diabetes. If you've never tried veal, the Classic Veal Stew with Mushrooms, Carrots, Shallots & Beer on page 267 is a tasty dish low in calories and loaded with protein. Let each family member pick out a new food to try each month.

Live Well > This Year

Over the course of a year of cooking better and eating right, you should be able to notice a few changes. You'll likely have more energy, have dropped a few pounds, and avoided more blood-sugar spikes and plunges than in previous years. But you don't have to guess how you're doing. If you've kept a food diary, your progress will be right there in black and white for you to celebrate.

Live Well > Forever+

Managing diabetes over the long haul means avoiding the peaks and valleys of weight gain and the highs and lows of blood sugar. When you develop an attitude of moderation with all foods, you'll have lifelong control over your condition. That moderation means you'll never again have to deprive yourself of an occasional sweet treat. When you have smart desserts such as Old-Fashioned Secret Ingredient Chocolate Cake (p.280) or Lemon Blueberry Cheesecake (p. 285), you can live your life with just the right amount of sweet.

Fruity Nutty Granola

This nutritious mix with a touch of sweetness makes for guaranteed good mornings.

Makes 5 servings

3 cups old-fashioned or quick-cooking oats

½ cup coarsely chopped walnuts

2 tablespoons wheat germ

2 tablespoons sesame seeds

¼ teaspoon salt

⅓ cup honey

1 tablespoon light brown sugar

1 tablespoon extra-light olive oil

1 teaspoon vanilla

1 cup dried cranberries

ONE Preheat oven to 300°F. Combine oats, walnuts, wheat germ, sesame seeds, and salt in a 13- by 9-inch baking pan. Bake until oats and nuts are toasted and fragrant, about 30 minutes. Remove pan from oven. Increase oven temperature to 350°F.

TWO Meanwhile, combine honey, brown sugar, and oil in a small skillet over medium heat. Cook until the sugar has melted, about 1 minute. Remove from heat and stir in vanilla.

THREE Drizzle honey mixture over oat mixture and stir to coat. Return to oven and bake, stirring occasionally, until oats are crispy, about 10 minutes.

FOUR With a spoon, break up any clumps. Stir in cranberries. Store in airtight container.

Per serving: 154 calories, 5 g total fat, 0.5 g saturated fat, 25 g carbohydrates, 4 g protein, 3 g fiber, 0 mg cholesterol, 41 mg sodium

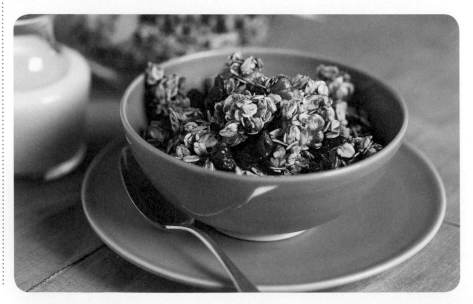

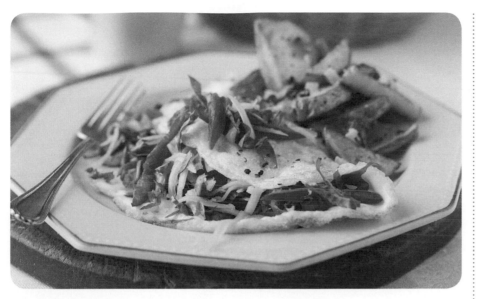

Egg-White Omelet with Vegetable-Cheddar Filling

Don't save this lovely dish for weekends—it goes from mixing bowl to table in just 10 minutes! Enjoy a savory, low-fat, low-carbohydrate, low-cholesterol start to the day.

Makes 1 serving

3 egg whites

2 teaspoons chopped fresh dill (optional)

⅛ teaspoon salt

⅛ teaspoon freshly ground black pepper

½ cup loosely packed, thinly sliced fresh spinach

1 plum tomato, chopped

2 tablespoons shredded nonfat cheddar cheese

Nonstick cooking spray

ONE Whisk egg whites, 1 teaspoon water, dill (if using), salt, and pepper in medium bowl until soft peaks form. Toss spinach, tomato, and cheddar in small bowl.

TWO Lightly coat omelet pan or small skillet with nonstick cooking spray and set over medium heat 1 minute. Pour egg mixture into pan and cook until eggs begin to set on bottom.

THREE Spread filling over half of omelet, leaving ½-inch border and reserving 1 tablespoon mixture for garnish. Lift up omelet at edge nearest handle and fold in half, slightly off-center, so filling peeks out. Cook 2 minutes. Slide omelet onto plate and garnish with reserved filling.

Per serving: 109 calories, 0.5 g total fat, 0 g saturated fat, 8 g carbohydrates, 18 g protein, 1 g fiber, 3 mg cholesterol, 906 mg sodium

Grab 'n' Go Muffins

No time for breakfast? Bake these yummy muffins on Sunday, and enjoy one at your desk for breakfast on Monday morning. Sweetened with cider, raisins, carrots, and just a touch of brown sugar, these muffins are easy, delectable treats.

Makes 12 servings

Nonstick cooking spray

⅓ cup golden raisins or currants

¼ cup apple cider or orange juice

¾ cup rye flour

¾ cup whole wheat flour

¾ cup cornmeal

2 teaspoons baking powder

1 teaspoon baking soda

½ teaspoon salt

1 cup plain low-fat yogurt

2 tablespoons dark brown sugar

1 large egg

1 large egg white

2 medium-size carrots, peeled and shredded (1½ cups)

2 tablespoons coarsely chopped pecans or walnuts

ONE Preheat the oven to 400°F. Lightly coat twelve 2½-inch muffin cups with nonstick cooking spray or insert cupcake liners. In a small bowl, soak the raisins in the cider for 15 minutes. Meanwhile, in a large bowl, stir together the rye flour, whole wheat flour, cornmeal, baking powder, baking soda, and salt. Make a well in the center.

TWO In a small bowl, stir together the yogurt, sugar, egg, and egg white until blended. Stir in the carrots, raisins, and cider just until combined. Pour the mixture into the dry ingredients and stir just until combined. Do not over mix.

THREE Spoon ¼ cup batter into each muffin cup and sprinkle with the nuts. Bake for 18 to 20 minutes or until golden and a toothpick inserted in the center comes out clean.

Per serving: 137 calories, 2 g total fat, 0.5 g saturated fat, 26 g carbohydrate, 5 g protein, 2 g fiber, 19 mg cholesterol, 242 mg sodium

Multigrain Waffles
with Apple-Raspberry Sauce

Hot, crisp waffles hit the spot for breakfast or brunch. Sweetened mainly with fruit and apple cider, these are low-fat, thanks to the buttermilk.

Makes 8 servings

1 cup apple cider

2 red or green apples, cut into ½-inch chunks

½ teaspoon vanilla

1 cup fresh raspberries

¼ cup flaxseeds

¼ cup whole wheat flour

¼ cup buckwheat flour

¼ cup all-purpose flour

2 teaspoons brown sugar

2 teaspoons baking powder

¼ teaspoon salt

1 large egg, separated, plus 2 large egg whites

1 cup buttermilk

Nonstick cooking spray

ONE Bring apple cider to a boil in medium skillet over high heat and cook 1 minute. Add apples and simmer until firm-tender, about 4 minutes. Remove from heat and let cool to room temperature. Stir in vanilla and raspberries.

TWO Place flaxseeds in a spice grinder or mini-food processor and grind to the consistency of coarse flour. Transfer to a large bowl and add whole wheat flour, buckwheat flour, all-purpose flour, brown sugar, baking powder, and salt. Stir to mix well.

THREE Combine egg yolk and buttermilk in small bowl. Beat 3 egg whites in large bowl until stiff peaks form. Make a well in center of dry ingredients and stir in egg-yolk mixture. Gently fold in egg whites.

FOUR Spray a waffle iron (with two 4- to 4½-inch squares) with nonstick cooking spray. Preheat iron. Spoon batter into iron, ½ cup per waffle. Cook until golden brown and crisp, about 2 minutes. Repeat with remaining batter. Serve warm with apple-raspberry sauce.

Per serving: 130 calories, 3 g total fat, 0.5 g saturated fat, 22 g carbohydrates, 5 g protein, 4 g fiber, 28 mg cholesterol, 187 mg sodium

Gulf Coast Hot Crab Dip

Lumps of crab in a spicy sauce make a wonderful and festive appetizer. But savor this treat only in small amounts—limit yourself to two or three crackers with dip.

Makes 24 servings

12 ounces fresh lump crabmeat or 2 cans (6 ounces each) crabmeat, drained

8 ounces fat-free cream cheese, softened

1 cup nonfat sour cream

1 small onion, finely chopped

1 tablespoon prepared horseradish

2 teaspoons Worcestershire sauce

¼ teaspoon hot red-pepper sauce

3 tablespoons plain dry bread crumbs

½ teaspoon paprika

4½ ounces baked low-sodium thin wheat crackers (about 72)

ONE Preheat oven to 350°F. Coat gratin dish or deep-dish pie plate with nonstick cooking spray. Pick through crabmeat; discard any shells and cartilage. Rinse crabmeat and drain.

TWO Stir cream cheese in medium bowl until smooth. Blend in sour cream, onion, horse-radish, Worcestershire sauce, and hot-pepper sauce. Gently fold in crabmeat. Spoon into baking dish; smooth top.

THREE Combine bread crumbs and paprika and sprinkle evenly over crabmeat mixture. Bake until bubbly, about 20 minutes. Serve piping hot with crackers.

Per serving: 57 calories, 1 g total fat, 0.5 saturated fat, 6 g carbohydrates, 5 g protein, 0 g fiber, 12 mg cholesterol, 129 mg sodium

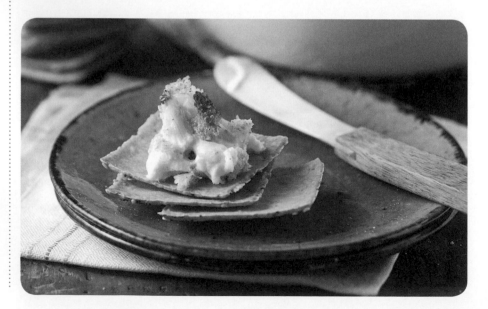

Parmesan Breadsticks

You'll wow friends and family alike with these crisp, savory twists. Perfect for healthy nibbling—or serve them to complete a delicious soup or salad meal.

Makes 40 servings

3¼ cups all-purpose flour

1 cup freshly grated Parmesan cheese

2 teaspoons chopped fresh rosemary or ½ teaspoon dried

2 teaspoons salt

1 teaspoon pepper

1 teaspoon rapid-rise dry yeast

1¼ cups very warm water (120° to 130°F)

¼ cup semolina flour or cornmeal

1 teaspoon olive oil

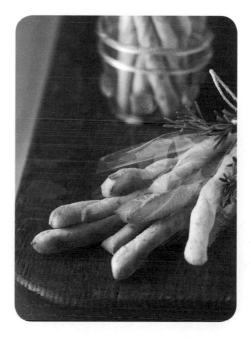

ONE Mix 1½ cups all-purpose flour, Parmesan, rosemary, salt, pepper, and yeast in a large bowl. Blend in water. Add 1½ cups more flour to form a soft dough. Dust work surface with flour. Turn dough onto floured surface and knead until smooth and elastic (or, use dough hook of your food processor or standing mixer), about 10 minutes, working in remaining flour to keep dough from sticking. Divide dough into two equal pieces. Cover with a damp kitchen towel and let rest 10 minutes.

TWO Sprinkle two 16- by 12-inch sheets of waxed paper with 1 tablespoon semolina each and pat dough pieces into 10- by 6-inch rectangles. Brush with oil and cover with a kitchen towel. Let rise in a warm place until doubled, about 30 minutes. Refrigerate 1 piece of dough.

THREE Preheat oven to 400°F. Line two baking sheets with parchment paper and sprinkle with half of remaining semolina. Cut unrefrigerated dough crosswise into 20 equal strips, each about 8 inches long. Hold dough strips by the ends, twisting and stretching until about 12 inches long. Place twists 1 inch apart on baking sheets. Let rise, uncovered, 10 minutes.

FOUR Lightly coat breadsticks with nonstick cooking spray. Bake 10 minutes. Remove breadsticks from oven and lightly coat again with cooking spray. Bake until golden and crisp, about 8 minutes longer. Transfer to a wire rack and cool completely. Repeat with the remaining dough.

Per serving: 56 calories, 1 g total fat, 0.5 g saturated fat, 9 g carbohydrate, 2 g protein, 0 g fiber, 2 mg cholesterol, 163 mg sodium

Rosemary Marinated Olives

A fruity olive oil marinade, infused with fresh herbs and citrus juices, pumps up the olive flavor. When served with colorful chunks of red and yellow bell peppers and little cherry tomatoes, these look and taste fabulous.

Makes 8 servings

7 ounces olives, preferably a mixture of black and green

2 tablespoons extra virgin olive oil

1 tablespoon lemon juice

1 thin-skinned orange, scrubbed but not peeled, cut into small chunks

2 sprigs fresh rosemary

1 fresh green chile pepper, seeded and thinly sliced

1 red bell pepper, seeded and cut into small chunks

1 yellow bell pepper, seeded and cut into small chunks

½ cup halved cherry tomatoes

ONE Place the olives in a large bowl and add the olive oil, lemon juice, chunks of orange, rosemary sprigs, and chile pepper. Stir together, then cover. Place in the refrigerator.

TWO For the next 2 days, every 12 hours or so, take the olive mixture from the fridge, uncover, and stir. Cover again and return to the fridge to continue marinating.

THREE When ready to eat, combine the marinated olives with the red and yellow bell peppers and tomatoes, and stir well.

Per serving: 83 calories, 6 g total fat, 1 g saturated fat, 7 g carbohydrate, 1 g protein, 2 g fiber, 0 mg cholesterol, 218 mg sodium

Babaganoush (Eggplant Dip)

This classic Mediterranean dip is delicious and extravagantly flavor-packed. Make it once for a dinner party or potluck, and your friends will beg you to make it again and again.

Makes 4 to 6 servings

1 lb. eggplant

1 tablespoon chopped fresh cilantro

1 to 2 garlic cloves, crushed

1 tablespoon lemon juice

4 to 6 tablespoons nonfat Greek yogurt

Salt and black pepper, to taste

ONE Heat oven to 400°F. Roast the eggplant for 15 minutes, or until the skin is blistered and charred, turning it over halfway through.

TWO Place the eggplant in a bowl, seal with plastic wrap and leave to cool for 10 minutes. Peel off the skin, then place the flesh in a sieve and press lightly to squeeze out any excess liquid. Transfer the flesh to a mixing bowl.

THREE Mash the eggplant thoroughly with a fork or potato masher, stir in the cilantro, garlic, lemon juice, and yogurt and blend well. Season to taste and add a little more crushed garlic, if desired.

Per serving: 39 calories, 0 g total fat, 0 g saturated fat, 8 g carbohydrate, 3 g protein, 4 g fiber, 0 mg cholesterol, 8 mg sodium

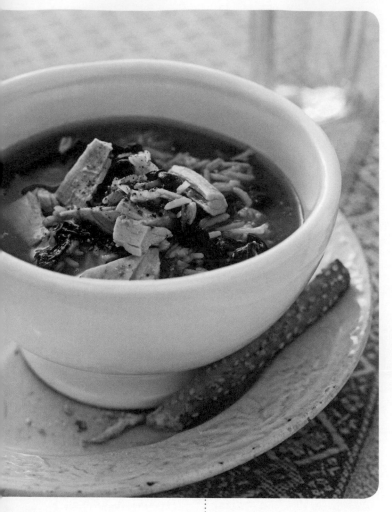

Turkey, Spinach, and Rice in Roasted Garlic Broth

This Grecian-inspired soup is soul-soothing on a crisp fall day—and is also the ideal meal when you or a loved one has a cold or the flu.

Makes 4 servings

2 medium whole heads garlic, unpeeled

2 tablespoons tomato paste

2 cans (14½ ounces each) reduced-sodium, fat-free chicken or turkey broth

1 cup cooked turkey cubes

1 cup cooked long-grain white rice

¾ pound spinach, stemmed and coarsely chopped

¼ teaspoon black pepper

¼ teaspoon hot pepper flakes, or to taste

1 tablespoon fresh-squeezed lemon juice

ONE Preheat oven to 400°F.

TWO Cut top third off garlic heads. Wrap each head in foil. Bake until very soft, about 50 minutes. Let cool. Remove foil. Squeeze out pulp into small bowl.

THREE In a large saucepan, stir together garlic pulp and tomato paste. Stir in broth. Bring to a boil. Add turkey, rice, spinach, pepper, and pepper flakes. Simmer, uncovered, 8 minutes. Just before serving, stir in lemon juice.

Per serving: 197 calories, 4 g total fat, 1 g saturated fat, 24 g carbohydrate, 19 g protein, 3 g fiber, 30 mg cholesterol, 208 mg sodium

Zesty Gazpacho

This delectable cold soup is a great way to get your entire family to enjoy their veggies. If you like it spicier, add dashes of hot sauce.

Makes 6½ cups

3 ounces crusty French or Italian bread

1 large red or green bell pepper, coarsely chopped

1 red onion, coarsely chopped

1 small cucumber, peeled, seeded, and sliced

8 ounces plum tomatoes, cored and quartered

¼ cup packed basil or parsley

1 clove garlic, finely chopped

2 tablespoons olive oil

2 tablespoons red or white wine vinegar

3 cups reduced-sodium tomato juice

⅛ teaspoon freshly ground black pepper

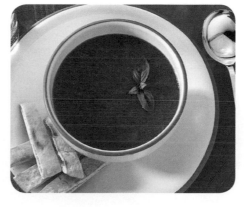

ONE Remove the crusts from the bread and tear the bread into pieces. Place in a bowl and cover with water. Let stand at least 5 minutes. Drain some of the water from the bowl and, with your hands, squeeze out most of the remaining water from the bread. Set aside the soaked bread.

TWO Place the bell pepper, red onion, and cucumber in a food processor and process until very finely chopped. Pour the mixture into a large bowl.

THREE Place the tomatoes and basil in the food processor and pulse until very finely chopped but not totally pureed. Add to the pepper mixture in the bowl.

FOUR Place garlic, oil, wine vinegar, soaked bread, and tomato juice in the food processor and process until blended. Stir into the soup until combined. Add black pepper. Cover the bowl and refrigerate the soup for at least 1 hour before serving.

Per serving: 129 calories, 5 g total fat, 1 g saturated fat, 19 g carbohydrate, 3 g protein, 3 g fiber, 0 mg cholesterol, 167 mg sodium

Chicken-Kale Soup

You'll make this soup a family standard. With kale—the perfect soup green for its flavor and texture—and pureed sweet red peppers, this rich potage is perfect for chilly days.

Makes 4 servings

1¼ pounds skinless, boneless chicken thighs, cut into 1-inch chunks

4 carrots, thinly sliced

3 large red onions, cut into ½-inch chunks

6 garlic cloves (5 minced, 1 whole)

2 tablespoons finely chopped fresh ginger

1 teaspoon cayenne pepper

¾ teaspoon salt

2 red bell peppers, cored, seeded, and cut lengthwise into flat pieces

1 tablespoon hulled roasted pumpkin seeds

1 tablespoon flaxseed oil

¼ cup orzo pasta

8 cups shredded kale

ONE In a large saucepan or soup pot over high heat, combine 4 cups water, chicken, carrots, onions, minced garlic, ginger, cayenne, and salt. Bring to boil, then reduce heat and simmer, partially covered, 25 minutes.

TWO Preheat broiler. Place peppers skin side up on a broiler pan and broil 6 inches from heat 10 minutes or until skin is well charred. Transfer peppers to a small paper bag and close the top for 10 minutes or so. When cool enough to handle, peel and transfer to a food processor or blender with pumpkin seeds, oil, and whole garlic clove. Cover and puree until smooth.

THREE Add orzo to pot with chicken and cook, uncovered, 5 minutes. Stir in kale and cook 5 minutes or until tender. Serve with roasted pepper puree.

Per serving: 445 calories, 12 g total fat, 2 g saturated fat, 50 g carbohydrate, 39 g protein, 9 g fiber, 118 mg cholesterol, 686 mg sodium, 273 mg calcium

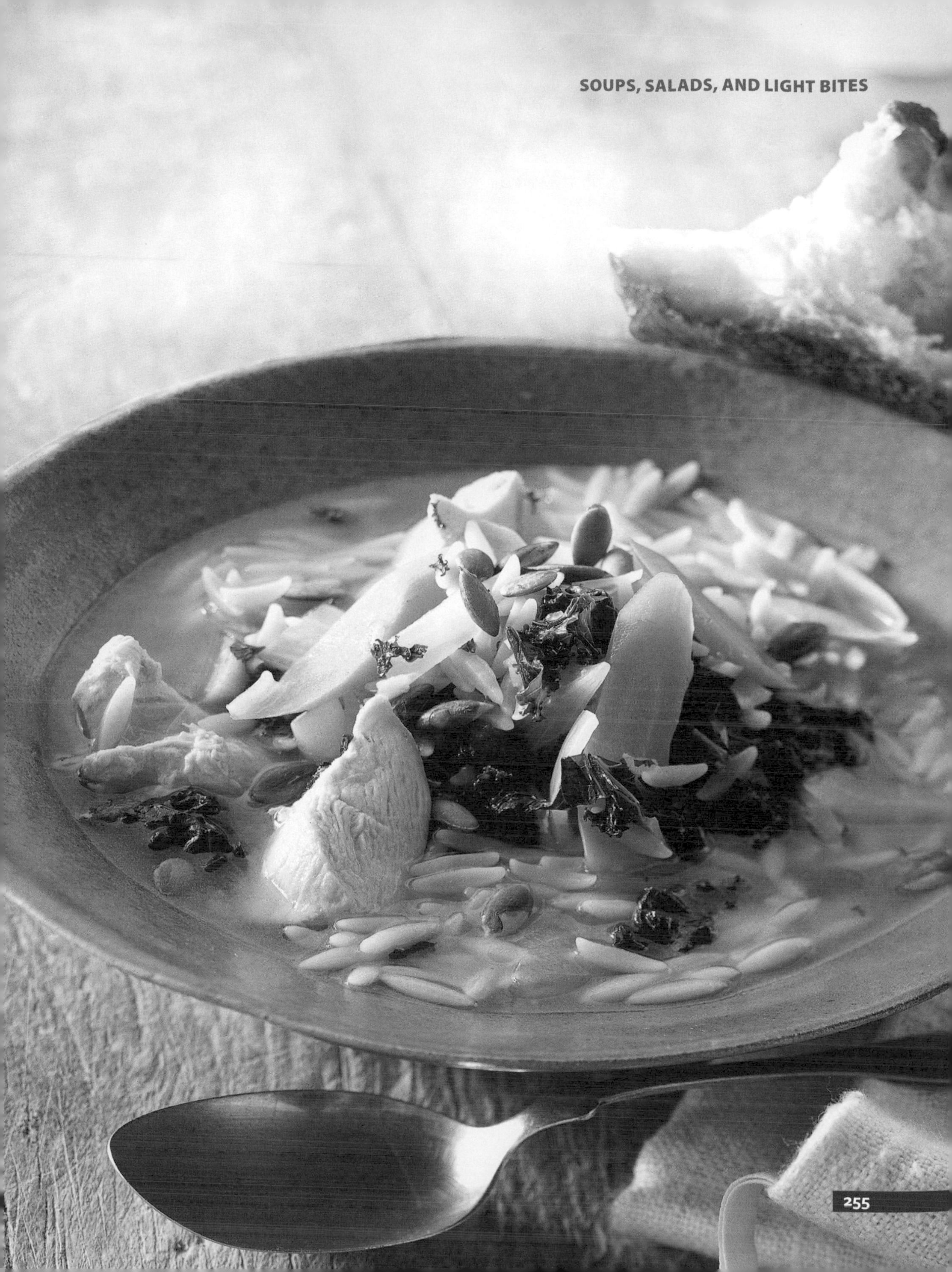

Russian Vegetable Soup

Serve this hearty, delicious, bursting-with-nutrition soup with thin pumpernickel or dark rye toast.

Makes 4 servings

½ cup dried mushrooms

2 tablespoons olive oil

1 large onion, finely chopped

4 garlic cloves, minced

1 large carrot, peeled and thinly sliced

1 large parsnip, peeled and thinly sliced

1 small head green cabbage, shredded

1¼ cups frozen baby lima beans

⅓ cup chopped fresh dill

⅓ cup tomato paste

¼ cup red wine vinegar

¾ teaspoon salt

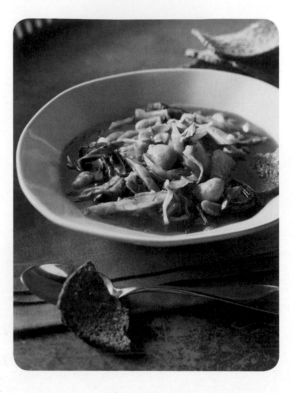

ONE In a small bowl, combine mushrooms and 1½ cups boiling water. Let stand until softened, about 20 minutes, then remove mushrooms, reserving liquid. Trim stems from mushrooms and coarsely chop caps. Strain liquid through a fine-mesh sieve or coffee filter into a small bowl.

TWO Heat oil in large saucepan or Dutch oven over medium heat. Add onion and garlic and sauté at least 5 minutes or until onion is golden. Add carrot and parsnip and sauté 5 minutes or until carrot is crisp-tender.

THREE Stir in cabbage and cook, covered, 5 minutes or until beginning to wilt. Stir in 3 cups water, mushrooms, soaking liquid, lima beans, dill, tomato paste, vinegar, and salt. Bring to boil, then reduce heat and simmer, covered, 25 minutes or until soup is richly flavored.

Per serving: 336 calories, 8 g total fat, 1 g saturated fat, 53 g carbohydrate, 14 g protein, 14 g fiber, 0 mg cholesterol, 685 mg sodium, 176 mg calcium

Tuscan Three-Bean Soup

In the Tuscany region of Italy, cooks focus on the freshest local ingredients and simple cooking techniques. Wonderful bean soups like this one are standard fare for lunches and light suppers.

Makes 6 servings

1 tablespoon olive oil

2 medium onions, coarsely chopped

2 medium carrots, coarsely chopped

2 celery stalks, chopped

2 cans (14½ ounces each) low-sodium chicken broth

1 can (28 ounces) crushed tomatoes in puree

½ cup chopped fresh basil

2 tablespoons chopped fresh oregano or 1 teaspoon dried oregano

1 can (15½ ounces) red kidney beans, drained and rinsed

1 can (15½ ounces) cannellini beans, drained and rinsed

1 can (15½ ounces) chickpeas, drained and rinsed

6 tablespoons freshly grated Parmesan cheese

ONE Heat oil in a large nonstick Dutch oven or soup pot over medium-high heat. Add onions, carrots, and celery and sauté 5 minutes or until soft. Add broth, tomatoes, basil, and oregano and bring to boil. Reduce heat and simmer, partially covered, 10 minutes

TWO Stir kidney beans, cannellini beans, and chickpeas into pot and simmer 10 minutes. Remove from heat.

THREE Using a handheld blender, coarsely puree about a quarter of soup (or transfer 2 cups to a food processor or blender, cover, puree coarsely, and return to pot). Garnish each 2-cup serving with 1 tablespoon Parmesan.

Per serving: 226 calories, 5 g total fat, 1 g saturated fat, 34 g carbohydrate, 13 g protein, 9 g fiber, 4 mg cholesterol, 481 mg sodium

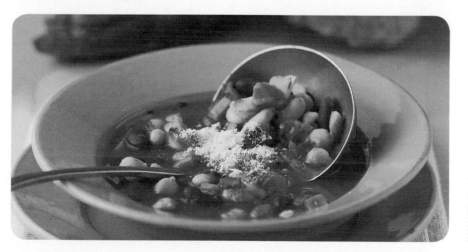

Pita Pizzas

These yummy little pizzas make for an easy light lunch or a terrific after-school snack.

Makes 4 servings

½ cup thinly sliced roasted red bell peppers

¼ teaspoon crushed fennel seeds or dried oregano, crumbled

¼ teaspoon salt

⅛ teaspoon black pepper

1 ounce reduced-fat mozzarella cheese, shredded (about ¼ cup)

½ ounce Gruyère or Jarlsberg cheese, shredded (about 2 tablespoons)

2 whole-wheat pita breads (4 inches)

8 teaspoons bottled tomato sauce or pizza sauce

½ small red onion, thinly sliced

ONE Preheat broiler.

TWO In small bowl, combine red peppers, fennel or oregano, salt, and pepper. In second bowl, combine mozzarella and Gruyère.

THREE Separate each pita bread into 2 flat rounds. Place rounds, rough side up, on baking sheet. Broil 4 inches from heat until golden brown around edges, about 1 minute. Remove from broiler.

FOUR Spread 2 teaspoons sauce over each pita, covering edges. Spoon 2 tablespoons red pepper mixture over each pita. Sprinkle with cheese, dividing equally, then add onion in rings.

FIVE Broil until cheese is melted and pizzas are hot, about 2 minutes.

Per serving: 137 calories, 3 g total fat, 2 g saturated fat, 23 g carbohydrate, 7 g protein, 3 g fiber, 7 mg cholesterol, 475 mg sodium

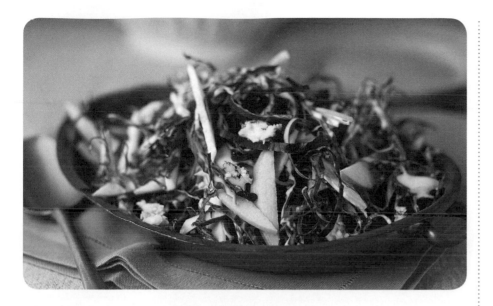

Cabbage-and-Apple Slaw with Blue-Cheese Dressing

It's almost too good to be true—this pretty show-stopping salad features a velvety, low-fat blue-cheese dressing!

Makes 8 servings

⅔ cup fat-free sour cream

⅔ cup plain fat-free yogurt

¼ cup cider vinegar

1 tablespoon low-fat mayonnaise

4 teaspoons sugar

1 teaspoon hot red-pepper sauce

1 teaspoon salt

⅓ cup crumbled blue cheese (2 ounces)

8 cups finely shredded red and/or green cabbage

4 Granny Smith apples, cut into thin wedges

2 red bell peppers, slivered

ONE Whisk together the sour cream, yogurt, vinegar, mayonnaise, sugar, hot-pepper sauce, and salt in a large bowl. Stir in blue cheese.

TWO Add cabbage, apples, and red peppers to bowl and toss to combine. Serve at room temperature or chilled.

Per serving: 150 calories, 3 g total fat, 1 g saturated fat, 30 g carbohydrate, 5 g protein, 5 g fiber, 5 mg cholesterol, 441 mg sodium

Tabbouleh

Made from bulgur—or steamed, dried, and crushed wheat berries—tabbouleh is a Middle Eastern delight. For people with diabetes, dishes made with bulgur are a great sub for rice, thanks to its higher fiber content and lower glycemic load. Delicious, satisfying, and a snap to prepare, tabbouleh keeps for four days in the fridge (if you use radishes, add them just before serving).

Makes 6 servings

Boiling water

¾ cup bulgur

1 medium-size red onion, chopped (1 cup)

1 medium-size tomato, coarsely chopped, with its juice (1 cup)

½ cucumber, seeded and coarsely chopped (½ cup)

4 large radishes, slivered (optional)

1 cup flat-leaf parsley, coarsely chopped

2 tablespoons minced fresh mint or 2 teaspoons mint flakes, crumbled

1 tablespoon olive or canola oil

1 teaspoon grated lemon rind

4 tablespoons lemon juice

¾ teaspoon salt

8 to 10 drops hot red-pepper sauce

ONE In a large heatproof serving bowl, pour 1 cup of boiling water over the bulgur and let stand for 20 minutes or until the water is absorbed. Meanwhile, in a small bowl, pour just enough boiling water over the onion to cover and let stand for 10 minutes. Drain.

TWO Add the onion, tomato, cucumber, radishes (if using), parsley, mint, oil, lemon rind, lemon juice, salt, and red-pepper sauce to the bulgur. Toss until well combined. Refrigerate, covered, for 6 hours or until chilled. Serve cold or at room temperature.

Per serving: 153 calories, 4 g total fat, 1 g saturated fat, 28 g carbohydrates, 5 g protein, 8 g fiber, 0 mg cholesterol, 418 sodium

Green Vegetable Salad with Garlic and Ginger

This sweet-salty salad is an easy, tasty way to eat your veggies—and to get your family to eat theirs!

Makes 4 servings

½ pound broccoli

½ pound small bok choy, or other Chinese leaves

4 scallions

¼ pound sugar snaps, trimmed

1 small clove garlic, crushed

1 teaspoon finely grated ginger

1 teaspoon dark-brown sugar

1 tablespoon Thai fish sauce

ONE Fill steamer pot with water to just below basket. Bring water to a boil.

TWO Cut broccoli into small florets, trimming stalks to about ½ inch. Peel remaining stalk and cut diagonally into ½-inch slices. Trim bok choy and slice stems. Trim scallions and cut diagonally into thin slices.

THREE In large bowl, combine broccoli, bok choy, scallions, and sugar snaps. Add garlic and ginger and toss well. Transfer to steamer basket, cover, and steam until vegetables are tender-crisp, 3 to 4 minutes.

FOUR In small cup, combine sugar and fish sauce, stirring until sugar dissolves. Arrange vegetables in serving dish and drizzle with this dressing. Serve hot, or let cool, then refrigerate until 10 minutes before serving.

Per serving: 50 calories, 0 g total fat, 0 g saturated fat, 9 g carbohydrate, 4 g protein, 3 g fiber, 0 mg cholesterol, 400 mg sodium

Stir-Fried Chicken with Snow Peas and Baby Corn

You can put this tasty family-pleasing dish on the table in just minutes—and it's special enough for company too!

Makes 4 servings

4 teaspoons reduced-sodium soy sauce

4 teaspoons dark sesame oil

1 tablespoon rice wine, dry sherry, or rice vinegar

1 pound skinned and boned chicken breasts, cut into 1-inch cubes

½ cup low-sodium chicken broth mixed with 2 teaspoons cornstarch

1 tablespoon vegetable oil

1 tablespoon minced fresh ginger

1 tablespoon minced garlic

4 scallions, white part only, sliced (⅓ cup)

4 ounces snow peas, trimmed (1 cup)

1 can (14 ounces) baby corn, drained and rinsed

ONE In a medium-size bowl, mix 2 teaspoons each of the soy sauce and sesame oil with the wine. Add the chicken and marinate for 30 minutes. In a small bowl, combine the stock-cornstarch mixture with the remaining 2 teaspoons each of soy sauce and sesame oil.

TWO In a 12-inch nonstick skillet, heat the vegetable oil over moderately high heat. Add the ginger, garlic, and scallions and stir-fry for 30 seconds. Add the chicken and stir-fry for about 2 minutes or until no longer pink on the outside. Add the snow peas and corn and stir-fry 2 minutes more.

THREE Add the cornstarch-stock mixture to the skillet, lower the heat, and simmer, stirring, for 2 to 3 minutes or until the sauce is slightly thickened and the juices run clear, not pink, when the chicken is pricked with a fork.

Per serving: 302 calories, 11 g total fat, 2 g saturated fat, 23 g carbohydrate, 31 g protein, 2 g fiber, 66 mg cholesterol, 536 mg sodium

Turkey Piccata

The enticing aroma of this elegant entrée sets the stage for a great meal. Turkey is a healthy—and less expensive—substitute for veal in this classic recipe. What's more, it's high in protein and low in both fat and carbohydrates.

Makes 4 servings

1 tablespoon olive oil

4 turkey cutlets (4 ounces each)

2 tablespoons flour

2 cloves garlic, minced

1 teaspoon grated lemon zest

¼ cup lemon juice

1 cup reduced-sodium, fat-free chicken broth

1 teaspoon cornstarch blended with 1 tablespoon water

1 tablespoon capers, rinsed and drained

2 tablespoons chopped parsley

1 lemon, sliced thin and seeded, for garnish (optional)

ONE Heat oil in a large nonstick skillet over medium heat. Dredge turkey in flour, shaking off excess. Sauté turkey until golden brown and cooked through, about 2 minutes per side. With tongs or a slotted spoon, transfer turkey to a plate; cover loosely with foil to keep warm.

TWO Add garlic to pan and cook, stirring, until tender, about 1 minute. Add lemon zest, lemon juice, and chicken broth to pan and bring to a boil. Boil 1 minute.

THREE Stir in cornstarch mixture and capers, and cook until slightly thickened, about 1 minute. Stir in parsley. Serve turkey with sauce spooned on top. Garnish with thinly sliced lemons, if desired.

Per serving: 187 calories, 4 g total fat, 1 g saturated fat, 6 g carbohydrate, 30 g protein, 0.5 g fiber, 70 mg cholesterol, 178 sodium

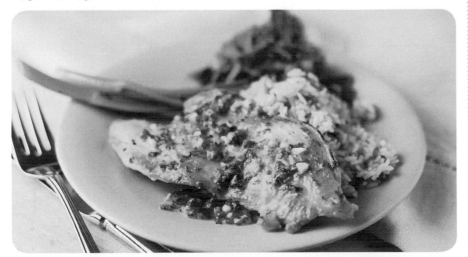

Turkey and Black Bean Enchiladas

Next time you get a hankering for a fast-food Mexican meal, try this zippy guilt-free variation—all of the flavor and very little fat.

Makes 4 servings

2½ cups medium salsa

¼ cup chopped cilantro

1 teaspoon ground cumin

8 corn tortillas (6 inches)

8 ounces cooked turkey breast, shredded

1 cup canned black beans, rinsed and drained

1 small red onion, finely chopped

1 cup shredded reduced-fat Cheddar cheese (about 4 ounces)

Nonstick cooking spray

ONE Preheat oven to 350°F. Coat a 7- by 11-inch baking dish with nonstick cooking spray.

TWO Combine salsa, cilantro, and cumin in a shallow bowl at least 6 inches in diameter.

THREE Working with one at a time, dip tortilla in salsa mixture, coating it completely. Place on plate or sheet of waxed paper. Top each tortilla with 2 tablespoons salsa mixture. Top with one-eighth of turkey, beans, and red onion. Sprinkle with 1 tablespoon cheese. Roll tortilla up and place seam side down in baking dish. Repeat filling and rolling with remaining tortillas.

FOUR Spoon remaining salsa mixture over enchiladas and sprinkle with remaining ½ cup cheese. Bake until bubbling, about 15 minutes.

Per serving: 369 calories, 7 g total fat, 3.5 g saturated fat, 45 g carbohydrate, 34 g protein, 9 g fiber, 62 mg cholesterol, 880 mg sodium

Herb-Roasted Beef

This lean cut of roast beef is company-ready and full of flavor. Serve a generous portion of vegetables with a smaller piece of meat for a nutritionally balanced meal.

Makes 6 servings

2 pounds lean boneless beef rib roast

Salt and pepper to taste

1 cup mixed fresh herbs, such as parsley, basil, sage, rosemary, thyme, and chives, or 1½ tablespoons dried of each

2 tablespoons Dijon mustard

1 tablespoon olive or canola oil

3 large onions, cut into eighths

6 small zucchini, cut into thirds

1 cauliflower, cut into florets

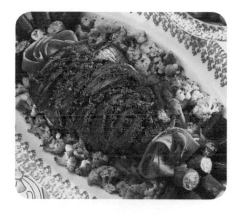

ONE Preheat the oven to 350°F. With a sharp knife, trim all the fat and cartilage from the beef roast. Season the meat with salt and pepper.

TWO Place the fresh herbs and mustard in a food processor and process to chop herbs fine and combine mixture. Scraping down the sides of the bowl, transfer mixture to a small bowl. Mix dry herbs and mustard in bowl.

THREE Spoon the herb mixture onto the roast, spreading it evenly to cover all sides. Coat the bottom of a large roasting pan with the oil. Place the meat in the pan and roast, uncovered, for 30 minutes.

FOUR Arrange the onions, zucchini, and cauliflower around the meat in the roasting pan and toss the vegetables to coat them thoroughly in the oil.

FIVE Roast the meat and vegetables about 1 hour or until a thermometer inserted in the center of the meat reads 150°F (for medium). Turn the vegetables occasionally so that they cook evenly.

SIX Remove pan from the oven. With a slotted spoon, transfer the vegetables to a serving dish and keep them warm. Transfer the roast to a carving platter, and let stand for 10 minutes. Slice beef and serve with vegetables.

Per serving: 317 calories, 10 g total fat, 3 g saturated fat, 20 g carbohydrate, 5 g protein, 7 g fiber, 82 mg cholesterol, 278 mg sodium

Beef, Scallion & Asparagus Roll-Ups

Here's a delicious variation on the Japanese dish called negamaki. You'll be surprised to discover how easy, not to mention yummy, it is to make at home. Tip: This meal is a real kid pleaser.

Makes 4 servings

8 asparagus stalks, trimmed to 6-inch lengths

8 thin slices sirloin steak (¼ pound total)

4 scallions, trimmed to 6-inch lengths

2 teaspoons vegetable oil

3 tablespoons bottled teriyaki sauce

1 tablespoon sesame seeds, toasted

1 tablespoon chopped cilantro

ONE Heat saucepan of water to a boil. Cut each asparagus stalk in half. Blanch in boiling water 1 minute, and then drain.

TWO Meanwhile, pound sirloin slices to ⅛-inch thickness. Cut each scallion into two 3-inch pieces.

THREE Place 2 pieces of asparagus and 1 piece scallion near one end of each beef strip. Roll beef around middle of vegetables to form 8 bundles.

FOUR In large nonstick skillet over medium-high heat, heat oil. Add rolls. Brown 2 minutes, turning rolls frequently. Add teriyaki sauce, lower heat to medium, and boil 3 minutes.

FIVE Transfer rolls to serving platter. Sprinkle with sesame seeds and cilantro.

Per serving: 98 calories, 6 g total fat, 1 g saturated fat, 5 g carbohydrate, 7 g protein, 1 g fiber, 14 mg cholesterol, 536 mg sodium

Stir-Fried Beef with Broccoli, Snow Peas, Peppers & Shiitake Mushrooms

Why spend money on unhealthy Chinese take-out when a nutritious and delicious dish like this is oh so easy to make right in your own kitchen?

Makes 4 servings

3 tablespoons reduced-sodium soy sauce

2 teaspoons packed dark-brown sugar

1 pound beef round steak, cut across grain into ⅛-inch-thick strips

1 small head broccoli, cut into 4-inch-long florets (about 2 firmly packed cups)

2 tablespoons vegetable oil

2 cups sliced shiitake mushroom caps

1 red bell pepper, seeded and thinly sliced

1 cup snow peas, stems and strings removed

4 scallions, cut diagonally into ¼-inch pieces

1 tablespoon minced garlic

1 tablespoon finely chopped, peeled fresh ginger

Pinch red pepper flakes

⅓ cup reduced-sodium, fat-free chicken broth

1 tablespoon balsamic vinegar

2 teaspoons cornstarch

ONE In medium bowl, stir together 1 tablespoon of the soy sauce and brown sugar. Add beef. Toss to coat. Marinate at room temperature 20 minutes.

TWO Steam broccoli until crisp-tender, 3 to 4 minutes. Cool under cold running water. Drain.

THREE In large nonstick skillet or wok over high heat, heat oil. Add meat. Stir-fry just until pink, about 2 minutes. Transfer from skillet with slotted spoon.

FOUR Add mushrooms, bell pepper, snow peas, scallions, garlic, ginger, and pepper flakes to skillet. Stir-fry until snow peas are crisp-tender, 3 to 4 minutes.

FIVE Stir together broth, remaining 2 tablespoons soy sauce, vinegar, and cornstarch in small bowl until smooth. Add to skillet. Bring to a boil (mixture will be very thick). Add broccoli. Cook just until heated through, about 2 minutes.

SIX Drain beef. Add to skillet. Heat through, about 30 seconds. Serve immediately.

Per serving: 276 cal, 12 g total fat, 3 g saturated fat, 13 g carbohydrate, 30 g protein, 3 g fiber, 74 mg cholesterol, 392 mg sodium

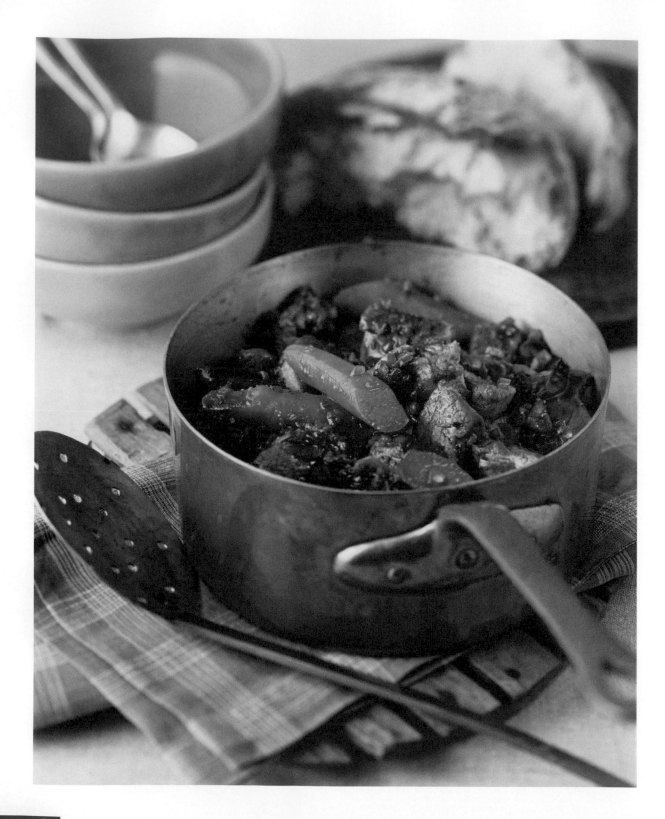

Classic Veal Stew with Mushrooms, Carrots, Shallots & Beer

Perfect for a cold winter's evening, this wonderful stew packs a lot of flavor into each serving. Cook with a beer you enjoy drinking because its flavor will infuse the dish.

Makes 4 servings

1 pound stewing veal, cut into 1-inch pieces

¾ teaspoon salt

¼ teaspoon black pepper

2 tablespoons vegetable oil

2 portobello mushrooms, stems removed and caps cut into 1-inch dice

8 large shallots (or 1 onion), finely chopped

2 tablespoons all-purpose flour

1 bottle dark beer

1 tablespoon white wine vinegar

½ teaspoon dried thyme, crumbled

1 pound large carrots, peeled and cut into 2-inch lengths

ONE Pat veal dry. Season with ¼ teaspoon of the salt and pepper. In large flameproof casserole over high heat, heat oil. Working in batches, add veal and brown on all sides, 3 to 4 minutes per batch. Transfer veal to plate.

TWO Lower heat to medium. Add mushrooms and shallots to casserole. Sauté until shallots are just golden, about 5 minutes. Stir in flour. Add veal, beer, vinegar, thyme, and remaining ¼ teaspoon salt. Bring to a boil. Add carrots. Cover. Lower heat. Simmer until veal is tender, about 1¼ hours.

THREE Transfer veal, carrots, and mushrooms to serving dish. Boil sauce to reduce to about 1¼ cups. Pour over veal.

Per serving: 317 calories, 10 g total fat, 2 g saturated fat, 24 g carbohydrate, 27 g protein, 4 g fiber, 94 mg cholesterol, 626 mg sodium

Pork Tenderloin with Honey-Mustard Sauce

This quick-and-easy dish is delightfully tangy and also low in calories and fat.

Makes 4 servings

1 tablespoon chopped fresh rosemary or 1 teaspoon dried

2 garlic cloves, minced

1 teaspoon grated lemon zest

½ teaspoon salt

1 pork tenderloin (about 1 pound), trimmed

⅓ cup fresh lemon juice

¼ cup honey

3 tablespoons coarse Dijon mustard

½ cup nonfat half-and-half

1 tablespoon all-purpose flour

ONE Preheat oven to 400°F. Line small roasting pan with foil. Combine rosemary, garlic, lemon zest, and salt in small bowl and rub evenly over pork tenderloin; transfer pork to pan. Mix lemon juice, honey, and mustard in small bowl. Transfer half to small saucepan and set aside.

TWO Brush pork with 2 tablespoons honey-mustard sauce. Roast pork until glazed and golden brown or until instant-read thermometer reads 160°F, about 25 minutes, basting 2 or 3 times with remaining sauce.

THREE Meanwhile, put half-and-half in small bowl and whisk in flour until smooth. Warm reserved honey-mustard sauce in small saucepan over low heat. Gradually whisk in half-and-half mixture and cook, whisking constantly, until sauce thickens, about 3 minutes. Serve over the pork.

Per serving: 247 calories, 5 g total fat, 1 g saturated fat, 25 g carbohydrate, 25 g protein, 1 g fiber, 74 mg cholesterol, 525 mg sodium

Grilled Shrimp
with Mustard Dipping Sauce

A pound of shrimp and six seasonings, and you're in for great healthy, low-fat grilling.

Makes 4 servings

2½ tablespoons Dijon mustard

1½ tablespoons fresh lemon juice

2 teaspoons ground coriander

2 teaspoons ground cumin

½ teaspoon pepper

½ teaspoon salt

1 pound (about 24) large shrimp, peeled and deveined

ONE Stir together mustard, lemon juice, ½ teaspoon coriander, ½ teaspoon cumin, and ¼ teaspoon pepper in small bowl. Set mustard dipping sauce aside.

TWO Combine salt with remaining 1½ teaspoons coriander, 1½ teaspoons cumin, and ¼ teaspoon pepper in large bowl. Add shrimp, tossing to coat.

THREE Preheat grill to medium. Thread shrimp onto four long skewers. Place shrimp on grill and cook until opaque throughout, about 1 minute per side. Serve at room temperature or chilled with mustard dipping sauce.

Per serving: 88 calories, 2 g total fat, 0.5 g saturated fat, 3 g carbohydrate, 15 g protein, 1 g fiber, 135 mg cholesterol, 684 sodium

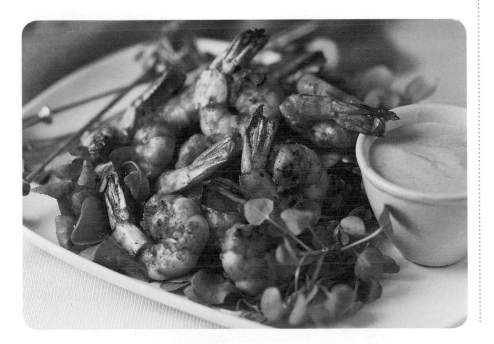

Stuffed Fish with Corn Salsa

Stuffing a whole fish with a zesty vegetable or fruit salsa in place of traditional bread stuffing adds plenty of flavor without the fat.

Makes 4 servings

1 tablespoon olive or canola oil

1 onion, finely chopped

1 clove garlic, finely chopped

2 stalks celery, sliced thick

½ teaspoon chili powder

1 cup fresh or frozen corn kernels, thawed

1 small cucumber, peeled, seeded, and diced

1 fresh or canned jalapeño pepper, chopped

3 tablespoons chopped fresh parsley or 1 tablespoon dried

2 tablespoons lime juice

⅛ teaspoon each salt and pepper

1 or 2 pan-dressed mild fish, such as snapper, perch, or trout (2 pounds total)

ONE Preheat the oven to 450°F. In a nonstick skillet, heat the oil over moderate heat. Sauté the onion and garlic, stirring, about 5 minutes or until soft but not browned. Add the celery and chili powder; cook 3 to 4 minutes longer.

TWO Transfer the onion mixture to a large bowl. Add the corn, cucumber, jalapeño pepper, parsley, lime juice, salt, and pepper, and toss gently to combine.

THREE Coat a baking sheet with vegetable oil cooking spray. Using a spoon, stuff the fish cavity with salsa mixture and transfer to the baking sheet.

FOUR Bake 40 to 55 minutes or until fish flakes easily when tested with a fork.

Per serving: 268 calories, 6 g total fat, 1 g saturated fat, 17 g carbohydrate, 37 g protein, 3 g fiber, 63 mg cholesterol, 202 mg sodium

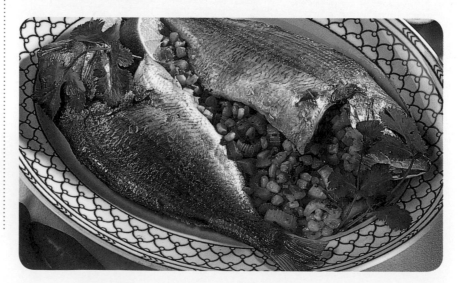

Steamed Fish with Ginger and Sesame

Master the art of steaming and you'll be a whiz at tasty, quick, low-fat meals. Steamed fish, infused with spices and other seasonings, is utterly delicious. Any white-fleshed fish filet will work well in this recipe.

Makes 4 servings

2 tablespoons grated fresh ginger

3 cloves garlic, minced

½ teaspoon grated lime zest

½ cup chopped cilantro

4 tilapia fillets (5 ounces each)

½ teaspoon salt

2½ teaspoons dark sesame oil

2 tablespoons fresh lime juice

½ cup water

1 teaspoon cornstarch blended with 1 tablespoon water

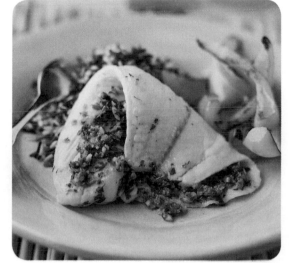

ONE Combine ginger, garlic, lime zest, and ¼ cup of cilantro in small bowl. Lay fillets skinned side up on work surface and sprinkle with salt and cilantro mixture. Fold fillets in half. Drizzle sesame oil over folded fish, and place fish on a heatproof plate.

TWO Place a cake rack in a skillet large enough to hold plate of fish and add water to just fall short of cake rack. Cover and bring to a simmer.

THREE Carefully place plate of fish on rack over simmering water. Cover and steam until cooked through, about 5 minutes. With slotted spatula, transfer fish to a platter and cover loosely to keep warm.

FOUR Pour cooking liquids on plate used for steaming into a small saucepan. Add lime juice and water and bring to a boil. Stir in cornstarch mixture and cook, stirring, until sauce is slightly thickened, about 1 minute. Stir in remaining ¼ cup cilantro. Pass sauce at the table in a small serving bowl.

Per serving: 182 calories, 6.5 g total fat, 1 g saturated fat, 3 g carbohydrate, 27 g protein, 0 g fiber, 120 mg cholesterol, 107 mg sodium

Eggplant Lasagna

Need to feed a roomful of vegetarians? Or just looking to satisfy the gang with a low-fat, low-calorie variation of their favorite Italian dinner? This sumptuous lasagna will definitely please everyone at the dinner table.

Makes 12 servings

2 tablespoons olive oil

1 large onion, chopped

2 cloves garlic, minced

1 tablespoon Italian seasoning

2 cans (14 ounces each) diced tomatoes

1 can (28 ounces) tomato sauce

1 small eggplant, peeled and cut into 1-inch pieces

¼ teaspoon salt

1 container (16 ounces) light silken tofu, drained

2 large eggs

1 cup freshly grated Parmesan cheese

9 no-boil lasagna noodles

1 package (8 ounces) shredded part-skim mozzarella cheese

ONE Preheat the oven to 400°F. Heat the oil in a large saucepan over medium-high heat. Add the onion and cook until tender, about 5 minutes. Add the garlic and Italian seasoning and cook for 1 minute. Add the tomatoes and tomato sauce and bring to a simmer. Reduce the heat to low and simmer until the flavors are blended, 40 minutes.

TWO Meanwhile, coat a baking sheet with sides with cooking spray. Add the eggplant, coat with cooking spray, and sprinkle with the salt. Roast, turning occasionally, until browned, 30 minutes.

THREE In a food processor or blender, combine the tofu, eggs, and Parmesan and puree until smooth.

FOUR Coat a 9- by 13-inch baking dish with cooking spray. Spread 1 cup sauce in the dish and arrange 3 lasagna noodles on top. Spread half of the tofu filling over the noodles, followed by half of the eggplant. Top with 1½ cups sauce and ½ cup mozzarella. Repeat with another layer, then top with the remaining noodles, sauce, and mozzarella.

FIVE Cover with foil and bake for 1 hour. Remove the foil and bake until heated through, about 15 minutes. Let cool slightly before serving.

Per serving: 229 calories, 10 g total fat, 4 g saturated fat, 23 g carbohydrate, 15 g protein, 3 g fiber, 51 mg cholesterol, 852 mg sodium

Barley Risotto with Asparagus and Mushrooms

This vegetarian entrée is so hearty and satisfying that we promise you'll never miss the meat!

Makes 4 servings

2 cans (14½ ounces each) reduced-sodium, fat-free chicken broth

2 tablespoons olive oil

1 onion, finely chopped

8 ounces mushrooms, preferably mixture of wild varieties, coarsely chopped

2 cloves garlic, minced

1 cup pearl barley

8 ounces asparagus, trimmed, and cut into bite-size pieces, leaving tips whole

½ cup grated Parmesan cheese

ONE In medium saucepan, heat broth and 2 cups water to just below a simmer. Cover; keep at a simmer.

TWO In large deep nonstick skillet over medium heat, heat oil. Sauté onion until slightly softened, about 3 minutes. Add mushrooms and garlic. Sauté until mushrooms are softened, about 5 minutes. Stir in barley. Stir in 2 cups hot broth mixture. Simmer, covered, 15 minutes.

THREE Meanwhile, blanch asparagus tips in the pot of hot broth for 2 minutes. Transfer with slotted spoon to plate.

FOUR Add more hot broth to barley mixture, ½ cup at a time, stirring frequently. Let each batch of liquid be absorbed before adding more. When adding the last batch of liquid, stir in asparagus stem pieces. Stir in Parmesan. Serve risotto topped with asparagus tips.

Per serving: 329 calories, 10 g total fat, 2 g saturated fat, 49 g carbohydrate, 15 g protein, 10 g fiber, 23 mg cholesterol, 743 mg sodium

Grilled Summer Vegetables

If you've never grilled veggies before, you're in for a treat. Even true carnivores will dive into a platter of these delicacies.

Makes 4 servings

2 small fennel bulbs (about 8 ounces each), trimmed

1 small eggplant (about 1 pound), cut lengthwise into 2 slices ½ inch thick

4 plum tomatoes, halved

3 large bell peppers (preferably 1 green, 1 red, 1 yellow),
cut into strips ½ inch wide

½ teaspoon salt

½ teaspoon pepper

2 tablespoons orange juice

8 basil leaves, slivered

1 garlic clove, minced

1 teaspoon grated orange zest

Nonstick vegetable spray

ONE Preheat grill to high. Prepare fennel: Cut off stalks with fronds and set aside. Peel bulbs and cut vertically into ½-inch slices. Coat fennel, eggplant, tomatoes, and bell peppers with nonstick cooking spray (preferably olive-oil flavored) and sprinkle with salt and pepper.

TWO Grill vegetables until tender and evenly browned, about 4 minutes on each side, turning once. Transfer to a serving platter and sprinkle with orange juice.

THREE Finely chop 1 tablespoon reserved fennel fronds and mix in small bowl with basil, garlic, and orange zest. Sprinkle over vegetables. Serve vegetables warm or at room temperature.

Per serving: 118 calories, 1 g total fat, 0 g saturated fat, 28 g carbohydrate, 4 g protein, 9 g fiber, 0 g cholesterol, 364 mg sodium

Lemony Sugar Snaps

Catch them while you can—sweet, succulent sugar snap peas have a short season, in early summer. Their crisp pods and bright flavor make them a delicious low-fat treat.

Makes 4 servings

1½ pounds sugar snap peas

2 teaspoons olive oil

3 shallots, thinly sliced

1 clove garlic, minced

1 tablespoon grated lemon zest

1 teaspoon salt

ONE Remove strings from both sides of sugar snap peas.

TWO Heat oil in large nonstick skillet over medium heat. Add shallots and garlic and cook, stirring, until shallots are softened, about 3 minutes.

THREE Add sugar snaps, lemon zest, and salt to skillet and cook, stirring, until peas are just tender, about 4 minutes.

Per serving: 99 calories, 2.5 g total fat, 0.5 g saturated fat, 15 g carbohydrate, 4 g protein, 5 g fiber, 0 mg cholesterol, 454 mg sodium

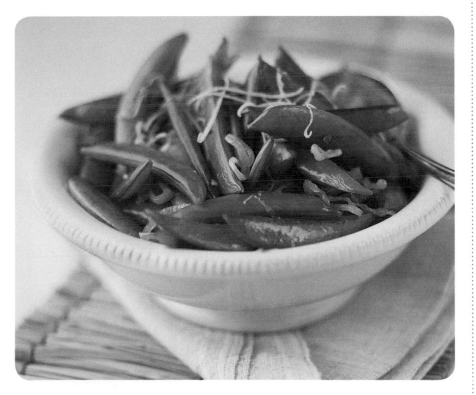

Braised Red Cabbage with Apples

Apples and red cabbage, both high in fiber, are appealing even without butter or oil. This makes a perfect side dish for pork and turkey entrées.

Makes 6 servings

1 medium-size head red cabbage (about 1¾ pounds), cored and thinly sliced

2 medium-size Granny Smith apples, peeled, cored, and grated (1½ cups)

1 tablespoon brown sugar

2 tablespoons all-purpose flour

¼ teaspoon black pepper

1 cup dry red wine or unsweetened apple juice

ONE In a large enameled or stainless-steel saucepan, mix the cabbage, apples, sugar, flour, and pepper. (Iron or aluminum will react with the cabbage and turn it brown.) Stir in the wine and bring to a boil over high heat.

TWO Lower the heat, cover, and simmer, stirring occasionally, for 25 to 30 minutes or until the cabbage is tender. Serve with pork chops or venison.

Per serving: 108 calories, 1 g total fat, 0 g saturated fat, 20 g carbohydrate, 2 g protein, 0 mg cholesterol, 40 mg sodium

Steamed Sesame Spinach

Simple, easy, and delicious. This Asian twist gives a whole new dimension to one of the healthiest veggies you can eat.

Makes 4 servings

1 pound spinach, stems removed

⅛ teaspoon red pepper flakes

½ teaspoon dark sesame oil

1 teaspoon salt

1 teaspoon fresh-squeezed lemon juice

1 tablespoon sesame seeds, toasted

ONE In medium saucepan, steam spinach with pepper flakes until tender, 3 to 5 minutes. Transfer to serving bowl.

TWO Add sesame oil, salt, and lemon juice to spinach. Toss to mix. Sprinkle with sesame seeds. Serve at once.

Per serving: 38 calories, 2 g total fat, 0 g saturated fat, 4 g carbohydrates, 3 g protein, 3 g fiber, 0 mg cholesterol, 43 mg sodium

Baked Sweet Potato Fries

Replace your french fries with these healthy beauties—we'll bet you won't miss them one bit.

Makes 4 servings

1 pound sweet potatoes, peeled and cut into ½-inch-thick fries

1 tablespoon vegetable oil

¼ teaspoon salt

¼ teaspoon black pepper

ONE Preheat oven to 425°F. Lightly coat baking sheet with nonstick cooking spray.

TWO In large bowl, combine sweet potatoes, oil, salt, and pepper. Toss to coat. Spread fries in single layer on baking sheet.

THREE Bake 10 minutes. Turn fries over. Continue baking until tender and lightly browned, about 10 minutes longer.

Per serving: 102 calories, 4 g total fat, 0 g saturated fat, 17 g carbohydrates, 1 g protein, 2 g fiber, 0 mg cholesterol, 152 mg sodium

Savory Green Beans

A little bacon goes a long way, giving plain old green beans the "wow" factor!

Makes 6 servings

4 cups fresh or frozen green beans, cut into 2 inch pieces

2 bacon strips, diced

1 medium onion, thinly sliced

½ cup white wine or apple juice

3 tablespoons sugar

3 tablespoons tarragon vinegar or cider vinegar

¼ teaspoon salt

2 teaspoons cornstarch

1 tablespoon cold water

ONE Place beans in a saucepan and cover with water; bring to a boil. Cook, uncovered, until crisp-tender, 8 to 10 minutes. Meanwhile, in a large nonstick skillet, cook bacon over medium heat until crisp. Remove to paper towels. Drain, reserving 1 teaspoon drippings.

TWO In the drippings, sauté onion until tender. Add wine or apple juice, sugar, vinegar, and salt. Combine cornstarch and cold water until smooth; add to the skillet. Bring to a boil; cook and stir until thickened, about 2 minutes. Drain beans; top with onion mixture. Sprinkle with bacon; toss to coat.

Per serving (¾ cup): 98 calories, 2 g total fat, 1 g saturated fat, 16 g carbohydrate, 2 g protein, 3 g fiber, 3 mg cholesterol, 140 mg sodium

Old-Fashioned Secret-Ingredient Chocolate Cake

Shhhh...don't let on that the secret in this delectable to-die-for cake is actually tomato juice, which adds surprising richness and moisture to the batter.

Makes 16 servings

Cake:

¾ cup tomato juice

¼ cup water

⅔ cup unsweetened cocoa powder

2¼ cups all-purpose flour

1 teaspoon baking soda

½ teaspoon baking powder

¼ teaspoon salt

1½ cups sugar

½ cup vegetable oil

3 large eggs

1½ teaspoons vanilla extract

Icing:

1 ounce unsweetened chocolate

2 tablespoons low-fat (1%) milk

1 tablespoon unsweetened cocoa powder

4 ounces one-third-less-fat cream cheese

2½ cups confectioners' sugar, sifted

½ cup seedless raspberry jam

ONE Preheat oven to 350°F. Coat two 9-inch round cake pans with nonstick cooking spray.

TWO In small saucepan, bring tomato juice and water to a boil. Whisk in cocoa powder until smooth. Remove from heat.

THREE In medium bowl, stir together flour, baking soda, baking powder, and salt.

FOUR In large bowl, beat together sugar, oil, eggs, and 1 teaspoon vanilla extract until combined. Beat in cocoa mixture. Beat in flour mixture just until evenly moistened. Divide batter between prepared pans.

FIVE Bake until toothpick inserted in centers of cakes comes out clean, 25 to 30 minutes. Transfer pans to wire rack. Let cool 10 minutes. Turn cakes out onto rack. Let cool completely.

SIX Prepare icing: In medium microwave-safe bowl, microwave together chocolate and milk on high power 1 minute. Stir until smooth. Whisk in cocoa powder until smooth. Whisk in cream cheese and ½ teaspoon vanilla extract. Stir in confectioners' sugar until combined.

SEVEN Place one cake layer on flat plate or platter. Spread top of this layer with jam. Place remaining layer over layer with jam on it. Spread icing over sides and top of cake.

Per serving: 283 cal, 11 g total fat, 3 g saturated fat, 44 g carbohydrate, 5 g protein, 2 g fiber, 39 mg cholesterol, 207 mg sodium

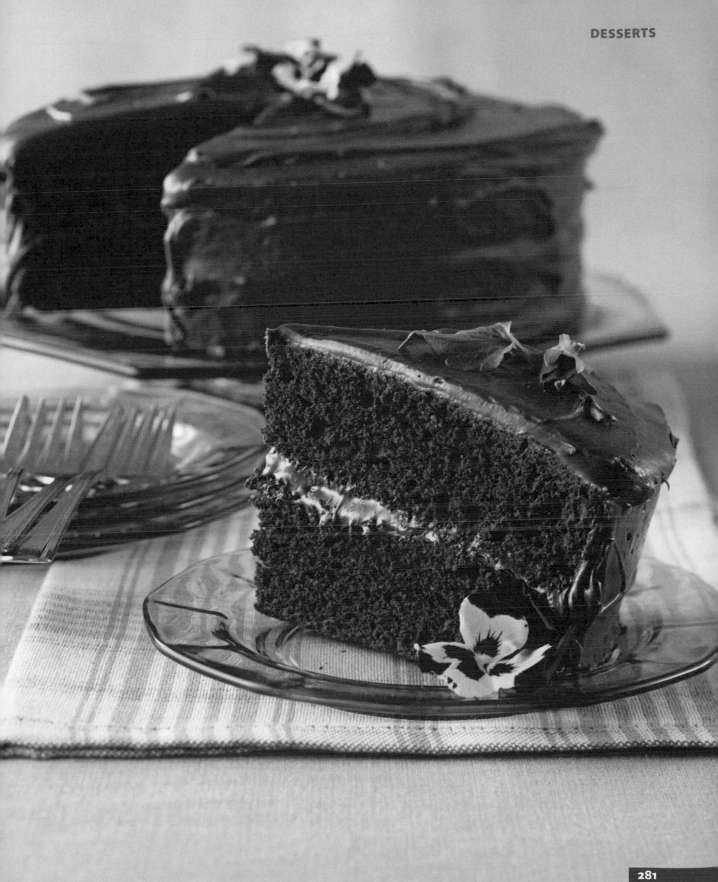

Daffodil Cake

A fragrant, delicate sponge cake with swirls of yellow and white in every slice, this festive, healthy treat is flavored with orange.

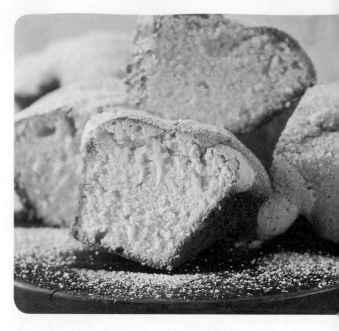

Makes 16 servings

10 large eggs, separated

1½ cups granulated sugar

2 teaspoons grated orange zest

1 tablespoon vanilla

Salt to taste

½ teaspoon cream of tartar

1⅓ cups sifted cake flour

⅓ cup sifted confectioners' sugar

ONE Preheat oven to 375°F.
Beat 4 egg yolks (reserve remaining 6 yolks for another recipe), ¼ cup granulated sugar, and orange zest in large bowl with electric mixer at high speed until batter is thick and lemon-colored, about 10 minutes. Scrape down bowl occasionally with spatula. Beat in vanilla.

TWO Beat all 10 egg whites and salt in separate large bowl with clean beaters at high speed until foamy. Add cream of tartar and beat until soft peaks form. Add remaining granulated sugar, 2 tablespoons at a time, beating at high speed until sugar has dissolved and stiff, glossy peaks form.

THREE Sift flour over egg whites, ⅓ cup at a time, gently folding in each addition with a wire whisk just until flour is no longer visible. Fold one-third of egg white mixture into yolk mixture.

FOUR Alternately spoon heaping tablespoons of yellow and white batters into a 9- or 10-inch tube pan. Swirl thin spatula or knife through batter to marbleize. Lightly swirl top of cake. Bake until cake springs back when lightly touched, about 35 minutes. Invert cake in pan onto bottle and cool completely. Run knife around pan to loosen cake. Remove cake from pan, place on serving plate, and sprinkle cake with confectioners' sugar.

Per serving: 175 calories, 3 g total fat, 1 g saturated fat, 32 g carbohydrate, 5 g protein, 0 g fiber, 113 mg cholesterol, 44 mg sodium

Old-Fashioned Fruit Cobbler

Pretty in pink, this springtime treat stars rhubarb and strawberries. Lucky you if these grow in your garden or if you have access to a good green market. The flaxseed and whole wheat flour make this dessert wholesome and healthy.

Makes 4 servings

Filling:

3 cups chopped (½-inch pieces) rhubarb

2 cups halved strawberries

¼ cup granulated sugar

3 tablespoons cornstarch

1½ teaspoons grated orange zest

Topping:

¼ cup whole flaxseed

⅓ cup whole wheat flour

⅓ cup all-purpose flour

¼ cup plus 1 teaspoon sugar

1 teaspoon baking soda

½ teaspoon baking powder

pinch of salt

2 ounces (¼ cup) reduced-fat cream cheese

2 tablespoons canola oil

¼ cup low-fat buttermilk

3 tablespoons sliced almonds

ONE Preheat the oven to 400°F. Coat an 8- by 8-inch baking dish with cooking spray.

TWO To make the filling: In a large bowl, combine the rhubarb, strawberries, sugar, cornstarch, and orange zest and mix. Spread in the baking dish.

THREE To make the topping: Grind the flaxseed into a coarse meal in a spice grinder or blender. Transfer to a large bowl. Add the flour, ¼ cup sugar, baking soda, baking powder, and salt and whisk to blend. Add the cream cheese and blend with a pastry blender or your fingers, until the mixture resembles coarse crumbs. Add the oil and toss with a fork. Gradually add the buttermilk, stirring with a fork until the dough clumps. Transfer to a lightly floured surface and knead several times. Pat into a ½-inch-thick square and cut into 9 pieces. Arrange the pieces over the fruit, leaving a little space between them. Sprinkle with the almonds and remaining 1 teaspoon sugar.

FOUR Bake until the fruit is bubbly and the biscuit is golden and firm, 35 to 40 minutes.

Per serving: 213 calories, 9 g total fat, 1 g saturated fat, 31 g carbohydrate, 4 g protein, 4 g fiber, 4 mg cholesterol, 258 mg sodium

Crispy Pumpkin Tartlets

A delicious, creative—and easy!—take on a Thanksgiving favorite, these tartlets are pretty and appealing.

Makes 8 servings

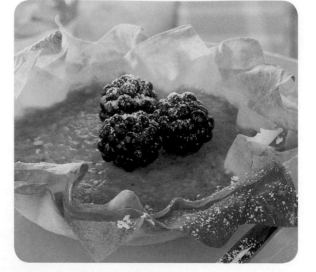

1 tablespoon vegetable oil

1 tablespoon butter

3 eggs

8 ounces reduced-fat evaporated milk

¼ cup light-brown sugar

¼ cup shredded coconut

Grated zest and juice of 1 orange

½ teaspoon each ground cinnamon, ground ginger, and grated nutmeg

1 can (15 ounces) solid-pack pumpkin puree

4 sheets phyllo pastry (20 by 11 inches each), thawed

½ pint blackberries

Confectioners' sugar for dusting

ONE Preheat oven to 375°F. In small saucepan, warm oil and butter together until butter melts. Remove from heat. Use a little of this mixture to lightly grease eight 3-inch individual pie or tart pans.

TWO In large bowl, whisk together eggs, milk, brown sugar, coconut, orange zest and juice, and spices until well combined. Stir in pumpkin puree.

THREE Cut 32 five-inch squares from phyllo pastry (8 from each sheet). Layer 4 phyllo squares in each prepared pan, brushing each with oil and butter mixture. Add squares at different angles for petal-edge effect. Spoon pumpkin filling into pastry-lined pans.

FOUR Bake tartlets until filling is set, 20 to 25 minutes. Transfer pans to wire rack to cool slightly. Just before serving, top tartlets with blackberries and dust lightly with confectioner's sugar.

Per serving: 172 calories, 8 g total fat, 4 g saturated fat, 21 g carbohydrate, 6 g protein, 4 g fiber, 76 mg cholesterol, 118 mg sodium

Lemon Blueberry Cheesecake

This lovely and lemony no-bake dessert is easy enough for a beginner and packs lots of sweet-tart flavor into very few calories.

Makes 12 servings

1 package (3 ounces) lemon gelatin

1 cup boiling water

2 tablespoons butter or stick margarine, melted

1 tablespoon canola oil

1 cup graham cracker crumbs (about 16 squares)

1 carton (24 ounces) fat-free cottage cheese

¼ cup sugar

Topping:
2 tablespoons sugar

1½ teaspoons cornstarch

¼ cup water

1⅓ cups fresh or frozen blueberries, divided

1 teaspoon lemon juice

ONE In a bowl, dissolve gelatin in boiling water; cool. Combine butter and oil; add crumbs and blend well. Press onto the bottom of a 9-inch springform pan. Chill. In a blender, process cottage cheese and sugar until smooth. While processing, slowly add cooled gelatin. Pour into crust; chill overnight.

TWO For topping, combine sugar and cornstarch in a saucepan; stir in water until smooth. Add 1 cup blueberries. Bring to a boil; cook and stir until thickened, about 2 minutes. Stir in lemon juice; cool slightly. Process in a blender until smooth. Refrigerate until completely cooled. Carefully run a knife around edge of pan to loosen cheesecake; remove sides of pan. Spread the blueberry mixture over the top. Top with remaining blueberries. Refrigerate leftovers.

Per serving: 171 calories, 4 g total fat, 1 g saturated fat, 27 g carbohydrate, 8 g protein, 1 g fiber, 8 mg cholesterol, 352 mg sodium

Blueberry Bavarian

This creamy dessert is a low-fat berried treasure—but we promise, you won't miss the extra calories!

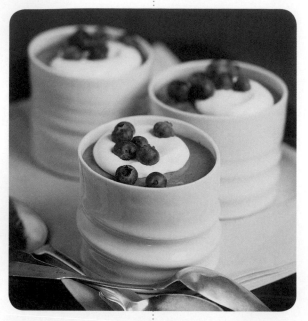

Makes 6 servings

1 cup low-fat (1%) milk

¼ cup fat-free dry milk

2 packages (12 ounces each) frozen blueberries, thawed

½ cup plus 1 tablespoon sugar

¼ teaspoon salt

1 cup fat-free sour cream

1 packet unflavored gelatin

¼ cup cold water

½ cup fresh blueberries

ONE Combine milk and dry milk in a small bowl and whisk until well blended. Place in freezer for up to 30 minutes.

TWO Combine frozen blueberries, ½ cup sugar, and salt in a medium saucepan over low heat. Bring to a simmer and cook until the sugar has dissolved, berries have broken up, and mixture has reduced to 2¼ cups, about 10 minutes. Let cool to room temperature. Stir in ⅔ cup sour cream.

THREE Sprinkle gelatin over cold water in heatproof measuring cup. Let stand 5 minutes to soften. Set measuring cup in small saucepan of simmering water and heat until gelatin has melted, about 2 minutes. Let cool to room temperature.

FOUR With a hand mixer, beat chilled milk until thick, soft peaks form. Beat in remaining 1 tablespoon sugar until stiff peaks form. Beat in gelatin mixture. Fold milk mixture into blueberry mixture.

FIVE Spoon into 6 dessert bowls or glasses. Chill until set, about 2 hours. At serving time, top each with a dollop of sour cream and fresh blueberries.

Per serving: 202 calories, 1 g total fat, 0.5 g saturated fat, 43 g carbohydrate, 7 g protein, 3 g fiber, 2 mg cholesterol, 178 sodium

Mixed Berry Tart

What a delectable way to get your berries! You can easily whip up this professional-looking dessert, even if you're a beginner.

Makes 12 servings

¼ cup ice water, without ice

3 tablespoons low-fat plain yogurt

1 cup whole-grain pastry flour

½ cup all-purpose flour

1 tablespoon plus ⅓ cup sugar

¼ teaspoon ground cinnamon

¼ teaspoon salt

7 tablespoons nonhydrogenated butter-replacement stick margarine

5 cups mixed berries, such as blueberries, raspberries, and strawberries

2 tablespoons cornstarch

1 tablespoon lemon juice

Confectioners' sugar (optional)

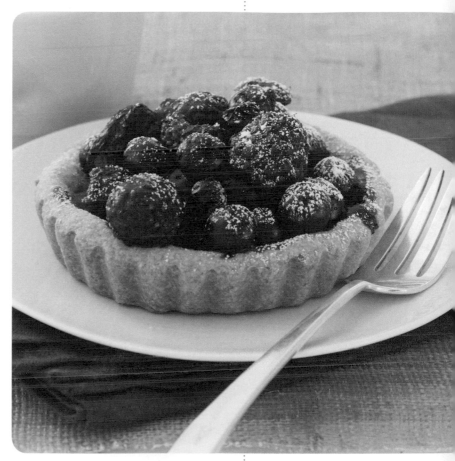

ONE In a measuring cup, whisk together the water and yogurt. In a food processor, combine the pastry and all-purpose flour, 1 tablespoon sugar, cinnamon, and salt. Add the margarine and pulse until the mixture resembles coarse crumbs. With the motor running, gradually add the yogurt mixture and process just until the ingredients come together. Gather the dough into a ball. Wrap in plastic and refrigerate for at least 2 hours.

TWO Preheat the oven to 350°F. In a large bowl, combine the berries, cornstarch, lemon juice, and sugar and toss gently.

THREE Shape dough into 6 small balls. Roll out each ball on a lightly floured work surface to about a 6-inch circle (tip: roll dough between 2 layers of plastic wrap). Using six 4-inch tartlet pans with removable bottoms, line the pans with the dough. Evenly distribute the fruit mixture into the pans.

FOUR Bake until the filling is bubbling and crust is browned, 15 to 20 minutes. Transfer to a rack for 15 minutes. Remove from pans and cool completely. Each tartlet is 2 servings. Dust with confectioners' sugar.

Per serving: 164 calories, 7 g total fat, 2 g saturated fat, 25 g carbohydrate, 2 g protein, 3 g fiber, 0 mg cholesterol, 124 mg sodium

Raspberry Frozen Yogurt

Here's a great way to use summer's bounty of ripe red raspberries. This refreshing homemade dessert has far less sugar than store-bought frozen yogurt.

Makes 8 servings

1 pound raspberries, rinsed

4 tablespoons seedless raspberry jam

2 tablespoons rose water (optional)

1 pound plain nonfat yogurt

3 tablespoons confectioners' sugar, or to taste

Raspberries for garnish

Fresh mint leaves for garnish

ONE Put the raspberries into a saucepan and add the raspberry jam. Warm over a low heat until the raspberries are pulpy, stirring occasionally, about 5 minutes.

TWO Press the raspberries and their juice through a sieve into a bowl; discard the seeds in the sieve. Stir in the rose water, if using. Whisk in the yogurt until smoothly blended. Taste the mixture and sweeten with the sugar.

THREE Pour into an ice cream machine and freeze according to the manufacturer's instructions. When you have a smooth and creamy frozen mixture, spoon it into a rigid freezer-proof container. Freeze for at least 1 hour. If you do not have an ice cream machine, pour the mixture straight into a large freezer-proof container and freeze until set around the edges, about 1 hour. Beat until the mixture is smooth, then return to the freezer. Freeze for 30 minutes, then beat again. Repeat the freezing and beating several times more until the frozen yogurt has a smooth consistency, then leave it to freeze for at least 1 hour.

FOUR If storing in the freezer for longer than 1 hour, transfer the frozen yogurt to the fridge 20 minutes before serving, to soften slightly. Decorate with raspberries and mint, if desired.

Per serving: 80 calories, 0 g total fat, 0 g saturated fat, 18 g carbohydrate, 3 g protein, 4 g fiber, 1 mg cholesterol, 36 mg sodium

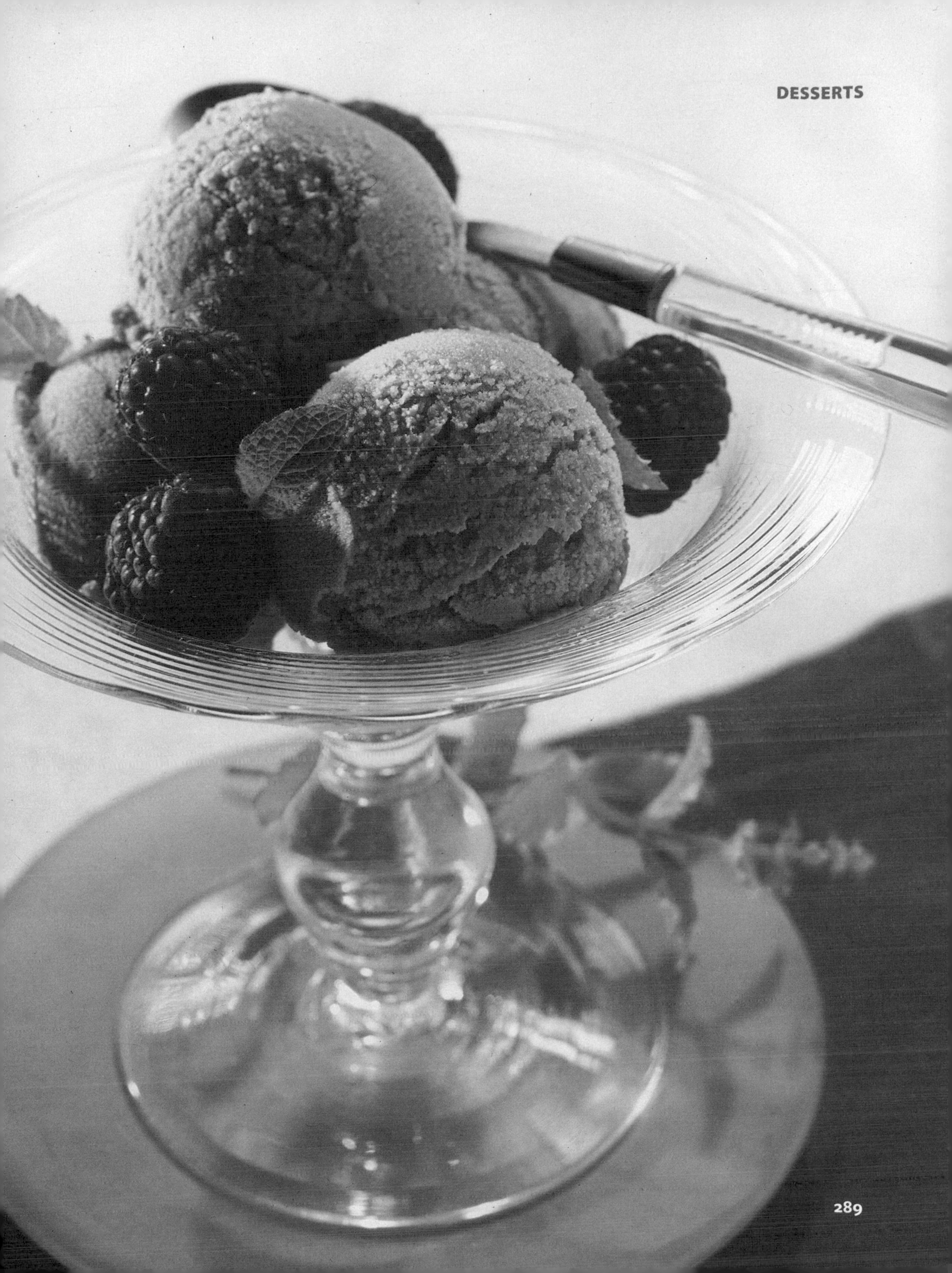

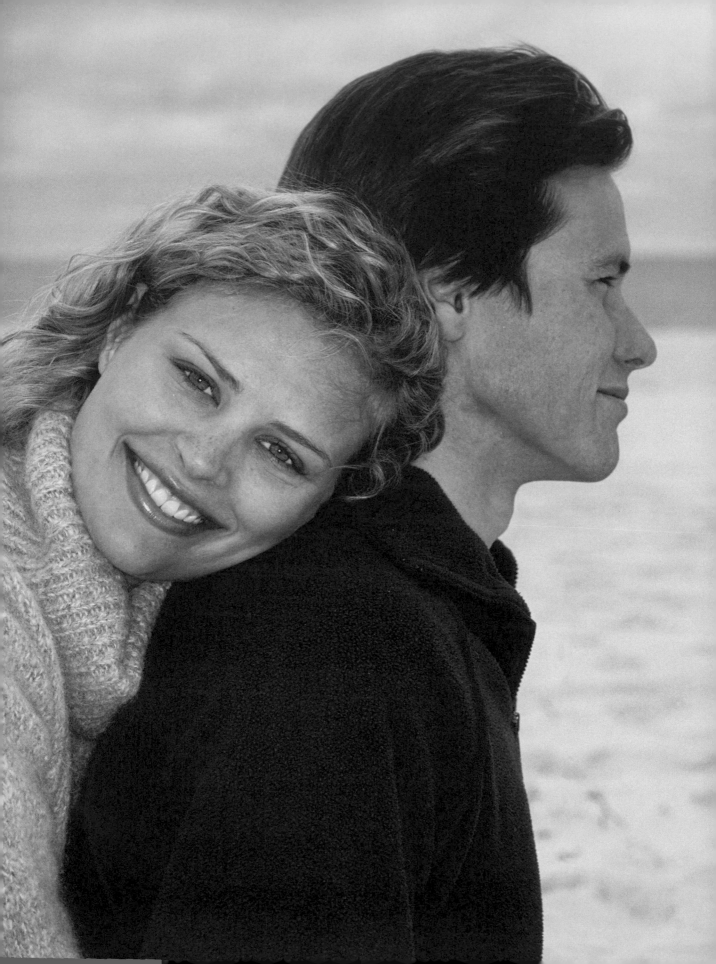

PART 6

Healthy Tools

As you begin your journey to reverse diabetes forever, lots of diet and lifestyle changes can seem abstract or overwhelming. But here, in the following pages, are hands-on tools to help you plan exercise, track diets, and ensure you're staying up to date on medical checkups. By using these tools, many of those abstract notions will become real. When you post your diet diary on your fridge, you'll see your progress from day to day. Time to get to work!

▼▼▼▼▼▼▼▼▼▼▼▼

Start Here: Your Food Diary

To be successful in reversing diabetes forever, it's essential to start by having a baseline of what you take in everyday. Write down everything you eat and drink, the estimated portion size, and the estimated calories (check the calorie counts at www.caloriecontrol.org). At the end of the week, look over your food diary for patterns and opportunities. Do you skip fruits or vegetables at breakfast or lunch? Do you snack late at night? Where are you overdoing the calories?

Copy these two pages to keep track week after week. In addition to any notes about food, feel free to include any other comments that can help you (and your doctor) look back to examine trends.

monday	tuesday	wednesday
breakfast		
lunch		
dinner		

thursday	friday	saturday	sunday

Reverse Diabetes Forever Daily Diet and Lifestyle Goals

Record what you eat for a week, then compare that to how you should eat. This diary provides an easy-to-use self-assessment. By circling a few numbers and checking some boxes, you can track your progress every day. The numbers in bold are the goal you should shoot for. Copy these pages and post them in a visible place for a daily diet and lifestyle record.

① monday

My numbers:

weight _____

blood sugar (time/level) _____ / _____
_____ / _____ • _____ / _____

Servings I ate today:

vegetables 0 1 2 3 4 **5 6 7**
fruit 0 1 2 **3**
whole grains 0 1 2 3 **4 5 6**
calcium-rich foods 0 1 **2 3**

Times I ate out of boredom, stress, or habit:

0 1 2 3 4 5

How I took charge:

eat right
☐ ate a healthy breakfast
☐ had protein at every meal
☐ avoided refined carbohydrates and sugary drinks
☐ swapped saturated fats for good fats

exercise more
☐ walked _____ minutes / _____ steps
☐ got other exercise _____

live well
☐ got enough sleep (_____ hours)
☐ kept TV time under 2 hours
☐ found time for relaxation and/or socializing

My attitude today:

☐ excellent
☐ pretty good
☐ not my best day; I'll do better tomorrow

① tuesday

My numbers:

weight _____

blood sugar (time/level) _____ / _____
_____ / _____ • _____ / _____

Servings I ate today:

vegetables 0 1 2 3 4 **5 6 7**
fruit 0 1 2 **3**
whole grains 0 1 2 3 **4 5 6**
calcium-rich foods 0 1 **2 3**

Times I ate out of boredom, stress, or habit:

0 1 2 3 4 5

How I took charge:

eat right
☐ ate a healthy breakfast
☐ had protein at every meal
☐ avoided refined carbohydrates and sugary drinks
☐ swapped saturated fats for good fats

exercise more
☐ walked _____ minutes / _____ steps
☐ got other exercise _____

live well
☐ got enough sleep (_____ hours)
☐ kept TV time under 2 hours
☐ found time for relaxation and/or socializing

My attitude today:

☐ excellent
☐ pretty good
☐ not my best day; I'll do better tomorrow

① wednesday

My numbers:

weight _____

blood sugar (time/level) _____ / _____

_____ / _____ • _____ / _____

Servings I ate today:

vegetables 0 1 2 3 4 **5 6 7**
fruit 0 1 2 **3**
whole grains 0 1 2 3 **4 5 6**
calcium-rich foods 0 1 **2 3**

Times I ate out of boredom, stress, or habit:

0 1 2 3 4 5

How I took charge:

eat right
☐ ate a healthy breakfast
☐ had protein at every meal
☐ avoided refined carbohydrates and sugary drinks
☐ swapped saturated fats for good fats

exercise more
☐ walked _____ minutes / _____ steps
☐ got other exercise _____

live well
☐ got enough sleep (_____ hours)
☐ kept TV time under 2 hours
☐ found time for relaxation and/or socializing

My attitude today:

☐ excellent
☐ pretty good
☐ not my best day; I'll do better tomorrow

① thursday

My numbers:

weight _____

blood sugar (time/level) _____ / _____

_____ / _____ • _____ / _____

Servings I ate today:

vegetables 0 1 2 3 4 **5 6 7**
fruit 0 1 2 **3**
whole grains 0 1 2 3 **4 5 6**
calcium-rich foods 0 1 **2 3**

Times I ate out of boredom, stress, or habit:

0 1 2 3 4 5

How I took charge:

eat right
☐ ate a healthy breakfast
☐ had protein at every meal
☐ avoided refined carbohydrates and sugary drinks
☐ swapped saturated fats for good fats

exercise more
☐ walked _____ minutes / _____ steps
☐ got other exercise _____

live well
☐ got enough sleep (_____ hours)
☐ kept TV time under 2 hours
☐ found time for relaxation and/or socializing

My attitude today:

☐ excellent
☐ pretty good
☐ not my best day; I'll do better tomorrow

1 friday

My numbers:

weight _____

blood sugar (time/level) _____ / _____
_____ / _____ • _____ / _____

Servings I ate today:

vegetables 0 1 2 3 4 **5 6 7**
fruit 0 1 2 **3**
whole grains 0 1 2 3 **4 5 6**
calcium-rich foods 0 1 **2 3**

Times I ate out of boredom, stress, or habit:

0 1 2 3 4 5

How I took charge:

eat right
☐ ate a healthy breakfast
☐ had protein at every meal
☐ avoided refined carbohydrates
   and sugary drinks
☐ swapped saturated fats for good fats

exercise more
☐ walked _____ minutes / _____ steps
☐ got other exercise _____

live well
☐ got enough sleep (_____ hours)
☐ kept TV time under 2 hours
☐ found time for relaxation and/or socializing

My attitude today:

☐ excellent
☐ pretty good
☐ not my best day; I'll do better tomorrow

1 saturday

My numbers:

weight _____

blood sugar (time/level) _____ / _____
_____ / _____ • _____ / _____

Servings I ate today:

vegetables 0 1 2 3 4 **5 6 7**
fruit 0 1 2 **3**
whole grains 0 1 2 3 **4 5 6**
calcium-rich foods 0 1 **2 3**

Times I ate out of boredom, stress, or habit:

0 1 2 3 4 5

How I took charge:

eat right
☐ ate a healthy breakfast
☐ had protein at every meal
☐ avoided refined carbohydrates
   and sugary drinks
☐ swapped saturated fats for good fats

exercise more
☐ walked _____ minutes / _____ steps
☐ got other exercise _____

live well
☐ got enough sleep (_____ hours)
☐ kept TV time under 2 hours
☐ found time for relaxation and/or socializing

My attitude today:

☐ excellent
☐ pretty good
☐ not my best day; I'll do better tomorrow

① sunday

My numbers:

weight _____

blood sugar (time/level) _____ / _____

_____ / _____ • _____ / _____

Servings I ate today:

vegetables 0 1 2 3 4 **5 6 7**

fruit 0 1 2 **3**

whole grains 0 1 2 3 **4 5 6**

calcium-rich foods 0 1 **2 3**

Times I ate out of boredom, stress, or habit:

0 1 2 3 4 5

How I took charge:

eat right

☐ ate a healthy breakfast

☐ had protein at every meal

☐ avoided refined carbohydrates and sugary drinks

☐ swapped saturated fats for good fats

exercise more

☐ walked _____ minutes / _____ steps

☐ got other exercise _____

live well

☐ got enough sleep (_____ hours)

☐ kept TV time under 2 hours

☐ found time for relaxation and/or socializing

My attitude today:

☐ excellent

☐ pretty good

☐ not my best day; I'll do better tomorrow

① the week in review

Successes and confessions

_____

_____

_____

_____

_____

_____

My numbers:

weight loss: _____ pounds

waist measurement: _____ inches

Next week's goals

eat right

Dinner should be 450-550 calories. This may be quite a bit less than you're eating now. To help bring your calories in line, start dinners this week with either a green salad or a bowl of clear soup to help fill you up.

exercise more

You should have started the walking plan by now. Next week, walk for 15 minutes at least 5 days a week. Put your walks on your calendar, and be sure to keep all your "appointments."

live well

Enlist a support team. Ask your spouse to join you in your walks next week. Tell all your friends and family that you've started to improve your diet and ask for their encouragement.

Weekly Blood-Sugar Log

Use this chart to log the results of your blood-sugar checks for an overall snapshot of your blood-sugar control over the course of a day and a week. Bring these log sheets to your doctor.

Beginning date: _____

Day	Medication	BLOOD-SUGAR LEVELS							
		Breakfast		Lunch		Dinner		Bedtime	Other
Sun.		Before	After*	Before	After*	Before	After*		

Day	Medication	Breakfast		Lunch		Dinner		Bedtime	Other
Mon.		Before	After*	Before	After*	Before	After*		

Day	Medication	Breakfast		Lunch		Dinner		Bedtime	Other
Tues.		Before	After*	Before	After*	Before	After*		

Day	Medication	Breakfast		Lunch		Dinner		Bedtime	Other
Wed.		Before	After*	Before	After*	Before	After*		

Day	Medication	Breakfast		Lunch		Dinner		Bedtime	Other
Thurs.		Before	After*	Before	After*	Before	After*		

Day	Medication	Breakfast		Lunch		Dinner		Bedtime	Other
Fri.		Before	After*	Before	After*	Before	After*		

Day	Medication	Breakfast		Lunch		Dinner		Bedtime	Other
Sat.		Before	After*	Before	After*	Before	After*		

*Take your after-meal readings two hours after the start of the meal.

Calories, Carbohydrates, and Fiber

Item	Amount	Calories	Carb grams	Fiber grams
BEEF				
Beef, chuck	3 oz	293	0	0
Corned beef	3 oz	213	0.8	0
Ground beef, 75% lean	3 oz	236	0	0
Ground beef, 85% lean	3 oz	213	0	0
Beef, rib	3 oz	304	0	0
Beef, bottom round	3 oz	210	0	0
Beef, top sirloin	3 oz	207	0	0
BEVERAGES				
Beer, light	12 fl oz	103	5.2	0
Beer, regular	12 fl oz	138	10.7	0
Chocolate milk	1 cup	226	31.7	1.1
Club soda	12 fl oz	0	0	0
Coffee	6 fl oz	2	0	0
Cola	12 fl oz	155	39.8	0
Diet cola	12 fl oz	4	0.4	0
Espresso	2 fl oz	1	0	0
Fruit punch	8 fl oz	117	29.7	0.5
Hot cocoa	1 cup	113	24	1
Ginger ale	12 fl oz	124	32.1	0
Instant coffee	6 fl oz	4	0.6	0
Lemonade	8 fl oz	112	34.1	0.2
Liquor (rum, gin, vodka, whiskey)	1.5 fl oz	110	0	0
Piña colada	4.5 fl oz	245	32	0.4
Soy milk	1 cup	127	12.08	3.2
Tea	6 fl oz	2	0.5	0
Wine, red	3.5 fl oz	74	1.8	0
Wine, white	3.5 fl oz	70	0.8	0
BREAD, BAGELS, ROLLS				
Bagel, plain	4"	245	48	2
Bagel, cinnamon raisin	4"	244	49	2
Bagel, egg	4"	247	47.2	2
Biscuit, buttermilk	4"	358	45.1	1.5
Bread, French	1/2" slice	69	13	0.8

Item	Amount	Calories	Carb grams	Fiber grams
Bread, Italian	1 slice	54	10	0.5
Bread, white	1 slice	67	12.7	0.6
Bread, wheat	1 slice	69	12.9	1.9
Bread, rye	1 slice	83	15.5	1.9
Bread, pumpernickel	1 slice	80	15.2	2.1
Bread, raisin	1 slice	71	13.6	1.1
Croissant	1	231	26.1	1.5
Corn bread	1 piece	173	28.3	1.4
Pita	4"	77	15.6	0.6
CEREALS				
All Bran	1/2 cup	79	23	9.7
Apple Cinnamon Cheerios	3/4 cup	118	25	1.6
Cap'n Crunch	3/4 cup	108	22.9	0.7
Cheerios	1 cup	111	22.2	3.6
Chex, Corn	1 cup	112	25.8	0.6
Chex, Honey Nut	3/4 cup	117	26	0.4
Chex, Multi-Bran	1 cup	165	41	6.4
Cornflakes	1 cup	101	24.4	0.7
Cream of Wheat	1 cup	126	26.9	1
Froot Loops	1 cup	118	26.2	0.8
Frosted Flakes	3/4 cup	114	28	1
Frosted Mini-Wheats	1 cup	173	42	5.5
Honey Nut Cheerios	1 cup	115	24	1.6
Life	3/4 cup	121	25	2
Oatmeal, regular	1 cup	147	25.3	4
Oatmeal, instant, apples and cinnamon	1 packet	130	26.5	2.7
Puffed Rice	1 cup	56	12.6	0.2
Puffed Wheat	1 cup	44	10	0.5
Raisin Bran	1 cup	195	46.5	7.3
Rice Krispies	1 1/4 cups	119	28	0.1
Special K	1 cup	117	22	0.7
Shredded Wheat	2 biscuits	155	36.2	5.5
Total	3/4 cup	105	24	2.6

Item	Amount	Calories	Carb grams	Fiber grams
Trix	1 cup	122	26	0.7
Wheaties	1 cup	107	26.7	3

DAIRY AND EGGS

Item	Amount	Calories	Carb grams	Fiber grams
Butter	1 Tbsp	102	0	0
Cheese food, American	1 oz	94	2.2	0
Cheese spread	1 oz	82	2.5	0
Cheese, blue	1 oz	100	0.7	0
Cheese, cheddar	1 oz	114	0.4	0
Cheese, cottage, regular	1 cup	216	5.6	0
Cheese, cottage, 2% milk fat	1 cup	203	8.2	0
Cheese, cottage, 1% milk fat	1 cup	163	6.2	0
Cheese, cream	1 Tbsp	51	0.4	0
Cheese, feta	1 oz	75	1.2	0
Cheese, mozzarella, part skim milk	1 oz	72	0.79	0
Cheese, mozzarella, whole milk	1 oz	85	0.6	0
Cheese, Muenster	1 oz	104	0.3	0
Cheese, Parmesan	1 Tbsp	22	0.2	0
Cheese, American	1 oz	106	0.5	0
Cheese, provolone	1 oz	100	0.6	0
Cheese, ricotta, part skim milk	1 cup	339	12.6	0
Cheese, ricotta, whole milk	1 cup	428	7.5	0
Cheese, Swiss	1 oz	108	1.5	0
Cream, half and half	1 Tbsp	20	0.7	0
Cream, heavy whipping	1 Tbsp	52	0.4	0
Cream, light	1 Tbsp	29	0.6	0
Cream, sour	1 Tbsp	26	0.5	0
Cream, sour, reduced-fat	1 Tbsp	20	0.6	0
Cream, sour, fat-free	1 Tbsp	12	2	0
Egg, whole	large	74	0.8	0
Egg, white	large	17	0.2	0
Egg, yolk	large	53	0.6	0
Eggnog	1 cup	343	34.3	0
Ice cream, chocolate	1/2 cup	143	18.6	0.8

Item	Amount	Calories	Carb grams	Fiber grams
Ice cream, vanilla, soft-serve	1/2 cup	191	19.1	0.6
Ice cream, vanilla	1/2 cup	133	15.6	0.5
Milkshake, vanilla	11 fl oz	351	55.6	0
Buttermilk	1 cup	98	11.7	0
Milk, condensed, sweetened	1 cup	982	166.5	0
Milk, evaporated, nonfat	1 cup	200	29.1	0
Milk, nonfat	1 cup	83	12.1	0
Milk, 1% milk fat	1 cup	102	12.2	0
Milk, 2% milk fat	1 cup	102	11.4	0
Milk, whole	1 cup	146	11	0
Yogurt, fruit, low-fat	8 oz	232	43.2	0
Yogurt, plain, low-fat	8 oz	143	16	0

FATS AND OIL

Item	Amount	Calories	Carb grams	Fiber grams
Lard	1 Tbsp	115	0	0
Margarine	1 Tbsp	102	0.1	0
Margarine-like spread	1 Tbsp	51	0	0
Mayonnaise, regular	1 Tbsp	99	0	0
Mayonnaise, fat-free	1 Tbsp	12	2	0.6
Oil, canola	1 Tbsp	124	0	0
Oil, olive	1 Tbsp	119	0	0
Oil, peanut	1 Tbsp	119	0	0
Oil, sesame	1 Tbsp	120	0	0
Oil, vegetable or corn	1 Tbsp	120	0	0
Shortening	1 Tbsp	113	0	0

FISH AND SHELLFISH

Item	Amount	Calories	Carb grams	Fiber grams
Catfish, breaded and fried	3 oz	195	6.8	0.6
Crab	3 oz	82	0	0
Flounder	3 oz	99	0	0
Haddock, baked	3 oz	95	0	0
Halibut	3 oz	119	0	0
Lobster	3 oz	83	1.1	0
Ocean perch	3 oz	103	0	0
Orange roughy	3 oz	76	0	0

Item	Amount	Calories	Carb grams	Fiber grams
Pollock	3 oz	96	0	0
Rainbow trout	3 oz	144	0	0
Raw clams	3 oz	63	2.2	0
Raw oysters	6 med	57	3.3	0
Salmon, baked or broiled	3 oz	184	0	0
Salmon, canned	3 oz	118	0	0
Sardines	3 oz	177	0	0
Scallops, breaded	6 large	200	9.4	0
Shrimp, breaded	3 oz	206	5.2	0.2
Swordfish	3 oz	132	0	0
Tuna, baked or broiled	3 oz	118	0	0
Tuna, chunk white	3 oz	109	0	0

FRUIT AND JUICES

Item	Amount	Calories	Carb grams	Fiber grams
Apple juice	1 cup	117	29	0.2
Apple	1	72	19.1	3.3
Applesauce, sweetened	1 cup	194	51	3.1
Applesauce, unsweetened	1 cup	108	28	2.9
Apricot	1	17	3.9	0.7
Apricots, dried	1/4 cup	96	25	3.6
Apricots, canned in heavy syrup	1 cup	214	55	4.1
Apricots, canned in juice	1 cup	117	30	3.9
Apricot nectar, canned	1 cup	141	36	1.5
Asian pear	1 small	51	13	4.4
Avocado	1 oz	47	2.5	1.9
Banana	1	105	27	3.1
Blackberries	1 cup	75	18	7.6
Blueberries	1 cup	83	21	3.5
Cantaloupe	1 cup	107	28	3
Cherries, sour	1 cup	88	22	2.7
Cherries, sweet	10	49	11	1.6
Cranberries, dried, sweetened	1/4 cup	92	24	2.5
Cranberry juice cocktail	8 fl oz	144	36.4	0.3
Cranberry sauce, canned	1 slice	86	22	0.6
Currants, dried	1/4 cup	102	26.7	2.4

Item	Amount	Calories	Carb grams	Fiber grams
Dates, chopped	1/4 cup	122	32.7	3.3
Figs, dried	1/4 cup	127	32.5	5.8
Figs, fresh	1	37	9.6	1.7
Grape juice	1 cup	154	37.9	0.3
Grapefruit	1/2	39	9.9	1.3
Grapefruit juice	1 cup	96	22.7	0.2
Grapes, red or green	1 cup	110	29	1.4
Kiwi	1	46	11.1	2.3
Honeydew melon	1 cup	60	16	1
Lemon juice	juice of 1 lemon	12	4	0.2
Lime juice	juice of 1 lime	10	3.2	0.2
Mandarin oranges, canned in light syrup	1 cup	154	41	1.8
Mango	1 cup	107	28	3.7
Nectarine	1	67	16.0	2.2
Orange juice	1 cup	112	25.8	0.5
Orange	1	62	15.4	3.1
Papaya	1 cup	55	29.8	2.5
Peach	1	38	9.4	1.5
Peaches, canned in heavy syrup	1 cup	194	52	3.4
Peaches, canned in juice	1 cup	109	29	3.2
Pear	1 pear	96	25.7	5.1
Pears, canned in heavy syrup	1 cup	197	51	4.3
Pears, canned in juice	1 cup	124	32	4
Pineapple juice	1 cup	140	34.5	0.5
Pineapple	1 cup	74	19.6	2.2
Pineapple, canned in heavy syrup	1 cup	198	51	2
Pineapple, canned in juice	1 cup	149	39	2
Plantain, raw	1	218	57	4.1
Plantain, cooked slices	1 cup	179	48	3.5
Plum	1	30	7.5	0.9

Item	Amount	Calories	Carb grams	Fiber grams
Plums, canned in heavy syrup	1 cup	230	60	2.6
Plums, canned in juice	1 cup	146	38	2.5
Prunes, dried	5	100	26	3
Prunes, stewed	1 cup	265	70	16.4
Prune juice	1 cup	182	44.7	2.6
Raisins	1/4 cup	108	28.7	1.3
Raspberries	1 cup	64	14.7	8
Strawberries	1 cup	53	12.8	3.3
Tangerine	1	31	7.8	1.6
Watermelon	1 cup	56	11.5	0.6

GRAINS AND PASTAS

Item	Amount	Calories	Carb grams	Fiber grams
Couscous	1 cup	176	36.5	2.2
Barley, pearled and cooked	1 cup	193	44	6
Bulgur	1 cup	151	33	8.2
Cornmeal	1 cup	444	94	8.9
Egg noodles	1 cup	213	39.7	1.8
Kasha (buckwheat groats)	1 cup	155	33	4.5
Oat bran (raw)	1 cup	231	62.3	14.5
Rice, brown	1 cup	216	45	3.5
Rice, white	1 cup	205	45	0.6
Rice, instant	1 cup	162	35	1
Rice, wild	1 cup	166	35	3
Pasta, regular	1 cup	197	40	2.4
Pasta, whole-wheat	1 cup	174	37	6.3
Wheat flour, bleached (white)	1 cup	455	95	3.4
Wheat flour, whole-grain	1 cup	407	87	14.6
Wheat germ	1 Tbsp	27	3	0.9

LAMB, VEAL, AND GAME

Item	Amount	Calories	Carb grams	Fiber grams
Lamb, leg	3 oz	219	0	0
Lamb, loin	3 oz	265	0	0
Lamb, shoulder	3 oz	294	0	0
Veal, leg	3 oz	179	0	0
Duck	1/2 duck	144	0	0

LEGUMES

Item	Amount	Calories	Carb grams	Fiber grams
Baked beans	1 cup	239	53.9	10.4
Black beans	1 cup	227	40.8	15
Chickpeas	1 cup	185	32.7	7.9
Great northern beans	1 cup	209	37.3	12.4
Lentils	1 cup	230	39.9	15.6
Navy beans	1 cup	255	47.4	19.1
Pinto beans	1 cup	245	44.8	15.4
Red kidney beans	1 cup	225	40.4	13.1

NUTS AND SEEDS

Item	Amount	Calories	Carb grams	Fiber grams
Almonds	1 oz	164	5.6	3.3
Brazil nuts	1 oz	186	3.5	2.1
Cashews	1 oz	163	9.3	1
Chestnuts	1 cup	350	75.7	7.3
Hazelnuts	1 oz	178	4.7	2.7
Macadamia nuts	1 oz	203	3.6	2.3
Peanuts	1 oz	166	6.1	2.3
Pecans	1 oz	196	3.9	2.7
Pistachios	1 oz	161	7.6	2.9
Pumpkin seeds	1 oz	148	3.8	1.1
Sesame seeds	1 Tbsp	47	1.2	1
Sunflower seeds	1 oz	165	6.8	2.9
Walnuts	1 oz	185	3.9	1.9

PORK

Item	Amount	Calories	Carb grams	Fiber grams
Pork sausage	1 patty	92	0	0
Bacon	3 slices	103	0.3	0
Ham, roasted	3 oz	207	0	0
Pork, loin chops	3 oz	235	0	0
Pork, roast	3 oz	217	0	0
Pork, shoulder	3 oz	280	0	0
Pork, spareribs	3 oz	337	0	0

Item	Amount	Calories	Carb grams	Fiber grams
POULTRY				
Chicken roll	2 slices	87	1.4	0
Chicken, breast w/o skin	1/2 breast	142	0	0
Chicken, dark meat w/o skin	1 drumstick	76	0	0
Chicken, thigh w/o skin	1 thigh	109	0	0
Chicken, breast w/ skin, batter-fried	1/2 breast	364	12.6	0.4
Chicken, dark meat w/ skin, batter-fried	1 drumstick	193	6	0.2
Chicken, thigh w/ skin, batter-fried	1 thigh	238	7.8	0.3
Turkey, roasted, dark	3 oz	157	0	0
Turkey, roasted, light	3 oz	132	0	0
SAUSAGE AND LUNCH MEAT				
Bologna	2 slices	175	3.1	0
Chicken, white meat	2 slices	72	1.3	0
Chicken breast, roasted, fat free	2 slices	48	0.9	0
Cooked salami	2 slices	142	1.3	0
Ham, regular	2 slices	91	2.1	0.7
Ham, extra lean	2 slices	60	0.4	0
Hard salami	2 slices	77	0.8	0
Sausage, pork or beef	2 links	103	0.7	0
Turkey breast	2 slices	55	1.8	0
Turkey breast, fat free	2 slices	47	2.52	0
Vienna sausage	1	37	0.4	0
SNACKS				
Chex Mix	1 oz	120	8.5	1.6
Cheese puffs	1 oz	157	15.3	0.3
Crackers, saltine	4	51	8.5	0.4

Item	Amount	Calories	Carb grams	Fiber grams
Granola bar, plain	1 bar	134	18.3	1.5
Olives	5 large	25	1.4	0.7
Pickles, dill	1	12	2.7	0.8
Popcorn, air-popped	1 cup	31	6.2	1.2
Popcorn, oil-popped	1 cup	55	6	1.1
Potato chips	1 oz	155	14.5	1
Pretzels	10	229	47.5	1.9
Rice cakes	1 cake	35	7.3	0.4
Tortilla chips	1 oz	142	17.8	1.8
SOUPS, GRAVIES, AND SAUCES				
Barbecue sauce	1 Tbsp	12	2	0.2
Beef bouillon	1 cup	29	1.8	0
Beef gravy	1/4 cup	31	2.8	0.2
Cheese sauce	1/4 cup	110	4.3	0.3
Chicken gravy	1/4 cup	47	3.2	0.2
Chicken noodle soup	1 cup	75	9.4	0.7
Country sausage gravy	1/4 cup	96	3.9	0.4
Cream of mushroom soup	1 cup	129	9.3	0.5
Hot pepper sauce	1 tsp	1	0.1	0
Lentil soup	1 cup	126	20.3	5
Manhattan clam chowder	1 cup	78	12.2	1.5
Minestrone	1 cup	82	11.2	1
Mushroom gravy	1/4 cup	30	3.3	0.2
New England clam chowder	1 cup	164	16.7	1.5
Onion soup	1 cup	27	5.1	1
Pasta sauce	1 cup	185	28.2	1
Pea soup	1 cup	165	26.5	2.8
Salsa	1 Tbsp	4	1	0.3
Teriyaki sauce	1 Tbsp	15	2.9	0
Tomato soup	1 cup	85	16.6	0.5

Item	Amount	Calories	Carb grams	Fiber grams
Turkey gravy	1/4 cup	30	3	0.2
Vegetable beef soup	1 cup	78	10.2	0.5

SWEETS

Item	Amount	Calories	Carb grams	Fiber grams
Brownies	1	227	35.8	1.2
Chocolate chip cookies	1 cookie	49	9.3	0.4
Cinnamon roll	1 roll	223	30.5	1.4
Cake, pound	1 piece	109	13.7	0.1
Cake, chocolate w/o frosting	1 piece	340	50.7	1.5
Coffee cake, crumb-type	1 piece	263	29	1.3
Doughnut, plain	1	198	23.4	0.7
Doughnut, glazed	1	242	26.6	0.7
Fudge	1 piece	70	13	0.3
Graham crackers	2	59	10.8	0.2
Hard candy	1 small piece	12	2.9	0
Jellybeans	10 large	106	26.5	0.1
Marshmallows	1 cup	159	40.7	0.1
Milk chocolate	1 bar	235	26.2	1.5
Pie, apple	1 piece	411	57.5	1.9
Pie, pecan	1 piece	503	63.7	4
Pie, pumpkin	1 piece	316	40.9	2.9
Pineapple upside down cake	1 piece	267	58	0.9
Pudding, chocolate	1/2 cup	154	27.8	0.6
Semisweet chocolate pieces	1 cup	805	106.1	9.9
Snickers	1 bar	266	36.8	1.4

VEGETABLES

Item	Amount	Calories	Carb grams	Fiber grams
Asparagus	4 spears	13	3.5	2.9
Beets	1 cup	75	16.9	3.4
Broccoli	1 cup	55	5.8	2.3
Brussels sprouts	1 cup	56	11	4.1
Cabbage	1 cup	17	3.9	1.6
Carrots	1 carrot	30	10.5	3.1
Cauliflower	1 cup	25	5.3	2.5
Celery	1 cup	17	3.6	1.9
Collard greens	1 cup	92	9	5.3
Corn	1 cup	133	31.7	3.9
Cucumbers	1 cup	16	3.8	0.8
Eggplant	1 cup	28	7	2.5
Endive	1 cup	9	2	1.6
Kale	1 cup	39	7	2.6
Leeks	1 cup	32	8	1
Lettuce, iceberg	1 cup	8	1.6	0.7
Lima beans	1 cup	170	32	9.9
Mushrooms	1 cup	15	2.3	0.8
Mustard greens	1 cup	21	3	2.8
Okra	1 cup	52	11	5.2
Onions	1 cup	67	16.2	2.2
Parsnips	1 cup	111	26.5	5.6
Potato w/ skin	1	118	27.4	2.4
Peas	1 cup	125	22.8	8.8
Peppers, green	1 cup	30	6.9	2.5
Radishes	1 radish	1	0.2	0.1
Red hot chili pepper	1	18	4	0.7
Romaine lettuce	1 cup	10	1.8	1.2
Soybeans	1 cup	254	20	7.6
Scallions	1 cup	32	7.3	2.6
Spinach	1 cup	7	1.1	0.7
Squash, summer	1 cup	18	3.8	2.5
Squash, winter	1 cup	76	18.1	2.5
Sweet potato	1	131	30.2	4.8
Tomatoes	1 cup	32	7.1	2.2
Turnips	1 cup	34	7.9	3.1
Water chestnuts	1 cup	70	17.2	3.5

Glycemic Loads

The glycemic load (GL) is a scale used to indicate how much one serving of a particular food raises a person's blood sugar. A GL of 10 or less is considered low. Check your blood sugar two hours after eating a food to find out how it affects your blood sugar, since your reaction might be different. The GL is closely tied to portion size; if you eat twice as much as the portion size indicated, the food will have double the effect on your blood sugar. (Keep in mind that these portion sizes aren't necessarily the same as those used in the food exchange system.) Work with your registered dietitian to figure out how to fit more low-GL foods into your eating plan.

LOW (GL = 10 OR LESS)

Breads, Tortillas, Grains	Serving size	GL
Coarse barley bread (75% intact kernels)	2 slices	10
Soy and flaxseed bread	2 slices	10
Whole-grain pumpernickel bread	2 slices	10
Pearled barley	1 cup	8
Popcorn	2 cups	8
Wheat tortillas	2 6-inch	6

Breakfast Cereals	Serving size	GL
Alpen Muesli	1/3 cup (1 oz)	10
Oatmeal, instant 1 cup prepared	(1 oz)	10
All-Bran	1/2 cup (1 oz)	9
Bran Buds	1/3 cup (1 oz)	7
Oatmeal made from rolled oats 1 cup prepared	(1 oz)	7

Legumes	Serving size	GL
Lima beans	1 cup	10
Pinto beans	1 cup	10
Chickpeas	1 cup	8
Baked beans	1 cup	7
Kidney beans	1 cup	7
Navy beans	1 cup	7
Butter beans	1 cup	6
Green peas	1 cup	6
Split peas, yellow	1 cup	6
Lentils, green or red	1 cup	5

Dairy and Soy Drinks	Serving size	GL
Low-fat yogurt with fruit and sugar	7 oz	9
Soy milk	1 cup (8 oz)	7
Low-fat chocolate milk, sweetened with aspartame	1 cup (8 oz)	3
Low-fat yogurt with fruit, sweetened with aspartame	7 oz	2

Fruits and Vegetables	Serving size	GL
Prunes, pitted, chopped	1/3 cup (2 oz)	10
Apricots, dried, chopped	1/3 cup (2 oz)	9
Peaches, canned in light syrup	1/2 cup (4 oz)	9
Grapes, medium bunch	(about 50) 4 oz	8
Mango, sliced	2/3 cup (4 oz)	8
Pineapple, diced	2/3 cup (4 oz)	7
Apple	1 small	6
Kiwifruit, sliced	2/3 cup (4 oz)	6
Beets, sliced	1/2 cup	5
Orange	1 small	5
Peach	1 small	5
Plums	2 small	5
Pear	1 small	4
Strawberries	about 6 medium	4
Watermelon, chopped	2/3 cup (4 oz)	4
Carrots, raw	1 large	3
Cherries	about 16 (4 oz)	3
Grapefruit	1/2	3

Beverages	Serving size	GL
Orange juice, unsweetened	3/4 cup (6 oz)	10
Grapefruit juice, unsweetened	3/4 cup (6 oz)	7
Tomato juice	3/4 cup (6 oz)	4

Sweets	Serving size	GL
M&Ms with peanuts	25 (1 oz)	6
Nutella (chocolate hazelnut spread)	4 Tbsp	4

Nuts	Serving size	GL
Mixed nuts, roasted	1/3 cup (1.5 oz)	4
Cashew nuts	about 13 (1.5 oz)	3
Peanuts	1/3 cup (1.5 oz)	1

MEDIUM (GL = 11–19)

Bread, Tortillas, Crackers, Chips	Serving size	GL
Coarse barley bread (50% intact kernels)	2 slices	18
High-fiber white bread	2 slices	18
Corn chips	2 oz	17
100% whole-grain bread	2 slices	14
Sourdough rye bread	2 slices	12
Stone-ground wheat thins	4	12
Corn tortillas	2 6-inch	11

Grains	Serving size	GL
Converted long-grain white rice	2/3 cup cooked	16
Brown rice	2/3 cup cooked	18
Quinoa	2/3 cup cooked	16
Wild rice	2/3 cup cooked	18
Bulgur	2/3 cup cooked	12

Pasta	Serving size	GL
Spaghetti (cooked 15 minutes)	1 cup	17
Whole-wheat spaghetti	1 cup	13
High-protein spaghetti	1 cup	12

Beverages	Serving size	GL
Low-fat chocolate milk	8 oz	12
Pineapple juice, unsweetened	6 oz	12
Apple juice	8 oz	8

Fruits, Vegetables, Beans	Serving size	GL
Sweet corn	1 cup	18
Sweet potato	1 medium (5 oz)	17
Figs, dried, chopped	1/3 cup (2 oz)	16
Banana	1 small (4 oz)	11
Black-eyed peas	1 cup	11

Breakfast Cereals	Serving size	GL
Nabisco Cream of Wheat, regular	1 cup prepared (1 oz)	17
Post Grape-Nuts	1/2 cup (1 oz)	16
Cheerios	1 cup (1 oz)	15
Life	3/4 cup (1 oz)	15
Special K	1 cup (1 oz)	14

HIGH (GL = 20 OR HIGHER)

Potatoes	Serving size	GL
Baked russet Burbank potato	1 medium	26
French fries	5 oz	22

Grains	Serving size	GL
Sticky white rice	2/3 cup cooked	31
Couscous	2/3 cup cooked	23
Long-grain white rice	2/3 cup cooked	23

Pasta	Serving size	GL
Udon Japanese noodles	1 cup cooked	25
Spaghetti (cooked 20 minutes)	1 cup	22

Breads	Serving size	GL
French baguette	2 slices	30
Middle Eastern flatbread	1 large	30
Italian white bread	2 slices	22
Hamburger roll	1	21
Mini-bagel (Lender's)	1	20
Wonder Bread	2 slices	20

Breakfast Cereals	Serving size	GL
Kellogg's Cornflakes	1 cup (1 oz)	24
Rice Chex	1 1/4 cups (1 oz)	23
Nabisco Cream of Wheat, instant	1 cup prepared (1 oz)	22
Rice Krispies	3/4 cup (1 oz)	22
Corn Chex	1 cup (1 oz)	21

Dried Fruit	Serving size	GL
Raisins	1/3 cup	28
Dates, dried, chopped	1/3 cup	25

Beverages	Serving size	GL
Ocean Spray Cranberry Juice Cocktail	12 oz	36
Coca-Cola	12 oz	24

Sweets	Serving size	GL
Mars Bar	2 oz	26
Jelly beans	20	22

Diabetes Testing and Doctor's Visit Schedule

AT EVERY DOCTOR'S VISIT (USUALLY 4 TIMES PER YEAR)

TEST	DATE	RESULT	DATE	RESULT	DATE	RESULT	DATE	RESULT
A1C (goal is lower than 7)								
Blood pressure (goal is lower than 130/80)								
Foot check								

TWICE A YEAR

TEST	DATE	DATE
Dental cleaning and exam		

YEARLY (ON ANNIVERSARY OF LAST TEST)

TEST	LAST YEAR'S DATE	LAST YEAR'S RESULT	THIS YEAR'S DATE	THIS YEAR'S RESULT
Microalbumin urine test (for kidney function)				
Eye exam (with dilation)				
LDL cholesterol*				
HDL cholesterol**				
Triglycerides***				
Foot exam (from a podiatrist)				
Flu shot				

*Goal is lower than 100 mg/dL or lower than 70 mg/dL if you have known cardiovascular disease.

**Goal is higher than 40 mg/dL for men and higher than 50 mg/dL for women.

***Goal is lower than 150 mg/dL.

Numbers to Know

GENERAL BLOOD-SUGAR TARGETS

Fasting or before meal glucose	90–130 mg/dL
After-meal glucose (two hours after the start of your meal)	>180 mg/dL
Bedtime glucose	100–140 mg/dL

HOW TO TRANSLATE A1C NUMBERS

A1C	Blood Glucose Level	
6.0%	135 mg/dL	7.5 mmol/L*
6.5%	153 mg/dL	8.5 mmol/L*
7.0%	170 mg/dL	9.5 mmol/L*
7.5%	188 mg/dL	10.5 mmol/L*
8.0%	205 mg/dL	11.4 mmol/L*
8.5%	223 mg/dL	12.4 mmol/L*
9.0%	240 mg/dL	13.3 mmol/L*
9.5%	258 mg/dL	14.3 mmol/L*
10.0%	275 mg/dL	15.3 mmol/L*
10.5%	293 mg/dL	16.3 mmol/L*
11.0%	310 mg/dL	17.2 mmol/L*
11.5%	328 mg/dL	18.2 mmol/L*
12.0%	345 mg/dL	19.1 mmol/L*

* Millimoles per liter, used outside the U.S.

HEALTHY WAIST CIRCUMFERENCE

Men	up to 40 inches
Women	up to 35 inches

If your waist is bigger than this, you are at increased risk for type 2 diabetes, high blood pressure, high cholesterol, and cardiovascular disease.

Plan for Your Next Doctor's Visit

Date and time of appointment: _____

Name of doctor: _____

Name of certified diabetes educator: _____

Name of registered dietitian: _____

I NEED TO BRING THE FOLLOWING TO MY APPOINTMENT:

☐ A list of my medications

☐ My glucose meter

☐ My weekly blood-sugar log sheets

☐ A record of any test or examination I had other than in my doctor's office

☐ My food diary

☐ My daily diet and lifestyle goals tracking sheets

☐ Other: _____

CHECK IF ANY TESTS NEED TO BE DONE PRIOR TO APPOINTMENT:

☐ A1C

☐ Urine test of protein to check kidney function

☐ Dilated eye exam

☐ Cholesterol and triglycerides

☐ Other: _____

QUESTIONS TO ASK:

1. _____

_____

_____

2. _____

_____

_____

3. _____

_____

_____

4. _____

_____

_____

Medication Record

Name: _____

What it's for: _____

Amount: _____ How often: _____

When to take: _____

Name: _____

What it's for: _____

Amount: _____ How often: _____

When to take: _____

Name: _____

What it's for: _____

Amount: _____ How often: _____

When to take: _____

Name: _____

What it's for: _____

Amount: _____ How often: _____

When to take: _____

Name: _____

What it's for: _____

Amount: _____ How often: _____

When to take: _____

Name: _____

What it's for: _____

Amount: _____ How often: _____

When to take: _____

Recipe Index

RECIPE INDEX

Subject Index

PHOTO CREDITS

Cover: Getty Images, **9:** Photodisc, **10:** Pixland, **11:** Photodisc, **12:** Photodisc, **17:** BananaStock, **21:** Garry Wade/Taxi, **26:** Rolf Bruderer/Blend Images, **29:** Photodisc, **32:** Photodisc, **35:** Comstock, **38:** Stockbyte, **41:** istockFree, **44:** Comstock, **47:** Photodisc, **51:** Corbis, **52:** Dougal Waters/Digital Vision, **56:** Image Source, **61:** Image Source, **63:** RD Images, **67:** Photodisc, **68:** Digital Vision, **69:** Food Collection, **72:** Andrea Sperling/Photolibrary, **75:** Photodisc, **76:** Digital Vision, **77:** Shutterstock, **78:** BrandX, **83:** fStop, **89:** Shutterstock, **90:** BrandX, **92:** RD Images, **93:** BrandX, **94:** RD Images, **97:** Food Collection, **99:** Photodisc, **100:** Food Collection, **101:** BrandX, **103:** Photodisc, **105:** Phillip Nealey/Photographer's Choice RF, **110:** Shutterstock, **112:** BrandX, **114:** Food Collection, **115:** Daniel Grill/Tetra Images, **117:** Steve McAllister/Workbook Stock, **118:** Shutterstock, **121:** Photodisc, **122:** Food Collection, **124:** Pixland, **129:** ThinkStock, **130:** Photodisc, **133:** istockFree, **135:** Rubberball, **141:** Photodisc, **144:** Photodisc, **147:** Shutterstock, **150:** BrandX, **154:** Photodisc, **155-158:** RD Images, **160:** Open Door Images, **165:** istockFree, **166:** Photodisc, **169:** PolkaDot Images, **170-191:** ©Jill Wachter, **182:** Thomas Barwick/Taxi, **197:** Photodisc, **198:** Image 102, **201:** Photodisc, **203:** Photodisc, **205:** Photodisc, **206:** Photodisc, **211:** ©Jill Wachter, **215:** Photodisc, **216:** Photodisc, **225:** Creatas, **228:** Photodisc, **230:** Photodisc, **235:** Photodisc, **240:** Platform, **242-289:** RD Images, **290:** Photodisc

Also Available from Reader's Digest

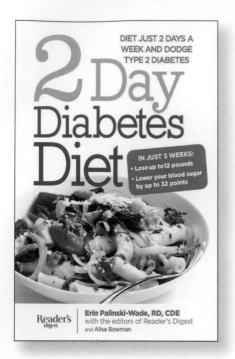

2 Day Diabetes Diet

Based on groundbreaking science, the *2 Day Diabetes Diet* makes it easy to prevent, treat, or even reverse type 2 diabetes. No forbidden foods. No carb-counting. Just restrict what you eat for 2 days a week. Featuring more than 150 meal options, including restaurant and frozen food options, and tension taming exercises to help you ward off cravings, the book will help you drop the pounds and stabilize your blood sugar levels.

Erin Palinski-Wade, RD, CDE, with the editors of Reader's Digest and Alisa Bowman
978-1-62145-271-3
$15.99 U.S. / paperback

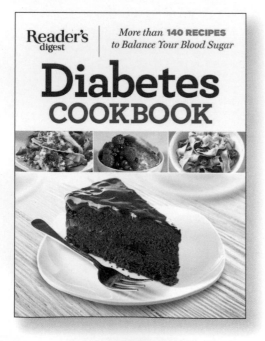

Diabetes Cookbook

Taking care of your diabetes has never been more delicious! Here are more than 140 recipes that have been carefully developed and proportioned to help you control your blood sugar levels. They are quick and easy to make, with budget-friendly options and recipes for two called out. Most importantly, they are scrumptious and satisfying!

From the Editors at Reader's Digest
978-1-62145-295-9
$17.99 U.S. / paperback